MACHIAVELLI AND THE POLITICS
OF DEMOCRATIC INNOVATION

CHRISTOPHER HOLMAN

Machiavelli and the Politics of Democratic Innovation

UNIVERSITY OF TORONTO PRESS
Toronto Buffalo London

ISBN 978-1-4875-0393-2

Library and Archives Canada Cataloguing in Publication

Holman, Christopher, 1979–, author
Machiavelli and the politics of democratic innovation / Christopher J. Holman.

Includes bibliographical references and index.
ISBN 978-1-4875-0393-2 (cloth)

1. Machiavelli, Niccolò, 1469–1527 – Criticism and interpretation.
2. Machiavelli, Niccolò, 1469–1527 – Political and social views.
3. Machiavelli, Niccolò, 1469–1527. Principe.   4. Machiavelli, Niccolò, 1469–1527.
Discorsi sopra la prima deca di Tito Livio.   I. Title.

JC143.M4H65 2018   320.1   C2018-902598-0

This book has been published with the help of a grant from the Federation
for the Humanities and Social Sciences, through the Awards to Scholarly
Publications Program, using funds provided by the Social Sciences
and Humanities Research Council of Canada.

University of Toronto Press acknowledges the financial assistance to its
publishing program of the Canada Council for the Arts and the Ontario
Arts Council, an agency of the Government of Ontario.

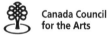

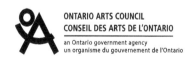

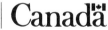

Contents

Acknowledgments

My thanks to the anonymous reviewers of earlier versions of this manuscript for their detailed critical commentary, which improved the final product immensely. I am grateful to the entire staff at the University of Toronto Press involved in the production of this book for their contributions, in particular Daniel Quinlan for providing his usual editorial expertise throughout the entire publication process. James Leahy, furthermore, provided comprehensive and detailed copy editing, greatly improving the readability of the book.

Material from this book has been presented at various meetings of the Western Political Science Association, the Canadian Political Science Association, and the International Herbert Marcuse Society, as well as the 2015 conference "Radical Democracy and Utopia" at the University of Paris Diderot, and the 2014 workshop "Moral Revolutions: Institutional and Ideational Dimensions" at Nanyang Technological University. The questions from many of the participants at these meetings were helpful in clarifying certain issues for me, and orienting the direction of the project.

Finally, my thanks to all of the usual friends, colleagues, and teachers from York University, Stony Brook University, NTU, and elsewhere with whom I have discussed Machiavelli and democratic theory over the years.

Abbreviated versions of chapters 1 and 2 appeared earlier as "Machiavelli's Constellative Use of History," *Theory and Event* 19, no. 2 (2016), and "Machiavelli's Philosophical Anthropology," *European Legacy* 21, no. 8 (2016): 769–90.

MACHIAVELLI AND THE POLITICS
OF DEMOCRATIC INNOVATION

Introduction

This book has a double aim. On the one hand, it looks to contribute to the history of political thought by providing a new interpretation of the political theory of Niccolò Machiavelli, whose perpetually studied works have garnerned even more recent attention as a result of the quincentenary of the production of several of them. On the other hand, it seeks to develop a new theoretical model and ethical defence of democratic practice, of radical democracy in particular. Specifically, the new method for thinking radical democracy will be mediated through a detailed consideration and reinterpretation of the texts of Machiavelli. The deployment of a five-hundred-year-old oeuvre for the sake of advancing a contemporary theoretical tradition that, even if it may trace its roots to ancient Athens has only emerged as a somewhat unified philosophical field recently, will no doubt strike some as a suspicious intellectual endeavour. The fact that this oeuvre is the Machiavellian one may only add to the suspicion. After all, the subject of Machiavelli studies is a notoriously partisan one. Claude Lefort does not overstate the case when he writes that here "the variety of interpretations and opinions, the depth of conflict, as well as the intensity of the critical passions, reach their highest degree."[1] The Machiavellian text is not so much an object of disinterested scholarly interpretation as a field in which contending forms and traditions of political thought, with their own ontological and normative assumptions regarding the being of politics, deploy the Florentine secretary in an effort to advance their particular commitments.

---

1 Claude Lefort, "L'oeuvre de pensée et l'histoire," in *Les formes de l'histoire: essais d'anthropologie politique* (Paris: Gallimard, 1978), 144.

I make no claims to being able to symbolically rise above this realm of appearance, with its conflicting images and perspectives, in order to touch the truth of Machiavelli's political thought. In this book I thus aim not at producing a systematic explication of the whole of Machiavelli's oeuvre, or an intellectual history schematically tracing the development of his thought through time, or a contextual situation of his work within the overall environment of the *Cinquecento*, and so on. On the contrary, I will adopt an interpretative methodology that I believe is much more consistent with Machiavelli's own approach to the doing of political theory, an approach that I argue is the very source of the intensity of the debates over Machiavellian meaning. Machiavelli's normative political theory proceeds mainly through an analysis of various historical events and personages drawn from ancient and modern Italian history, but focusing particulary on the ancient Roman republic and recent Florentine experience. As is often pointed out, however, Machiavelli's historical method is highly atypical. Rather than seek to represent the trajectory of past events in a linear and straightforward mode, he selectively alters, elides, and invents lessons and events in order to invest them with a specific political meaning, a meaning that is then redeployed in his own context for the sake of achieving a contemporary political goal: the unification and liberation of the Italian peninsula. Machiavelli's use of history is thus characterized by an imaginative and creative redistribution of historical meaning. This study asks what it means to read Machiavelli in the same way that Machiavelli read his historical sources, applying Machiavelli's method for the interpretative analysis of history to the interpretative analysis of Machaivelli. Just as Machiavelli's historical examples become, through their critical juxtaposition with one another, other than what they originally were, so too does Machiavelli become other than himself, depending on how we choose to read him in the moment. In this sense there are, potentially, innumerable Machiavellian moments.[2]

My emphasis will be on what Machiavelli has to contribute to democratic theory, specifically, to a radical democratic theory grounded in an affirmation of the universal capacity for creative innovation. There is certainly nothing original about suggesting that Machiavelli is capable

---

2 On the existence of more than one (if not innumerable) Machiavellian moments see Marie Gaille, *Machiavel et la tradition philosophique* (Paris: Presses Universitaires de France, 2007), 121–49.

of contributing important content to a theory of radical democracy. This has indeed been recognized for over forty years, such readings flourishing in particular in France and Italy.[3] Despite important contributions by figures such as Miguel Vatter, Filippo Del Lucchese, and others, however, within the Anglo-American world the democratic Machiavelli has come to be appreciated within mainstream political science only recently, in particular as a result of the many publications of John McCormick on the subject.[4] What I argue that existing democratic readers – radical and otherwise – have failed to fully appreciate, however, is the extent to which Machiavelli's normative commitment to a specific modality of political existence is ethically grounded in a particular understanding of the ontology of the human, and its relation to the form of existence of worldly being. In evaluating republican political life within the context of the affirmation of a precise philosophical anthropology, Machiavelli generates an entirely unique defence of democratic rule.

Just as Machiavelli creatively appropriates elements of ancient and modern history in order to articulate a new national project, so will I attempt to creatively appropriate elements of Machiavelli's thought in order to articulate a new model of democracy. Machiavelli is the ideal figure to work with in this respect because not only are there such elements in his work to be located, but also he is one of the few thinkers in the tradition of political thought to affirm the openness of political theory to such a form of investigation. Although I will draw extensively from Machiavelli's entire body of writing – including his major and minor political writings, historical studies, poetry, comedies, diplomatic

---

3 Perhaps the key point in this trajectory is the 1972 publication of Claude Lefort, *Le travail de l'oeuvre Machiavel* (Paris: Gallimard, 1986).

4 Although McCormick aims to articulate the participatory democratic commitments of Machiavelli, he explicitly contrasts his reading with those in the radical democratic tradition, which tend to de-emphasize the role of the institution in mediating democratic self-expression, locating the latter precisely in the interruption of instituted political forms. See, for example, John P. McCormick, "Defending the People from the Professors," ed. John Swadley, *The Art of Theory*, 27 September 2010, www.artoftheory .com/mccormick-machiavellian-democracy. Although I agree with McCormick that most radical democrats obscure the institutional form of Machiavelli's project, I will ultimately argue that it is possible to appreciate the radical content of his democratic theory by grasping the specific form of articulation of Machiavellian institutions, as institutions that are perpetually open to their own interrogation and interruption.

dispatches, personal correspondences, and more – at the heart of my analysis will be a reconsideration of the substance of and relationship between his two most well-known major political works, *The Prince* and the *Discourses on Livy*.[5] Without attempting to close off certain other readings, I will propose a new method for thinking the relationship between these two works, seeing each as one moment of a comprehensive normative project affirming a specific ethics of political creation. Each of the two works is aimed primarily at articulating a figure of thought that contributes to the revelation of the human capacity for creativity or innovation. The first figure is to be found in *The Prince*, Machiavelli here being concerned with presenting not only the mechanics of a certain type of regime, but also those elements that structure a specific model of human subjectivity: Machiavelli is telling the reader what it means to be a creative subject. In the *Discourses*, meanwhile, Machiavelli presents a second figure of thought, this one aimed at outlining a form of political regime that is capable of generalizing the model of human subjectivity detailed in *The Prince*. The Machiavellian republic can be read in democratic terms as the form of regime in which all citizens are able to actualize their potential for political creation. The difference in the objects of the two works does not express a discontinuity or non-correspondence, but rather is a manifestation of their very unity: *The Prince* as a treatise on what it means for an individual to be a creative subject, and the *Discourses* as a treatise on the possibility of conceptualizing a political regime in which this capacity for innovation is democratically institutionalized. Machiavelli's theoretical project can thus roughly be divided into two parts. On the one hand he develops a philosophical anthropology. Machiavelli radically destabilizes all

---

5 Throughout the study I will cite Niccolò Machiavelli, *Tutte le opere*, ed. Mario Martelli (Firenze: Sansoni Editore, 1971). I have also consulted the following English translations: Niccolò Machiavelli, *The Prince*, trans. Harvey C. Mansfield (Chicago: University of Chicago Press, 1998); Niccolò Machiavelli, *Discourses on Livy*, trans. Harvey C. Mansfield and Nathan Tarcov (Chicago: University of Chicago Press, 1996); Niccolò Machiavelli, *Florentine Histories*, trans. Harvey C. Mansfield and Laura F. Banfield (Princeton: Princeton University Press, 1988); Niccolò Machiavelli, *The Art of War*, trans. Christopher Lynch (Chicago: University of Chicago Press, 2003); Niccolò Machiavelli, *The Chief Works and Others, volumes 1–3*, trans. Allan Gilbert (Durham: Duke University Press, 1989); Niccolò Machiavelli, *Machiavelli and His Friends: Their Personal Correspondence*, ed. and trans. James B. Atkinson and David Sices (DeKalb: Northern Illinois University Press, 1996).

positive models of the human essence that attempt to outline a fixed structure of the human being, and instead interprets the essence of the latter negatively in terms of the ability to creatively shape the self and the world. Such a model of essence has been developed by a variety of the canonical thinkers in the history of political thought, but I will argue that Machiavelli is the first one who sees the actualization of this essence as being achieved primarily through political activity. Hence the second part of Machiavelli's project: the development of a political ontology in which he tries to think about a form of political life that is capable of affirming this fundamental human creativity. Machiavelli's ethical commitment to a form of democratic republic in which all citizens are capable of expressing their political will is a result of his perception of a universal human desire for creative self-expression. We are thus ultimately presented with a new normative foundation for democratic life, one grounded not in any judgment regarding the competency of popular decision making, nor one regarding the fundamental natural rights of individuals, but rather the orientation of individual beings toward creativity and innovation.[6]

As I have mentioned, the justification for such a reconstruction of the Machiavellian oeuvre is to be found in Machiavelli's own practice of writing. I thus begin in chapter 1 by providing a new analysis of what I take to be the unique character of Machiavelli's methodology, specifically his political deployment of ancient historical examples, and how it will inform my own reading of Machiavelli's texts. Although commentators have often pointed out the extent to which Machiavelli's affirmation of an active history oriented toward political creation is distinguished from a passive one in which historical events are treated merely as objects of contemplation, they have not gone far enough in describing how the precise form of Machiavelli's historiography is a necessary element of his valorization of political creation. I attempt to demonstrate how this is the case by arguing that Machiavelli's historical method can be thought of as an aesthetic practice of thinking in

---

6 Although he takes a different approach, Emmanuel Roux similarly interprets Machiavelli as initiating a new genealogy of democracy (which includes Spinoza, Montesquieu, and Rousseau), a genealogy that "does not speak of the individual, of natural right, of the separation of powers." Emmanuel Roux, *Machiavel, la vie libre* (Paris: Raisons d'agir, 2013), 16. Democracy, instead, is thought of in terms of mutation and perpetual change.

constellations, such as was most famously articulated in the twentieth century by Walter Benjamin. Machiavelli critically and selectively juxtaposes conceptual elements in order to generate figures of thought that reveal the potential to transcend the existing political organization of things. I argue that this method has important implications for how we think about both the means and ends of political theory, and my own approach to interpreting Machiavelli will take it as its model.

In part 2 I attempt to reconstruct from Machiavelli's thought a consistent philosophical anthropology. Chapter 2 details Machiavelli's rejection of positive models of human nature. This rejection is seen as a correlate of his theory of worldly being. Under the influence of the Epicurean philosophical tradition, Machiavelli provides a cosmological account of a world that is considered in terms of its fundamentally chaotic and indeterminate being, an account that rejects all transcendental attempts to absolutely ground the world and structure its being in a deterministic way, such as via theology, natural law, laws of history, and so on. This worldly indetermination also extends to the human being, and is represented in Machiavelli's rejection of the attempt to thematize human nature in terms of a perpetually fixed set of properties whose form could be objectively grasped and schematized. Such a rejection is demonstrated in two primary ways: through an account of the radical diversity of human forms of doing and being, and through an explanation of the fundamental openness of human being to change and alteration through subjection to processes of socialization. In the final instance Machiavelli theorizes a radical indetermination of human being, this indetermination being expressed in the multiplicity and non-identity of human desire, a fact that closes off in advance the potential for a stable reconciliation or harmonization of human interest. Human difference, and subsequently conflict, thus remain an ineradicable feature of social existence.

In chapter 3 I provide, through a reinterpretation of the mode of being of Machiavelli's ideal prince, an account of what I take to be Machiavelli's negative model of the human essence. Such negative models reject attempts to theorize all elements of human being in terms of a system of positive determinations, seeing one of the fundamental components of essence instead in the specifically human ability to transcend merely immediate and conventional forms of doing and being. A negative essence refers us, in other words, not to a specifically human content, but rather to a specifically human capacity, that is, the capacity for creativity, to generate new values and orders. The human being is that which is capable of perpetually remaking itself and its social world through its life activity. This capacity is expressed in Machiavelli's concept of ambition, which is identified in terms of a fundamental human striving to transgress existing forms and construct new realities. I argue that princely creation is exalted by Machiavelli to the extent that it is seen as providing a model for a political form of creative self-activity, for the realization of the human desire for value formation. What Machiavelli's idea of the new prince reveals, what the specific constellation of thought articulated through the juxtaposition of conceptual elements drawn from a variety of historical experiences and actors discloses, is the image of the prince as an ambitious creator: a model of the form of a fully realized human subjectivity.

According to my interpretation, Machiavelli's *Prince* may be read not only as a treatise on politics, but also as one on the nature of human subjectivity. In part three I turn to look more closely at the relation between this understanding of subjectivity and Machiavelli's conception of the being of politics. In chapter 4 I attempt to demonstrate that the psychic ambition which was seen in chapter 3 to stimulate virtuous political creation is one that belongs not only to princes and other social elites, but to all citizens. It is common for readers of Machiavelli – whether Straussian, republican, or democratic – to bifurcate human desire into two opposed poles: whereas the great or noble are seen as possessing a fundamental desire to dominate others through the expulsion of their ambition, the people are seen as passively desiring not to be dominated. I will argue that this distinction Machiavelli makes, however, does not refer us to an essential or originary opposition, but rather to two different forms of appearance of the single desire for ambitious creation. I show that, according to Machiavelli, all human beings, not just the great, possess ambition, as can be seen through a variety of episodes Machiavelli details that reveal the popular desire for creative self-expression. Machiavelli in fact goes to great lengths, both in the *Discourses* and in the *Florentine Histories* and the "Discourse on Florentine Affairs," to outline not only the popular desire to express ambition via participation in political modes and orders, but also a popular capacity to do so that is not differentiated in quality from that of any other groups in the city. There is not, in other words, a unique political skill, orientation, or knowledge that belongs to and can be exercised by only a minority of individuals. In recognizing both this political will and political capacity Machiavelli makes a simultaneous affirmation of a radical human freedom and equality, the latter residing not in the establishment of a self-identical common interest, but rather in the equal capacity of always distinct individuals to express their particular political desire in speech. The fact that particular individuals always remain particular, that human multiplicity is incapable of being effaced, renders the political sphere one of inevitable difference and conflict. Machiavelli's ultimate goal will be to think the means by which this difference and conflict may be agonistically expressed through democratic channels (as in the *Discourses*), as opposed to antagonistically and violently expressed (as in the *Florentine Histories*), or simply repressed (as in *The Prince*).

In chapter 5 I demonstrate how the full manifestation of human equality in the political sphere necessitates the establishment of concrete economic equality in the social sphere. The establishment of such economic equality depends on, above all, the elimination of the *grandi* as an organized social class embodying a particular shared humour, a unified desire directed toward command and oppression. If there is no essential distinction grounded in human nature between the people and the great, the contingency of the form of being of the *grandi* allows for the latter's elimination. Although Machiavelli only rarely acknowledges this potential, he nevertheless provides us with significant clues suggesting it remains a very condition of possibility for the institution of democratic life. Positioning myself against those democratic readers who understand popular freedom as being only articulated against an already existent desire to oppress, I show how the seemingly originary division between the people and the great may be overcome through the establishment of a general economic equality. Although it is impossible to structure a city such that insolent individuals never emerge, it is not impossible to structure a city in which these insolent individuals are incapable of consolidating themselves into a class that is able to leverage their disproportionate economic wealth for the sake of the advancement of their particular interests. For Machiavelli, humours – *umori* – do not have a natural biological foundation, but rather are the contingent result of the constitution of particular social relationships. To this degree the particular being of any social *umore* is not inexorable, even if the appearance of particular individual wills – be it a will to domination or otherwise – is. Theorizing the potential to terminate the conflict between the great and the people, furthermore, does not entail the termination of all conflict itself, for, as I show in chapter 2, human multiplicity is not exhausted by the division between the great and the people. Even if a social situation is instituted such as to militate against the emergence of those with a humour to oppress, such would not thereby instaurate a political site characterized by consensual relations, for human difference would continue to manifest itself inevitably in a variety of spheres and in a variety of modes.

Finally, in chapter 6 I turn to the question of the form of political regime that is capable of generalizing this creative self-expression, thus providing spaces for all citizens to have the opportunity to act on their innate ambition. The defence of democratic institutionalization is rooted in the recognition that all individuals share a negative human essence, an orientation toward political creation that is realized in the controlled expulsion of ambitious energy. The democratic ethical imperative is grounded in both the perception of the universality of the human desire for self-creation, but also the recognition of the need for the productive rechannelling of this desire into socially useful ends via a project of autonomous institutionalization. If the latter is not achieved, if desire is not institutionally mediated, the society will regress into a form such as is detailed in Machiavelli's *Florentine Histories*, where individuals attempt to advance their own private interests at the expense of other citizens, who are not seen as possessing a right to political self-expression. It is precisely because the human desire for creative expression is insatiable, however – that is, that the human is constantly redefining the nature of itself and its world through its self-activity – that the form of the political regime is never capable of becoming permanently fixed. Machiavelli's republic is thus unique in that it is oriented toward its own perpetual interrogation and possible overcoming. Machiavelli's project is to think a system of institutions that is capable, through harnessing the creative energy of the people who constitute the society, of continually calling itself into question, and through reinstituting itself provide a means for the actualization of that creative human desire that is detailed in *The Prince*. It is in this sense that the republic is, as Machiavelli says, the regime in which all the people "can, by means of their virtue, become princes."[7]

---

7 Machiavelli, "Discorsi sopra la prima Deca di Tito Livio," in *Tutte le opere*, bk. 2.2.

PART ONE

Methodology

Chapter One

Machiavelli and the Constellative Mode of Historical Appropriation

It is common for readers of Niccolò Machiavelli's political thought to begin their inquiries by noting the diversity of interpretative conclusions that have been drawn regarding his writings, as well as the multitude of oftentimes mutually irreconcilable philosophical and political positions that he has been forced into. It seems that the Machiavellian oeuvre can be deployed in the service of any number of theoretical paradigms.[1] And yet few of these readers attempt to critically scrutinize the foundation of such interpretative operations, assuming on the contrary that their own specific methodological modes – from precise contextual analyses of the historical environment in which Machiavelli's work was produced to deep textual readings emphasizing the esoteric or concealed content open to the eye of the sensitive interlocutor – are

---

1 See, for example, Rafael Major, "A New Argument for Morality: Machiavelli and the Ancients," *Political Research Quarterly* 60, no. 2 (2007): 172; Raymond Aron, "Machiavelli and Marx," in *Politics and History*, ed. and trans. Miriam Bernheim (New York: Free Press, 1978), 87. For a summary of just some of the modes of reading and appropriating Machiavelli see Felix Gilbert, "Machiavelli in Modern Historical Scholarship," *Italian Quarterly* 14, no. 3 (1970): 9–26; Mary Walsh, "Historical Reception of Machiavelli," in *Seeking Real Truths: Multidisciplinary Perspectives on Machiavelli*, ed. Patricia Vilches and Gerald Seaman (Leiden: Brill, 2007), 273–302; Victoria Kahn, "Machiavelli's Afterlife and Reputation to the Eighteenth Century," in *The Cambridge Companion to Machiavelli*, ed. John M. Najemy (Cambridge: Cambridge University Press, 2010), 239–55; Jérémie Barthas, "Machiavelli in Political Thought from the Age of Revolutions to the Present," in *The Cambridge Companion to Machiavelli*, ed. John M. Najemy (Cambridge: Cambridge University Press, 2010), 256–73; Giovanni Giorgini, "Five Hundred Years of Italian Scholarship on Machiavelli's Prince," *Review of Politics* 75, no. 4 (2013): 625–40.

capable of penetrating to the truth of Machiavelli.[2] It is curious that, as John Plamenatz observes, it seems as if "none of his interpreters writes about him as if he were seriously puzzled, or had come to his conclusions with difficulty or held to them tentatively."[3] It is thus, for example, not a problem for such a close reader of Machiavelli as Harvey Mansfield to write, in reference to the interpretative work of Leo Strauss, that "as far as I know, among hundreds of statements in *Thoughts on Machiavelli* susceptible of mistake, not one single mistake has yet been exposed."[4] The possibility of an objectively correct reading of the intrinsic meaning of the Machiavellian texts is not only achievable, but perhaps already achieved.

What I would like to suggest in this chapter, however, is that the very effort to read Machiavelli in terms of the schematic representation of a fixed meaning or intention itself constitutes a violation of the spirit of the Machiavellian project. Critical reflection on the nature of the Machiavellian methodology, specifically on Machiavelli's unique deployment of those historical examples that form the background to his political thought, opens up to us a unique vantage point from which to evaluate the meaning of his theoretical project. This chapter will attempt to reassess the well-known tension in Machiavelli's thought between the claim to novelty and the appeal to the wisdom of the ancients. Rather than implore the contemporary actor to uncritically repeat established

---

2 Yves Winter and Filippo Del Lucchese are two of several recent exceptions to this tendency. Winter, for example, recognizes that "the question of Machiavelli's 'true intentions' has no determinate answer, for the polysemy of his text makes securing a single meaning unfeasible." Yves Winter, "Plebeian Politics: Machiavelli and the Ciompi Uprising," *Political Theory* 40, no. 6 (2012): 738. On the variety of secondary interpretations of Machiavelli, meanwhile, Del Lucchese writes that "the diversity of points of view and perspectives is not only the work of the centuries; it was implied since the beginning in Machiavelli's methodology." Filippo Del Lucchese, *The Political Philosophy of Niccolò Machiavelli* (Edinburgh: Edinburgh University Press, 2015), 168. For a discussion of the multiple potentials contained within the Machiavellian oeuvre that are articulated within the context of the specifically Left appropriation of Machiavelli (Althusser's and Lefort's in particular), see Warren Breckman, "The Power and the Void: Radical Democracy, Post-Marxism, and the Machiavellian Moment," in *Radical Intellectuals and the Subversion of Progressive Politics*, ed. Gregory Smulewicz-Zucker and Michael J. Thompson (New York: Palgrave Macmillan, 2015), 237–54.

3 John Plamenatz, *Machiavelli, Hobbes, and Rousseau*, ed. Mark Philp and Z.A. Pelczynski (Oxford: Oxford University Press, 2012), 18.

4 Harvey C. Mansfield, "Strauss's Machiavelli," *Political Theory* 3, no. 4 (1975): 379.

modes of doing and being, Machiavelli encourages him or her to rede-
ploy the principle of creativity that lay at the source of those examples
that are highlighted for the sake of the stimulation of political activity
in the present. Aiming not at a literal representation of the sequence of
historical events, Machiavelli selectively reappropriates ancient and
modern examples and arranges them in specific organizations of
thought in order to affirm the uniquely human capacity for political
creation. This methodology, I suggest, is best thought of as a type of
thinking in constellations, such as was most significantly articulated in
the twentieth century by Walter Benjamin. This approach, whereby
Machiavelli imaginatively constructs universals through the juxtaposition of conceptual particulars, is considered by Benjamin as the most
effective strategy for countering the type of uncritical historicism that
assumes a determinate trajectory of events foreclosing the possibility of
meaningful human intervention in the world. Machiavelli's appeal to
the past is in the final instance made for the sake of a breaking free
from the past, for the sake of the affirmation of the human potential to
upset the order of things through the institution of the new.

Active vs Contemplative Historical Appropriation

It is by no means original to point out the apparent contradiction in
Machiavelli's use of history as a means to articulate a political ethos
that emphasizes the virtues of novelty and innovation. In the words of
Claude Lefort, "the thinker who was aware of innovating absolutely
and whom posterity has indeed judged to have opened a new path to
political thought, this man wished to erect Antiquity into a model."[5]
Hence in the Preface to the *Discourses on Livy* Machiavelli simultaneously proclaims his decision to "enter upon a road untrodden by anyone," and criticizes the inability of contemporary actors to properly
imitate ancient examples.[6] The contradiction between novelty and imitation in Machiavelli's exhortation to return to the study of ancient

---

5 Claude Lefort, "Machiavelli and the *Verità Effetuale*," in *Writing: The Political Test*, ed.
  and trans. David Ames Curtis (Durham: Duke University Press, 2000), 109. As Lefort
  writes elsewhere, "It is as though the discovery of the New and the Unknown coin-
  cides with the rediscovery of the past." Claude Lefort, "Machiavelli: History, Politics,
  Discourse," in *The States of Theory: History, Art, and Critical Discourse* (New York:
  Columbia University Press, 1990), 113.
6 Machiavelli, "Discorsi sopra la prima Deca di Tito Livio," in *Tutte le opere*, bk. 1, preface.

examples, of course, is only an apparent one, his return to antiquity never taking the form of a simple repetition. It constitutes rather, in the case of the *Discourses*, an imaginative reconstruction of the image of the Roman republic, made for the sake of the production of an alternative mental image of Rome that is capable of stimulating a practical imperative that stretches into a future marked by the production of the new.

Machiavelli thus contrasts his own critical and reflective form of engaging with antiquity with those of modes of appropriating the past which dominate the present day, and at which he can only "marvel and grieve."[7] Specifically, he will criticize those forms of historical appropriation that reduce Rome to a merely aesthetic object meant to be passively contemplated by a disinterested observer. Hence a typical mode of a contemporary Florentine's appreciation: "a fragment of an ancient statue has been bought at a high price for it to be near him, to honor his house and to be able to be imitated by those who delight in that art."[8] The goal is the extraction of a private pleasure that is achieved through the contemplation of the static form of the object. Such a passive appropriation is nothing less than a rejection of human virtue, for the great actors of the past – "kings, captains, citizens, legislators" – are "so much shunned by everyone in every little thing that no sign of that ancient virtue has remained with us."[9] The consequences of such a passive mode of historical appropriation can only be conformist. To the extent that it takes as its object a fixed image of the being of the city, an object that can be aesthetically contemplated to the degree that it is seen as complete and perpetual, it is fundamentally conservative, and hence an instrument for those who have an interest in the reproduction of the political status quo. The conservative reading of Rome that was dominant in the Florence of Machiavelli's time was an ideological representation that was oriented toward the symbolic maintenance of the current structure of the city, covering up the contingent fact of patrician domination.[10]

---

7 Ibid.
8 Ibid.
9 Ibid.
10 See, for example, Felix Gilbert, "Machiavelli's *Istorie Fiorentine*: An Essay in Interpretation," in *Studies on Machiavelli*, ed. Myron P. Gilmore (Firenze: G.C. Sansoni, 1972), 77; Martin Breaugh, *The Plebeian Experience: A Discontinuous History of Political Freedom*, trans. Lazer Lederhendler (New York: Columbia University Press, 2013), 47; John M. Najemy, "Baron's Machiavelli and Renaissance Republicanism," *American Historical Review* 101, no. 1 (1996): 127; Michelle T. Clarke, "Machiavelli and the Imagined Rome of Renaissance Humanism," *History of Political Thought* 36, no. 3 (2015): 452.

Machiavelli's rejection of the aesthetic mode of contemplation as the preferred form of historical engagement is thus a correlate of the rejection of the hypostatization of the existing organization of the city. The activation of the critical attitude and the critique of disinterested understanding functions to break up the unitary image of Rome as a perfectly unified and harmonious society that has achieved an ideal form of being, one that is reproduced in the present distribution of functions in the city. On the contrary, Machiavelli's consideration of Rome is novel in the degree to which it may be pressed into the service of critical political action, action that looks to the interruption of the existent and the reinstitutionalization of the social order. Machiavelli argues that those who treat the engagement with the classical histories in a disinterested and passive manner deny the specifically political potential that the former may open up for us, if we approach them with the proper spirit. The failure of historical imitation results "from not having a genuine understanding of histories, not drawing from reading them that sense nor savouring that flavour that they have in themselves."[11] Machiavelli here seems clear: his preferred form of imitation, that which reflects a "genuine understanding of histories," is not one that aims at the literal reproduction of the trajectory of historical events, but rather one that sensorially penetrates to the indeterminate soul of the work.[12] What this soul reveals to us is, as will be elaborated on in chapter 3 of this study, the specifically human potential to create the new through the exercise of *virtù*. What must be imitated is not a specific organization of events, but rather the critical spirit that animated the novel historical action. Machiavelli's use of history is thus an active one: what deserves to be remembered is that which reveals to us the potential for nondetermined political creation. Passive reflection on the humanistic tradition is subordinated to remembrance that looks to actualize political potential through the stimulation of practical activity in the world.

Commentators have usually interpreted this subordination in terms of Machiavelli's call both for a reactivation of an ethically oriented mode of critical thinking or reflective judgment, and for the pressing of

---

11 Machiavelli, "Discorsi sopra la prima Deca di Tito Livio," bk. 1, preface.
12 On the use that Machiavelli makes of bodily and sensory metaphors and the degree to which they can be seen as elements of a comprehensive political theory of sensation, see Davide Panagia, *The Political Life of Sensation* (Durham: Duke University Press, 2009), 74–95.

this mode into the service of a concrete political project aiming at the creation of a new form of political organization on the Italian peninsula. Such was classically recognized by Hegel, for example, in his 1802 essay "On the German Constitution," where he identifies Machiavelli's primary political concern as the self-constitution of a popular and independent Italian state. Hegel thus recognizes that Machiavelli, far from being an apologist for tyranny, is attempting to think the practical conditions for the unification of a dispersed people into a political mass: "this is his demand and the principle which he opposes to the misery of his country."[13] Machiavelli's theoretical project, articulated primarily through his historical juxtapositions, is thus unintelligible without consideration of what Louis Althusser will identify as his specific political conjuncture. The significance of Hegel's reading for Althusser lay in his recognition of the historical project of Machiavelli, as well as Machiavelli's appreciation of the conjunctural conditions from which this project must necessarily be launched: "A certain way of thinking about politics, not for its own sake, but in the shape of the formulation of a problem and the definition of a historical task – this is what surprises Hegel, and breaks open the empire of his own philosophical consciousness."[14] Machiavelli's historical use of antiquity, the form of the relationship that he establishes between the past and the present case, can be evaluated only within the context of the conjuncture: "Just as Machiavelli does not apply a general theory of history to particular concrete cases, so he does not apply antiquity to the present. Just as the general theory of history intervenes solely on condition of being determined by a series of 'negations' that have meaning only as a function of the central political problem, so too antiquity intervenes only under the determination of Rome, in order to illuminate the centre of everything – the political *vacuum* of Italy – and the task of filling it."[15]

---

13 G.W.F. Hegel, "The German Constitution," in *Political Writings*, ed. Lawrence Dickey and H.B. Nisbet, trans. H.B. Nisbet (Cambridge: Cambridge University Press, 2004), 81. For a short attempt to situate the last chapter of *The Prince* within the context of the emergence of a unified Italian national consciousness in the face of a renewed period of foreign invasion, see Felix Gilbert, "The Concept of Nationalism in Machiavelli's Prince," *Studies in the Renaissance* 1 (1954): 38–48.

14 Louis Althusser, *Machiavelli and Us*, ed. François Matheron, trans. Gregory Elliott (London: Verso, 1999), 10.

15 Ibid., 46–7. Original emphasis. Althusser, however, is hardly the only commentator to note the practical commitments that motivate the Machiavellian theoretical project,

We can begin to see here why Machiavelli, to the extent that he emphasizes the specificity of the individual case and the impossibility of conceptually subsuming this case in a standardized economy of thought through a process of derivation and identification, cannot be considered a scientific thinker in the traditional sense. His rejection of all systems of generalization includes the rejection of not only abstractly metaphysical utopian systems, but also those of the positive sciences. In Mikko Lahtinen's words, "The individual case cannot and should not be *subsumed* under any *general* law or theory. From the point of view of the man of action, this means that it is not possible to predict or govern the course of the individual case by means of some general law, theory or socially static utopia."[16] Machiavelli is far from being the founder of a modern political science, a system of causally connected rules and behaviours that can be generalized, and thus used as a universally valid explanatory instrument.[17] There is no system or science

---

and in particular the extent to which Machiavelli's use of history is critically deployed in order to advance this project. See, for just some examples, Martin Fleisher, "The Ways of Machiavelli and the Ways of Politics," *History of Political Thought* 16, no. 3 (1995): 331; Victoria Kahn, *Machiavellian Rhetoric: From the Counter-Reformation to Milton* (Princeton: Princeton University Press, 1994), 47; Bruce James Smith, *Politics and Remembrance: Republican Themes in Machiavelli, Burke and Tocqueville* (Princeton: Princeton University Press, 1985), 38; Jack D'Amico, "Machiavelli and Memory," *Modern Language Quarterly* 50, no. 2 (1989): 106; Joseph Khoury, "Machiavelli Manufacturing Memory: Terrorizing History, Historicizing Terror," in *Ars Reminiscendi: Minds and Memory in Renaissance Culture*, ed. Donald Beecher and Grant Williams (Toronto: Centre for Reformation and Renaissance Studies, 2009), 253.

16 Mikko Lahtinen, *Niccolò Machiavelli and Louis Althusser's Aleatory Materialism*, trans. Gareth Griffiths and Kristina Kolhi (Leiden: Brill, 2009), 140. Original emphasis.

17 Needless to say, there are plenty of commentators who insist on reading Machiavelli in this way, as a modern scientific or proto-scientific thinker of political technique. See, for example, Augustin Renaudet, *Machiavel: Étude d'histoire des doctrines politiques* (Paris: Gallimard, 1942), 193; James Burnham, *The Machiavellians: The Defenders of Freedom* (New York: John Day, 1943), 40; Leonardo Olschki, *Machiavelli: The Scientist* (Berkeley: Gillick Press, 1945), 25–6; Luigi Russo, *Machiavelli* (Bari: Laterza, 1949), 9; H. Butterfield, *The Statecraft of Machiavelli* (London: G. Bell and Sons, 1960); Anthony Parel, "Machiavelli's Method and His Interpreters," in *The Political Calculus: Essays on Machiavelli's Political Philosophy*, ed. Anthony Parel (Toronto: University of Toronto Press, 1972), 3, 5. For a much more plausible account of Machiavelli's "science," one that interprets the latter as a form of methodological anarchism such as was later articulated by Paul Feyerabend, see Megan K. Dyer and Cary J. Nederman, "Machiavelli against Method: Paul Feyerabend's Anti-Rationalism and Machiavellian Political 'Science,'" *History of European Ideas* 42, no. 3 (2016): 430–45.

of politics at play in his work. What motivates him is not the discovery of the form of the political most generally, but rather a specific political case, that of the crisis of Italian politics. There is no mode capable of uniting this case with all others in some sort of positive science, Machiavelli recognizing that the contingent dimension of human doing and being closes off any possibility of such universalization.

Although commentators have often stressed the degree to which Machiavelli's image of an active or critical history, a history practically oriented toward the generation of social and political change, is contrasted with a conservative history, a history which takes the form of the passive contemplation of complete and self-identical aesthetic objects, they have not gone far enough in articulating the precise form of the Machiavellian historiographical method and its implications for how Machiavelli understands the practice of political theory. An initial entry into this question can be developed through a consideration of the specificity of Machiavelli's use of Livy. It has been noted that there is nothing systematic in the method by which Machiavelli appeals to the authority of Livy.[18] Machiavelli is clearly not concerned with the simple reproduction of the Livian narrative, as evidenced by the perpetual tendency he has to divert from Livy via processes of elision, exaggeration, and on occasion fabrication. Markus Fischer, for example, provides two examples of Machiavelli's deliberate misreading of Livy:[19] in *The History of Rome* Livy reports that Romulus's murder of Remus was simply the culmination of a fit of rage and jealousy,[20] whereas Machiavelli roots it in Romulus's perception of the necessities of foundation;[21] and although Livy tries to demonstrate the degree to which the Roman violation of a peace agreement with the Samnites had a just origin,[22] Machiavelli uses this episode to demonstrate that states

---

18 J.H. Whitfield, "Machiavelli's Use of Livy," in *Livy*, ed. T.A. Dorey (Toronto: University of Toronto Press, 1971), 85.

19 Markus Fischer, "Machiavelli's Rapacious Republicanism," in *Machiavelli's Liberal Republican Legacy*, ed. Paul A. Rahe (Cambridge: Cambridge University Press, 2006), xxxvii.

20 Livy, *The Early History of Rome: Books I–V of The History of Rome from Its Foundations*, trans. Aubrey de Sélincourt (London: Penguin, 2002), bk. 1.7, 1.13–14.

21 Machiavelli, "Discorsi sopra la prima Deca di Tito Livio," bk. 1.9.

22 Livy, *Rome and Italy: Books VI–X of The History of Rome from Its Foundation*, trans. Betty Radice (London: Penguin, 1982), bk. 9.4–15.

need not keep promises that were made under duress.[23] And even when Machiavelli is relatively faithful to the Livian account of events, the interpretation of the political significance of these events is often greatly different. It would thus be fair to say that Machiavelli only "pretends to be a commentator,"[24] or even that "Machiavelli's Livy is a character of Machiavelli."[25] In the words of J.H. Whitfield, "the *Discorsi* are not an archaeological inquiry, or even a critical discussion of Livy, seen in historical perspective."[26] On the contrary, there is a "dual function of Livy and Machiavelli; the first constructs the past, makes it consist; the second seizes what is relevant, in the effort to construct the present, and to make the future consist."[27]

The consideration of Machiavelli's use of historical sources, and in particular of his use of Livy, like that between the claim of novelty and the appeal to imitation, presents us with another characteristic Machiavellian contradiction: the authority of Livy is affirmed as that most adequate to the extraction of meaning from the examples of Rome, and yet this authority is perpetually undermined through a highly selective and altered presentation of these examples, through the active misapplication of the Livian lessons. The second contradiction is merely a manifestation of the first, and is resolved in the same manner. Livy is of use in the contemporary political conjuncture to the extent that we are critically and reflectively able to represent elements of his histories which, through being combined in specific organizations of thought, reveal to us certain fundamental ethical and political imperatives relevant to the present. In this representation the Livian examples become other than what they originally were; they

---

23 Machiavelli, "Discorsi sopra la prima Deca di Tito Livio," bk. 3.42.

24 Smith, *Politics and Remembrance*, 54.

25 Leo Strauss, *Thoughts on Machiavelli* (Seattle: University of Washington Press, 1969), 141. Strauss also maintains that, to the extent that Machiavelli was not strictly concerned with the presentation of historical truth, he can be considered just as much an artist as an historian. Ibid., 45.

26 Whitfield, "Machiavelli's Use of Livy," 90.

27 Ibid., 84. It is certainly not difficult to locate additional inconsistencies in Machiavelli's deployment both of Livy and of examples drawn from other historical sources. See, for example, Felix Gilbert, *Machiavelli and Guicciardini: Politics and History in Sixteenth-Century Florence* (New York: W.W. Norton, 1984), 167; Maurizio Viroli, *Redeeming The Prince: The Meaning of Machiavelli's Masterpiece* (Princeton: Princeton University Press, 2014), 72; Michelle T. Clarke, "The Virtues of Republican Citizenship in Machiavelli's Discourses on Livy," *Journal of Politics* 75, no. 2 (2013): 322–3.

transcend their status as fixed statements regarding empirical patterns of behaviour, calling into question the very practice of historical representation, representation that seeks to organize the past into a complete object fit for contemplation. Machiavelli's selective approach to Livy is thus intended to overcome the conservatism of the Livian project.

Thinking in Constellations

Machiavelli's active engagement with the past, mediated through the texts of Livy in the case of the *Discourses*, is undertaken for the sake of the activation of Florentine political innovation in the present.[28] We thus see a triangulation of the terms of Rome, Florence, and Livy in "one unique time," where "neither the history of Rome, nor that of Florence, nor the Livian text is significant in itself: they have to be deciphered, as it were, reconstituted, through one another."[29] In *The Prince*'s dedicatory letter this dialectical relation between the past and the future, mediated through the deployed historical examples, is similarly affirmed as the ground from which emerges all practical political knowledge. Machiavelli proclaims that his specific historical understanding has been achieved relationally through his study of ancient things and his experience with modern ones.[30] If individuals and the world maintained an identical form across time, engagement in only one of the two modes would be necessary. But such is not the case; hence the necessity of Machiavelli's method. Given the nature of this method, it would be a mistake to judge the efficacy of the Machiavellian project on the basis of only one of its elements considered in its singularity. Most significantly, when evaluating Machiavelli's use of historical examples as a mode of communicating political ideals we must above all resist the temptation to interpret the legitimacy of the presentation in terms of the establishment of a strict correspondence

---

28 Needless to say, however, this method characterizes not only the Machiavelli of the *Discourses*. For an account of how Machiavelli reconfigures and redeploys historical examples in the *Florentine Histories* in order to stimulate a certain political sensibility, see Mauricio Suchowlansky, "Rhetoric and Violence in Machiavelli's *Florentine Histories*," *Shakespeare en devenir*, no. 5 (2011).

29 Lefort, "Machiavelli: History, Politics, Discourse," 114.

30 Machiavelli, "Il Principe," in *Tutte le opere*, chap. dedication.

between the Machiavellian discourse and the literal trajectory of events.[31]

It is insufficient to simply suggest, as several readers do, that the existence of a discontinuity between the images that Machiavelli constructs and the established historical record can be taken as evidence that Machiavelli does not intend his examples to be taken at face value.[32] To interpret Machiavelli according to such criteria of correspondence is to fail to appreciate Machiavelli's own historical methodology.[33] To borrow terms put forward by Edmund Jacobitti, we must be sensitive to the distinction between Machiavelli's rhetorical history and scientific history. Whereas the latter attempts to systematically recollect events as they actually occurred and order them in a straightforward representative manner, the former looks to imaginatively construct "external poetic universals" through the heuristic appropriation of past symbols and values, universals that the present historical actor may seize upon and apply in her own context in the effort to stimulate political change: "The task of the historian was to take situations, events, or characters from the past and make them fit current needs. If the actual record did not do so, if it was incomplete or silent, it simply needed to be embellished and recomposed in order to provide the examples."[34] Such a

---

31 Alkis Kontos, "Success and Knowledge in Machiavelli," in *The Political Calculus: Essays on Machiavelli's Political Philosophy*, ed. Anthony Parel (Toronto: University of Toronto Press, 1972), 94; Marie Gaille-Nikodimov, "An Introduction to *The Prince*," in *Seeking Real Truths: Multidisciplinary Perspectives on Machiavelli*, ed. Patricia Vilches and Gerald Seaman, trans. Gerald Seaman (Leiden: Brill, 2007), 25–6.

32 See, for example, Francesco Guicciardini, "Considerations on the *Discorsi* of Niccolò Machiavelli," in *The Sweetness of Power: Machiavelli's Discorsi and Guicciardini's Considerations*, trans. James B. Atkinson and David Sices (DeKalb: Northern Illinois University Press, 2002), 413; Catherine Zuckert, "The Life of Castruccio Castracani: Machiavelli as Literary Artist," *History of Political Thought* 31, no. 4 (2010): 577–603; John M. Najemy, "Machiavelli and Cesare Borgia: A Reconsideration of Chapter 7 of *Il Principe*," *Review of Politics* 75, no. 4 (2013): 539–56; Ryan Balot and Stephen Trochimchuk, "The Many and the Few: On Machiavelli's 'Democratic Moment,'" *Review of Politics* 74, no. 4 (2012): 559–88.

33 Hence Michael McCanles: "I am not concerned with Machiavelli's historical accuracy, with whether he rearranged historical events, or even if he made them up, because the text's meaning is not validated by the accuracy of its empirical reference." Michael McCanles, *The Discourse of Il Principe* (Malibu: Undena, 1983), xv.

34 Edmund E. Jacobitti, "The Classical Heritage in Machiavelli's Histories: Symbol and Poetry as Historic Literature," in *The Comedy and Tragedy of Machiavelli: Essays on the Literary Works*, ed. Vickie B. Sullivan (New Haven: Yale University Press, 2000), 180, 182.

method was, again, for the sake of the actualization of concrete political ends: "The actual events were secondary to the symbolic interpretation to which the events could be put. In short, the more Machiavelli infused mere empirical reality with poetic interpretation, that is, the farther he moved from chronological description of reality, the more instructive the writing became for use in reality."[35] Preceding Jacobitti, Federico Chabod identifies Machiavelli's mode of expression as being structured by an imaginative as opposed to a logical principle, and as being oriented toward the invention of new political norms through the reinterpretation of prior realities: "Machiavelli's imagination … accepts the legacy of the years, and converts it into a positive achievement – a new instrument, but still an imaginative one. On the other hand, it is nourished and illumined by an intense love of political invention – an obscure mental process by which a given situation is endowed with unsuspected possibilities."[36] This investment of the situation with new political potential is achieved through the critical redeployment of historical facts into new arrangements of thought: "Here is the true Machiavelli, assembling all the scattered elements of his experience and adapting them to another and more spacious form of existence with which they, viewed in the light of their individual, limited significance, would not appear commensurate."[37] The emergence of the new is the productive result of the creative and imaginative self-activity of the political theorist, a self-activity that takes the form of the reintegration of historical fragments, of past reflections and interpretations, into a new and "wholly unforeseen unity."[38] The end of historical analysis is not the reproduction of a fixed narrative, but the expression and extension of a fundamental imaginative capacity: "The value of what he says does not lie in the exactness of the detail. It lies in his inexhaustible creativeness, which even overlooks known facts, because it strives above all after continual self-development and self-renewal through an ever-widening experience."[39]

The significance of these two readings lies in their explicit identification of Machiavelli's creative deployment of historical examples with

---

35 Ibid., 186.
36 Federico Chabod, "An Introduction to *The Prince*," in *Machiavelli and the Renaissance*, trans. David Moore (London: Bowes and Bowes, 1960), 2–3.
37 Ibid., 9.
38 Ibid., 19–20.
39 Ibid., 11.

his normative concern with the affirmation of the new: the selective representation and juxtaposition of examples is seen as being not just oriented toward the stimulation of practical action in the world, but also a manifestation of the very principle of human creativity that makes possible political change. Nevertheless, the full significance of this identification is not grasped to the extent that both Jacobitti and Chabod ultimately reduce the general principles that are produced via the juxtaposition of examples to universal rules of behaviour. That is to say, the arrangement of examples x, y, and z is said to articulate the general maxim or rule a, a maxim or rule that is seen as being universally applicable across social contexts. Both readers succumb to the totalizing temptation to reduce the constructed figure of thought to a general unity that simply makes itself apparent in the concrete-specific case through the mode of comparison. Hence Chabod claims that Machiavelli "in any single event detects the ever-recurring workings of a universal process that is part and parcel of the human story."[40] The general idea which is illumined by the critical reconstruction of the arrangement of particulars is seen as being eternally manifest in each of these particulars prior to their arrangement in thought. Here it seems as if the eternal simply resides in the being-itself of the particular, such that "Between *to-day*, i.e. the passing moment with its particular problems, and *the eternal*, i.e. the great and ever-valid laws of politics, there certainly remains a continuing connection, we might even say reciprocity."[41] This image of the relation between particular and universal, where the former simply bears the latter in various apparent ways, is not able to fully grasp the Machiavellian concept of novelty. Rather than interpret the particular as a derivation of the universal, I believe that we would do better to interpret the universal as the productive consequence of a specific organization of particulars, recognizing that the universal lacks an independent being prior to this organization. Machiavelli's engagement with the particular example does not aim at the organization of such examples in a conceptual system structured by any sort of rational law.[42] I will argue that Machiavelli, to the extent that

---

40 Federico Chabod, "Machiavelli's Method and Style," in *Machiavelli and the Renaissance*, trans. David Moore (London: Bowes and Bowes, 1960), 129.

41 Ibid., 136.

42 In François Regnault's words, "Example is opposed to model." François Regnault, "La pensée du prince," *Cahiers pour l'analyse*, no. 6 (1967): 36. On his reading, Machiavelli's materialism "[proves] by example that there are only examples." Ibid., 41.

he establishes this relationship between universal and particular, anticipates a methodological mode which in the twentieth century would be
most famously developed by Walter Benjamin, and which can be
labelled thinking in constellations.[43]

Constellative thinking is distinct from traditional forms of comparative analysis that attempt to vertically relate concepts through the identification and isolation of the latter's common derivation from a higher
principle or term that remains static or fixed. Constellations challenge
conceptual understandings that have ossified into second natures
through the demonstration of the historical being of the phenomena
under consideration. To place a concept in a constellation is to be able
to take what was previously seen to be the content of the concept, *a*, and

---

43 Reading Machiavelli in light of Benjamin, even if only methodologically, may initially seem strange. There is some precedent, though, for thinking certain common-
alities between Machiavelli and members or associates of the Frankfurt School. Most
notably, Victoria Kahn argues that Machiavelli can be seen as a sort of kindred spirit
to Adorno and Horkheimer, with the latter in fact being able to help us appreciate the rhetorical dimensions of the former's thought: "Adorno and Horkheimer's
exemplary resistance to the traditional distinction between literary and philosophical or political texts can help us not only to see how literary and political notions
of representation and imitation are inextricable in Machiavelli's work but also to
recover the rhetoric in his political theory." Victoria Kahn, "Reduction and the Praise
of Disunion in Machiavelli's *Discourses*," *Journal of Medieval and Renaissance Studies*
18, no. 1 (1988): 2. What Machiavelli resists, most notably expressed in the *Discourses*'
praise of disunion, is the "lure of harmony and totality." Ibid. Despite his generally
critical view of Machiavelli (see, for example, Martin Jay, *The Dialectical Imagination:
A History of the Frankfurt School of Social Research, 1923–1950* [Berkeley: University of
California Press, 1973], 257), this at least was recognized by Horkheimer, for whom
Machiavelli was one of the "somber writers of the bourgeois dawn … who decried
the egotism of the self, acknowledged in so doing that society was the destructive
principle, and denounced harmony before it was elevated as the official doctrine
by the serene and classical authors. The latter boosted the totality of the bourgeois
order as the misery that finally fused both general and particular, society and self,
into one." Max Horkheimer and Theodor Adorno, *Dialectic of Enlightenment*, trans.
John Cumming (New York: Continuum, 2000), 90. In addition to Kahn's article, also
relevant in this respect is the following paper by Brian Harding, which suggests
that "we can note the similarity between Machiavelli's approach and that of critical theory: both look to history, rather than metaphysics, for an understanding of
political possibilities." Brian Harding, "Machiavelli's Politics and Critical Theory of
Technology," *Argumentos de Razón Técnica*, no. 12 (2009): 37–57. The specific possibility that critical theory is concerned with is the sublation of late capitalism, and that
which Machiavelli is concerned with is the liberation of the Italian peninsula.

recognize that it is, dependent upon its critical juxtaposition with other concepts, also *b, c, d,* and so on. The concept thus becomes both more and less than itself through the recognition of its internal difference and relation with other concepts. Although it is certainly the case that concepts have a content, constellative thinking aims to demonstrate that this content does not exhaust the being of the object. Concepts can only ever represent fragmented parts of the empirical world. Those parts available to consciousness vary, depending on the precise form of subjective mediation, on the specificity of the conceptual relation or the idea of which they are an element. By being rearranged through their constellative juxtaposition, concepts are capable of delivering to consciousness hitherto unrecognized contents.

The theory of the constellation would be given its classic expression in Benjamin's *The Origin of German Tragic Drama*. Benjamin here distinguishes between knowledge and truth, between philosophical representation and mathematical representation: "The more clearly mathematics demonstrate that the total elimination of the problem of representation – which is boasted by every didactic system – is the sign of genuine knowledge, the more conclusively does it reveal its renunciation of that area of truth towards which language is directed."[44] Philosophy must be oriented toward the representation of truth, as opposed to the acquisition of knowledge, which is characterized always by possession. Phenomena are capable of participating in truth only to the extent that they are able to elude assimilation into a system of acquired knowledge, only to the extent that their unity is broken up and their meaning multiplied. This multiplication is made possible through the empirical phenomenon's representation in a concept placed in a specific historical constellation: "Through their mediating role concepts enable phenomena to participate in the existence of ideas. It is this same mediating role which fits them for the other equally basic task of philosophy, the representation of ideas."[45]

As concepts are to knowledge, ideas are to truth. Truth, however, the representation of the idea, is not the representation of any determinate content, but rather the arrangement of the system of concepts: "For ideas are not represented in themselves, but solely and

---

44 Walter Benjamin, *The Origin of German Tragic Drama*, trans. John Osborne (London: Verso, 1998), 27.

45 Ibid., 34.

exclusively in an arrangement of concrete elements in the concept: as the configuration of those elements."[46] Whereas concepts delineate the nature of the empirical, ideas relate concepts to one another, truth lying in this contingent interrelatedness of concepts. To the extent that the arrangement of concepts in the idea is the foundation of the representative substance, neither concepts nor ideas present themselves as thematizable. The idea is simply the arrangement of such concepts, an arrangement that does not look toward the identification of static and singular contents: "When the idea absorbs a sequence of historical formulations, it does not do so in order to construct a unity out of them, let alone to abstract something common to them all."[47] Concepts are not extracted from ideas of which they participate a priori, but rather ideas are constructed historically through the critical arrangement of conceptual elements. Benjamin writes that "ideas are to objects as constellations are to stars."[48] The meaning of its perception, the way in which a star is appropriated by a viewing subject, is dependent upon the vantage point from which the subject perceives, upon the constellation within which the star is seen to exist at the moment of perception. Similarly, the way in which the object is to be represented depends upon the critical arrangement of concepts in a particular constellation: "The history locked in the object can only be delivered by a knowledge mindful of the historic positional value of the object in its relation to other objects – by the actualization and concentration of something which is already known and is transformed by that knowledge."[49] The form of subjective cognition thereby structures the objectivity of that which the subject appropriates, opening the seemingly closed world of the object to a multiplicity of meanings or realities.

Subjective mediation thus has the potential to break up perceived truths that have hardened into dogmas, the concept being dereified through the affirmation of the historical specificity of knowledge. In constructing a constellation, then, one does not simply aim to construct a new system, to supplant an old systematic doctrine with a

---

46 Ibid.
47 Ibid., 46.
48 Ibid., 34.
49 Theodor Adorno, *Negative Dialectics*, trans. E.B. Ashton (New York: Continuum, 1973), 163.

new one. Rather, one looks to reveal a previously hidden potentiality, bringing to light a new content without hypostatizing it, without invalidating the potential of the concept to enter into other relations. To put it more concretely, the image of Rome that results from Machiavelli's particular arrangement of conceptual elements drawn from Livy is one constellative possibility, just as is the conservative patrician image. Similarly, in emphasizing and juxtaposing particular elements of Machiavelli's political theory in deliberate ways, I produce a unique image of his thought. That production, however, is certainly not meant to instaurate an analytical closure that would bar the possibility of alternative readings via the construction of different constellative arrangements, be they democratic, Cambridge School, Straussian, and so on.

Perspectival Analysis and Constellative Thinking

In light of the above discussion, it is of the utmost significance that in *The Prince* Machiavelli begins his investigation into the nature of the virtuous political actor by affirming the necessity of recognizing the perspectival character of knowledge. In his dedicatory letter he will highlight the degree to which the acquisition of particular knowledges is structured by the observer's objective position in a circumscribed field that delimits understanding: "because just as those who design landscapes place themselves low on the plain in order to consider the nature of mountains and high places, and to consider the low place themselves high on the mountains, similarly, to know well the nature of peoples one must be a prince, and to know well the nature of princes one must be of the people."[50] Throughout Machiavelli's political work we are continually confronted with this theme of perspectivism, the virtuous political actor being identified as one who is capable of representing to him or herself a multiplicity of different perspectives, recognizing the extent to which the shift in perspective fundamentally alters the concept: one's perception of the nature of the object that is being

---

50 Machiavelli, "Il Principe," chap. dedication. Alejandro Bárcenas argues that Machiavelli "took the artist, not the *condottiere* as his model for the analysis of politics," precisely because we live in a world of multiple perspectives, and the artist is the one most adept at viewing from a plurality of angles. Alejandro Bárcenas, *Machiavelli's Art of Politics* (Leiden: Brill, 2015), 43.

observed.[51] This is most notably expressed, for example, in Machiavelli's exhortation to military leaders to privilege the study of the variance of sites and terrains, and how the occupation of different strategic locations strongly influences understanding.[52] Hence the subject matter of *Discourses* 3:39, in which Machiavelli writes that "among the other things that are necessary to a captain of armies is understanding of sites and of countries, for without this general and particular understanding a captain cannot carry out anything properly. And because all knowledges demand experience if one is to possess them well, this is one that requires very great experience."[53] The key form of such experience – that aiming at the refinement of the capacity for critical perspectival analysis – is hunting: "One cannot acquire this understanding of countries in any other suitable way than via hunting, because hunting makes he who uses it particularly knowledgeable of that country where he trains. And once one is properly familiar with a region, he then comprehends with ease all new countries, because every country and every member of these have some conformity with one another, so that understanding of the one easily passes to understanding of the other."[54]

We must not be misled here by Machiavelli's seeming suggestion that perspectival analysis generates in the prudent actor fixed standards of behaviour that are capable of being applied in necessarily identical contexts. Such forms of perspectival study are not valued to the degree that they result in the acquisition of a positive knowledge that can be referred to when one encounters equivalent situations. On the contrary, Machiavelli's emphasis is not on a content, but a capacity,

---

51 For recognitions of this fact see Charles D. Tarlton, "*Fortuna* and the Landscape of Action in Machiavelli's *Prince*," *New Literary History* 30, no. 4 (1999): 737; Kenneth C. Blanchard Jr, "Being, Seeing, and Touching: Machiavelli's Modification of Platonic Epistemology," *Review of Metaphysics* 49, no. 3 (1996): 598; Sebastián Torres, "Tempo e politica: una lettura materialista di Machiavelli," in *The Radical Machiavelli: Politics, Philosophy, and Language*, ed. Filippo Del Lucchese, Fabio Frosini, and Vittorio Morfino (Leiden: Brill, 2015), 179.

52 E.g., Machiavelli, "Dell'Arte della guerra," in *Tutte le opere*, 334.

53 Machiavelli, "Discorsi sopra la prima Deca di Tito Livio," bk. 3.39. Such a process of generalization is noted by Laura Janara, who perceives that the prince's success is grounded in his ability to imaginatively represent the diverse standpoints that exist in the political field. Laura Janara, "Machiavelli, Elizabeth I and the Innovative Historical Self: A Politics of Action, Not Identity," *History of Political Thought* 27, no. 3 (2006): 464.

54 Machiavelli, "Discorsi sopra la prima Deca di Tito Livio," bk. 3.39.

one being better equipped to critically confront the radically new situation when one is familiar with various forms of perspectival representation. This becomes clear in Machiavelli's discussion of the topic in chapter 14 of *The Prince*. Once again the significance of hunting is affirmed, it being maintained that the actor should "learn the nature of sites, learn about how mountains rise, how valleys descend, how plains lie, and understand the nature of rivers and marshes – and in this place the greatest care."[55] Machiavelli will go on to suggest, however, that better learning the layout of your land is not for the sake of the construction of a fixed schema that is universally applicable across multiple times and spaces, but for the sake of the development of a critical skill or capacity that can be deployed in necessarily unique circumstances. Thus he writes, "understanding of and experience with those sites facilitates understanding of any other new site that it is necessary to examine."[56]

The potential to refine this skill or capacity, furthermore, is potentially perpetual, as is revealed through the case of the Greek prince Philopoeman. Machiavelli will note that whenever Philopoeman was out with others he would always interrogate the landscape, asking, "If the enemy were up on that hill and we were here with our army, which of us would have the advantage? How could we advance, while maintaining order, to meet them? If we wanted to withdraw, how ought we to? If they were withdrawing, how ought we pursue them?"[57] The practical questioning of Philopoeman illustrates to Machiavelli the non-possibility of ever achieving a critical mastery that would terminate the need for perspectival study. But once again, the fact that it is not possible to abstract such practical activity from historical study is revealed in the manner in which Machiavelli concludes chapter 14, stressing again the dialectical relation between theory and practice, between the ancient and the present, through the reaffirmation of the actor's need to supplement the study of terrains with the exercise of the mind via the reading of histories and critical reflection on the deeds of past actors: "above all to do as some excellent man has done in the past, who has taken to imitate whosoever before him was praised and glorified, and who has always held these acts and deeds near himself, as it is said that

---

55 Machiavelli, "Il Principe," chap. 14.
56 Ibid.
57 Ibid.

Alexander the Great imitated Achilles; Caesar, Alexander; Scipio, Cyrus."[58] This common theme in Machiavelli, that great "men almost always walk on the paths beaten by others and proceed in their actions by imitation,"[59] that the prudent political actor will attempt to imitate the modes of clearly virtuous individuals in the past, refers us to a very precise form of imitation. It would be a mistake, for example, to think of imitation in terms of the static reproduction of prior particulars, such as is done by Francis Bacon, for whom "the form of writing which of all others is fittest for this variable argument of negotiation and occasions is that which Machiavel chose wisely and aptly for government; namely, discourse upon histories or examples. For knowledge drawn freshly and in our view out of particulars, knoweth the way best to particulars again."[60] On the contrary, Machiavelli is advocating not the imitation of inert particulars whose beings are stable prior to their arrangement in thought – not fixed and immobile patterns of behaviour – but rather a creative and critical mode of being, a reflective orientation toward the world that allows one to respond to the emergence of contingency in always unique ways. If the actor learns from these modes a form of flexibility and reflexivity, when fortune changes, he or she will be ready to resist.[61]

Machiavelli writes that "one who considers present and ancient things easily knows how in all cities and in all peoples there are the same desires and the same humours, and how there always have been."[62] It is this fact that allows prudent actors to anticipate the emergence of future problems and initiate activity that looks to their resolution. Although such remedies may on occasion necessitate a reproduction of past modes, they may also be rooted in the innovative generation of entirely new modes. Thoughtful reflection on history may allow the actor facing new problems to apply "those remedies that were used by the ancients, or, not finding any that were used, to *imagine new ones*, through the similarity of accidents."[63] This notion of

---

58 Ibid.
59 Ibid., chap. 6.
60 Francis Bacon, "The Advancement of Learning," in *Bacon's Advancement of Learning and the New Atlantis* (Oxford: Benediction Classics, 2008), 196.
61 Machiavelli, "Il Principe," chap. 14.
62 Machiavelli, "Discorsi sopra la prima Deca di Tito Livio," bk. 1.39.
63 Ibid. Emphasis added.

imitation as innovation is particularly well articulated in *Discourses* 2:16, where Machiavelli recalls the first battle of the Latin War. The armies of the Romans and the Latins, Machiavelli tells us, were identical in all respects, possessing an equivalent skill, size, and obstinacy. This likeness was achieved as a consequence of the similar education of each: "having served a long time together in the military, they were alike in speech, order, and arms."[64] The fundamental difference between the two armies, according to Livy, was the greater virtue among the Roman captains. And how did this virtue manifest itself? Crucially, for Machiavelli it was expressed through the Roman captains' abilities to utilize a mode of creative imitation in order to respond to the emergence of unexpected contingencies. Specifically, "in the managing of this battle there emerged two accidents that had not arisen before and of which afterwards there have been few examples: of the two consuls, to keep the spirits of the soldiers firm, obedient to their commands, and determined to fight, one killed himself and the other his son."[65] The actions of the Roman consuls Decius, who killed himself, and Torquatus, who killed his son, adequately hardened the spirits of the Romans, separating them from their enemies and providing them with the energy needed to prevail. In light of the objective identity of the opposing forces, the Romans could be elevated only through some extraordinary thing, but some thing which was absolutely singular and without prior existence. Virtue was not located in the repetition of a past good and timeless example, but rather lay in a creative bringing forth of a completely new mode. Indeed, Machiavelli maintains that this openness to innovation is in fact the source of all Roman virtue: "Titus Livy shows, in showing this equality of forces, the whole order that the Romans maintained in armies and in fighting."[66] Virtue lay not in literal imitation, but in the imitation of a creative capacity that is deployed in always unique situations and which results in always unique modes.

This account, furthermore, appears immediately before Machiavelli seemingly advocates a more traditional form of imitation, appealing to modern leaders to repeat specific ancient orders and patterns, in this case through the arrangement of the *astati, principi,* and *triari* in battle.

---

64 Ibid., bk. 2.16.
65 Ibid.
66 Ibid.

There is no contradiction in the chapter, however, for once again what Machiavelli admires in this latter example is the arrangement's openness to change, the fact that this mode of fighting gives itself three opportunities before it is defeated. Modern armies are incapable of structuring themselves such that they are open to this multiplicity of chance, preferring instead to interpret their initial fate as the ultimate one, closing off any future possibility for a change of trajectory: "whoever cannot resist but on the first push, as all the Christian armies today, can easily lose, because any disorder, any middling virtue, can take victory away from them."[67] To the extent that they eschew a willingness to organize themselves so as to allow for creative adaptation in response to changing fortune, the Christian armies affirm a one-sided and literal imitation of things, as opposed to a critical and reflective imitation of capacities. What is to be affirmed, in other words, is a critical orientation that is able to prudently recognize the need for behavioural adaptation should innovative activity be perpetuated and new realities generated.[68]

What Machiavelli hopes to reveal to his reader through these examples is the possibility for unprecedented human action. He wishes to preserve the memory of those events that break the seemingly

---

67 Ibid. On the fact that Machiavelli prioritizes the managing of accidents in battle see John P. McCormick, "Pocock, Machiavelli and Political Contingency in Foreign Affairs: Republican Existentialism Outside (and Within) the City," *History of European Ideas* 43, no. 2 (2017): 180. Compare my reading here to that of Felix Gilbert, who understands Machiavelli's call for a reappropriation of ancient lessons of warfare in terms of literal imitation. Felix Gilbert, "Machiavelli: The Renaissance of the *Art of War*," in *Makers of Modern Strategy: From Machiavelli to the Modern Age*, ed. Peter Paret (Princeton: Princeton University Press, 1986), 22.

68 Eugene Garver, arguing that Machiavelli never advocated slavish imitation of past modes, notes that "*The Prince* is filled with examples of princes going wrong by imitating examples; these must alert the prince to the paradoxical task of learning, through imitation, to become an innovator." Eugene Garver, "Machiavelli's *The Prince*: A Neglected Rhetorical Classic," *Philosophy and Rhetoric* 13, no. 2 (1980): 101. The examples Machiavelli provides are not meant to be strictly imitated, but on the contrary to stimulate prudent reflection; "examples do not function as instances of truths already ascertained." Ibid., 104. Elsewhere Garver will distinguish between the stylistic imitation of the hereditary prince and the rhetorical invention of the new prince, the straightforward or literal imitation of the latter being identified as necessarily antithetical to political creation. Eugene Garver, "Machiavelli and the Politics of Rhetorical Invention," *CLIO* 14, no. 2 (1985): 158.

determinate flow of history, thus revealing the fact that time is not sequential, but rather open to the radical emergence of the new.[69] It is within the context of Machiavelli's theorization of the event, of the human potential for historical creation, that we must understand the well-known concept of the *verità effettuale della cosa*. Distinguishing between his own historical approach, which takes off from the political potential germinating within the concrete here and now, and those abstractly utopian political projects ungrounded in consideration of the constraints of life in an empirical world, Machiavelli writes: "since my intention is to write something useful to one who understands it, it seemed the most suitable to go after the effectual truth of the thing rather than the fantasy of it. And many have fantasized about republics and principalities that have never been seen or known to exist in reality; for there is so much distance between how one lives and how one should live that he who gives up what is done for what should be done learns his ruin rather than his preservation."[70] The *verità effettuale* does not refer us to any sort of absolute truth or reality that would pre-structure the direction of our action, but rather to the truth of the possibility for the virtuous actor to generate new political realities – events – through the critical analysis of worldly potential. In the words of Barbara Godorecci, the *verità effettuale* expresses a "conception of truth whose identity is tied to the event ('lo evento della cosa'), to the process of living that is a constant becoming. In practical terms, Machiavellian *verità effettuale* rejects programming, if by 'program' one intends a pre-established goal to be achieved by pre-established methods (a rejection, therefore, of any specific form of methodology)."[71]

As I will argue in chapter 3 in my discussion of the relationship between *virtù* and *fortuna*, to recognize the *verità effettuale* is to recognize the contextual situation of your action within a non-teleological historical stream which you act into and which acts upon you, such interaction producing a multiplicity of unforeseeable and undetermined events. In

---

69 There is once more a strong parallel between Machiavelli and Benjamin here, given the latter's critique of historicism. See especially Walter Benjamin, "Theses on the Philosophy of History," in *Illuminations: Essays and Reflections*, ed. Hannah Arendt, trans. Harry Zohn (New York: Schocken Books, 1968), 253–64.

70 Machiavelli, "Il Principe," chap. 15.

71 Barbara J. Godorecci, *After Machiavelli: "Re-Writing" and the "Hermeneutic Attitude"* (West Lafayette: Purdue University Press, 1993), 134.

order to articulate such singularities, to further highlight the political significance of major historical events, Machiavelli theoretically pushes them to their most extreme points. For Benjamin "Ideas are timeless constellations, and by virtue of the elements' being seen as points in such constellations, phenomena are subdivided and at the same time redeemed; so that those elements which it is the function of the concept to elicit from phenomena are most clearly evident at the extremes."[72] It is thus that "the concept has its roots in the extreme."[73] Machiavelli's much-noted method of exaggeration can here be thought in terms of a form of thinking at the extreme, used in order to affirm the capacity to initiate the new.[74]

Just as Machiavelli pushes to the extreme his ancient sources in order to affirm the innovative capacity, in what remains of this work I will attempt to extract and push to the extreme those conceptual elements in Machiavelli that speak to the potential for radically democratic political creation. I have argued in this chapter that not only, as is commonly pointed out, does Machiavelli's appeal to the wisdom of the ancients not contradict his claim regarding his theoretical novelty, but also that this appeal is a deliberate methodological strategy that upholds a broad affirmation of novelty most generally. The lessons Machiavelli would

---

72 Benjamin, *The Origin of German Tragic Drama*, 34–5.

73 Ibid., 35.

74 It is especially notable that a recently inaugurated book series on the thought of Machiavelli takes as its title "Thinking in Extremes." For its first contribution see Filippo Del Lucchese, Fabio Frosini, and Vittorio Morfino, eds, *The Radical Machiavelli: Politics, Philosophy and Language* (Leiden: Brill, 2015). For different interpretations of the function of Machiavelli's exaggeration see Strauss, *Thoughts on Machiavelli*, 82; Gilbert, *Machiavelli and Guicciardini*, 166; Victoria Kahn, "*Virtù* and the Example of Agathocles in Machiavelli's *Prince*," in *Machiavelli and the Discourse of Literature*, ed. Albert Russell Ascoli and Victoria Kahn (Ithaca: Cornell University Press, 1993), 200; Pierre Manent, *An Intellectual History of Liberalism*, trans. Rebecca Balinski (Princeton: Princeton University Press, 1995), 13. On the relationship between thinking at the extreme and political creation see Emmanuel Terray, "An Encounter: Althusser and Machiavelli," in *Postmodern Materialism and the Future of Marxist Theory: Essays in the Althusserian Tradition*, ed. and trans. Antonio Callari and David F. Ruccio (Hanover: Wesleyan University Press, 1996), 258; Louis Althusser, "Is It Simple to Be a Marxist in Philosophy?," in *Essays in Self-Criticism*, trans. Grahame Lock (London: New Left Books, 1976), 170.

have us draw from the past are not to be found in our one-sided imitation of prior modes of doing and being, but rather in our critical recognition of the singularity of these past events, events that reveal to us the specifically human capacity for political innovation. Machiavelli's mode of historical appropriation aims at, through the creative reinvestment of the meaning of events through their selective juxtaposition in specific figures or constellations of thought, the articulation of this innovative potential. The recognition of this potential is then seen to provide a ground from which the interested political actor is able to launch a historical endeavour aimed at the transformation of the world. For Machiavelli such is the only legitimate mode of historical practice.

I would suggest that the implications of Machiavelli's project for political theory, and in particular the history of political thought, are potentially far-reaching. What would it mean to read Machiavelli, for example, in the same way that Machiavelli reads Livy? To begin to answer this question would be to begin to explain the staggering diversity of interpretations that characterize the field of Machiavelli studies, which might be initially divided into two broad categories. As is noted, for example, by Eric Weil and Miguel Abensour, we may distinguish between an academic Machiavelli who exists only as an object of scholarship, and a political Machiavelli who emerges in the present historical context in order to assist us in articulating the being of the contemporary political conjuncture. In Abensour's words, "The question is no longer to address the topic called Machiavelli, but to think Machiavelli through, or better to think *with* Machiavelli the political issues of the present."[75] This distinction between a scholarly and a political Machiavelli can be mapped onto Machiavelli's distinction between a contemplative and an active history. Just as Machiavelli's historical examples become, through their critical juxtaposition with one another, other than what they originally were, so might Machiavelli become other than himself depending upon how we choose to read him in the moment. Once we begin to read Machiavelli in our time, in our own here and now, we find that, in the words of Weil, "other moments emerge and give a new life to he who, until then, was

---

75 Miguel Abensour, *Democracy against the State: Marx and the Machiavellian Moment*, trans. Max Blechman and Martin Breaugh (London: Polity Press, 2011), 4. Original emphasis.

but one author among others."[76] The fact that Machiavelli was responding to his specific historical-political situation in no way delimits his potential to intervene in our own.[77] In opposition to the wide variety of contextualist and esoteric readings of Machiavelli, I would suggest that our goal should be not exclusively examining what it is that Machiavelli thought and why, but in addition, considering what it is that Machiavelli can do for us today, if we adopt the same approach to reading him as he did to his ancient sources.

---

76 Eric Weil, "Machiavel aujourd'hui," in *Essais et conférences*, vol. 2: *Politique* (Paris: Librairie Philosophique J. Vrin, 1991), 190.

77 On this point see, for example, Carlos Frade, "An Altogether New Prince Five Centuries On: Bringing Machiavelli to Bear on Our Present," *Situations* 5, no. 1 (2013): 60; Gopal Balakrishnan, "Future Unknown: Machiavelli for the Twenty-First Century," *New Left Review* 32 (April 2005): 20.

PART TWO

Philosophical Anthropology

Chapter Two

The Contingency of Being: On Worldly and Human Indetermination

In this chapter I will attempt to extract from Machiavelli's writings a general philosophy of being that is composed of two related elements: a theory of worldly being and a theory of human being. Machiavelli will theorize both external and internal nature in terms of a radical indetermination unhinged from any absolute structural foundations that would transcendentally ground them, as well as any determinable logics of development that would orient their movement in a rational or causal manner. Machiavelli's rejection of totalizing forms of philosophical investigation is well-known. Nevertheless, the lack of any trace of systematization is certainly no justification for suggesting that Machiavelli rejects all forms of philosophical investigation.[1] Machiavelli's rejection of static structures of Being, whether grounded in an affirmation of a positive natural law, cosmology, or theology, must not lead us to conclude that he rejects all ontological effort as such. On the contrary, he most notably gives us a very precise ontology of the human being, specifically one grounded in a consideration of its creative political power.[2] Machiavelli's philosophy does contain a specific ontology, a specific theory of human being in the world. It is just that for Machiavelli this question of being does not refer us to any positive metaphysic,

---

1 See, for example, Dante Germino, "Second Thoughts on Leo Strauss's Machiavelli," *Journal of Politics* 28, no. 4 (1966): 815. For a study of Machiavelli's relation to the philosophical tradition and the degree to which he can be situated in it see Gaille, *Machiavel et la tradition philosophique.*

2 As Agnès Cugno notes, "The thought of Machiavelli takes the human as its theme, but in the very specific mode of *homo politicus*." Agnès Cugno, "Machiavel et le problème de l'être en politique," *Revue philosophique de la France et de l'étranger* 189, no. 1 (1999): 19.

to any surplus reality beyond that which we are capable of experiencing as sensuous beings. In particular, Machiavelli is interested in the question of the form of political action as a modality of human creation.

I argue in this chapter and the following one that Machiavelli provides us with a very precise model of the human essence. His concept of human essence, however, is a negative as opposed to a positive one. A positive essence would refer us to a perpetually fixed set of natural human properties whose objective contours could be determined and mapped in systematic fashion, thus producing an architectonic model of humanity. A negative essence, on the contrary, rejects attempts to theorize all elements of human being in terms of such positive determinations, seeing one of the fundamental components of essence instead in the specifically human ability to transcend many merely immediate and conventional forms of doing and being. A negative essence refers us, in other words, not to a specifically human content, but rather a specifically human capacity, that is, the capacity for creativity. The human being is that which is capable of, through its life activity, perpetually remaking itself and its social world, although in a form that is obviously delimited by certain biological and historical constraints. Negative models of essence that emphasize the creative potential of human beings to shape their own nature have been developed in different ways by a variety of the canonical thinkers of the tradition of modern political thought. The significance of Machiavelli, however, lies in the fact that he was the first to interpret such creation as manifesting itself in the specifically political field, providing a model of an explicitly political form of the realization of the negative human essence. In chapter 3 I will examine in more detail this political form of realization through a study of the ethics of creation as articulated in *The Prince*. In this chapter, however, I will first provide an overview of those philosophical assumptions that for Machiavelli provided the conceptual background for the theorization of the human being in terms of a fundamental creativity. In the first part of the chapter I will detail Machiavelli's thoughts on the contingent and chaotic structure of the world. This structure of the world, lacking any positive organizing form, is mirrored in the indetermination of the individual human being. In the second part of the chapter I will thus begin to provide an initial account of this indetermination, specifically as it is represented for Machiavelli in both the diversity of modes of human doing and being, and the openness of human being to change and alteration.

Worldly Indetermination and the Rejection of Metaphysics

It has become increasingly common for readers of Machiavelli to stress the extent to which he not only engaged with but was significantly influenced by the Epicurean philosophical tradition, whose rediscovery in the Florentine context took on an especially acute form.[3] Machiavelli was very familiar with the Epicurean tradition, having transcribed Lucretius's *De rerum natura* and having known Diogenes Laertius's *Lives of Eminent Philosophers*, as revealed for example in his redeployment of various of the statements found in this text in "The Life of Castruccio Castracani."[4] Paul Rahe notes that "by 1517 or so, if not well before, Machiavelli had made Lucretius' repudiation of religion and his rejection of natural teleology his own."[5] In this section I will be concerned with outlining the main contours of this rejection of natural teleology, demonstrating how Machiavelli theorizes the fundamentally inconstant, irregular, and chaotic form of being of the world. This outline will certainly not be sufficient to construct a comprehensive philosophy of world in Machiavelli, a philosophy that he clearly never attempted to analytically define, but will hopefully suffice to demonstrate the extent to which Machiavelli understands temporal being in

---

3 See, for example, Alison Brown, *The Return of Lucretius to Renaissance Florence* (Cambridge: Cambridge University Press, 2010); Ada Palmer, *Reading Lucretius in the Renaissance* (Cambridge: Harvard University Press, 2014).

4 Machiavelli, "La vita di Castruccio Castracani da Lucca," in *Tutte le opere*, 613–28. On Machiavelli's annotations of *De rerum natura* see Palmer, *Reading Lucretius in the Renaissance*, 81–8.

5 Paul A. Rahe, "In the Shadow of Lucretius: The Epicurean Foundations of Machiavelli's Political Thought," *History of Political Thought* 28, no. 1 (2007): 44. For further studies of the influence of Lucretius on Machiavelli see Louis Althusser, "The Underground Current of the Materialism of the Encounter," in *Philosophy of the Encounter: Later Writings, 1978–87*, ed. François Matheron and Oliver Corpet, trans. G.M. Goshgarian (London: Verso, 2006), 163–207; Vittorio Morfino, "Tra Lucrezio e Spinoza: la 'filosofia' di Machiavelli," in *Machiavelli: immaginazione e contingenza*, ed. Filippo Del Lucchese, Luca Sartorello, and Stefano Visentin (Pisa: Edizioni Ets, 2006), 67–110; Rahe, "In the Shadow of Lucretius"; Robert J. Roecklein, *Machiavelli and Epicureanism: An Investigation into the Origins of Early Modern Political Thought* (Lanham: Lexington Books, 2012); Alison Brown, "Lucretian Naturalism and the Evolution of Machiavelli's Ethics," in *The Radical Machiavelli: Politics, Philosophy, and Language*, ed. Filippo Del Lucchese, Fabio Frosini, and Vittorio Morfino (Leiden: Brill, 2015), 105–27; Del Lucchese, *The Political Philosophy of Niccolò Machiavelli*, 32–6.

terms of non-determination, such non-determination being ultimately the very condition of possibility of human freedom.[6]

I am thus attempting to provide an alternative to those readings of Machiavelli that locate in his thought an affirmation of a natural or ontological stability that gives a consistency and uniformity to temporal being.[7] It is certainly true that there seem to be some passages in the Machiavellian texts that suggest the belief in the type of patterned order that certain commentators perceive. One chapter commonly cited, for example, is *Discourses* 3:43, where Machiavelli writes that "anyone who wants to see what has to be considers what has been; for all the things of the world, in every time, have their counterpart in ancient times."[8] Nevertheless, Machiavelli's seeming affirmation of the constancy of the world through time is immediately problematized, as he goes on to make clear that such constancy is by no means the product of natural movement, but rather is socially constituted and highly contextual. Speaking of the identity of past worldly being and present worldly being, he continues: "This arises because, being caused by men, who have and always have had the same passions, they of necessity result in the same effect. It is true that their works are now in this province more virtuous than in that, and in that more than in this, according to the

---

6 This relationship between worldly contingency and free human action that this contingency has opened has, as Maurice Merleau-Ponty has noted, puzzled many of Machiavelli's readers. Maurice Merleau-Ponty, "A Note on Machiavelli," in *Signs*, trans. Richard C. McCleary (Evanston: Northwestern University Press, 1964), 218. The extent to which the latter leans upon the former, however, has certainly been noticed by some commentators. See, for example, Miguel Vatter, *Between Form and Event: Machiavelli's Theory of Political Freedom* (Dordrecht: Kluwer Academic Publishers, 2000), 133. Antonio Negri, *Insurgencies: Constituent Power and the Modern State*, trans. Maurizia Boscagli (Minneapolis: University of Minnesota Press, 1999), 38. Dick Howard, *The Primacy of the Political: A History of Political Thought from the Greeks to the French and American Revolutions* (New York: Columbia University Press, 2010), 199.

7 Anthony J. Parel, *The Machiavellian Cosmos* (New Haven: Yale University Press, 1992); Sammy Basu, "In a Crazy Time the Crazy Come Out Well: Machiavelli and the Cosmology of His Day," *History of Political Thought* 2, no. 2 (1990): 213–39; John H. Geerken, "Elements of Natural Law Theory in Machiavelli," in *The Medieval Tradition of Natural Law*, ed. Harold J. Johnson (Kalamazoo: Medieval Institute Publications, 1987), 37–65; Graham Maddox, "The Secular Reformation and the Influence of Machiavelli," *Journal of Religion* 82, no. 4 (2002): 539–62; Mark Hulliung, *Citizen Machiavelli* (Princeton: Princeton University Press, 1983), 154.

8 Machiavelli, "Discorsi sopra la prima Deca di Tito Livio," in *Tutte le opere*, bk. 3.43.

form of education in which those people have taken their mode of liv-ing."[9] The affirmation of stability of worldly being, however, is not here simply displaced onto another register, the fixity of the world being a consequence of the fixity of the universal nature of the species, as rep-resented in the claim regarding the identity of the passions. On the con-trary, Machiavelli makes clear that in this discussion he is presuming a continuity in the precise forms of education and socialization that a community utilizes through time: "It is easy to know the things to come from the past, if a nation for a long time keeps the same customs, being continually avaricious or continually fraudulent, or having some other similar vice or virtue."[10] As I will argue in chapter 6, the republic is that form of regime that is capable of breaking out of this continuity and institutionalizing innovation, thus making it possible to reflectively and self-consciously remake the world. The identity and constancy of worldly things as presented in 3:43 is historically contingent, an artifi-cial result of a precise form of social organization, one which in the final instance Machiavelli will reject on normative grounds. Indeed, in this chapter Machiavelli will proceed to associate the impoverishment of the contemporary Florentine political situation with that type of uncrit-ical approach to history that generates the very sense of temporal uni-formity. Machiavelli says that in their dealings with external nations the Florentines, criticized for being avaricious and lacking in faith, failed to learn from past lessons, failed to recognize the modes which these nations have historically acted in. He writes, "if Florence had not been compelled by necessity or overcome by passion, and had read and understood the ancient customs of the barbarians, it would have been deceived by them neither this nor many other times, since they have always been in one mode and have always used with everyone the very same terms."[11] Florentine virtue would here lie precisely in the aboli-tion of the presumption of historical constancy, perpetually affirmed by its enemies. The Florentines' own corruption would be overcome through the transcendence of the belief in the continuity of time. Their recognition of the universality of the modes of others is the means by which the Florentines might overcome their own current, although by no means natural or inevitable, nature.

---

9 Ibid.
10 Ibid.
11 Ibid.

Although initially it might suggest a belief in the stable being of the form of the world, 3:43 in the end actually affirms the opposite. There are many other passages in the *Discourses* that lend further evidence to the argument that Machiavelli thinks of the being of the world in terms of contingent movement and flux. Here I will highlight just some of these passages, although in a necessarily, given Machiavelli's own form of presentation, non-systematic way.[12] The most notable such passage is 2:5, where, according to Antonio Negri, Machiavelli "tries to define the Heraclitean flux of becoming as an experience of freedom."[13] The title of 2:5 is "That the variation of sects and languages, together with the accident of floods or plague, extinguishes the memories of things." This title points us toward a dual concern with both conventional human variation and physical worldly variation via accidental natural events, and hence a simultaneous affirmation of natural and social flux. Indeed, Machiavelli begins the chapter by stating: "To those philosophers who determined that the world was eternal, I believe that one could reply that if such antiquity were true it would be reasonable that there should be memory of more than five thousand years, except it is seen how the memories of times is extinguished by diverse causes, of which part come from men, part from heaven."[14] First, the diversity of human beings is located in "the variations of sects and of languages."[15] Sectarian division here refers us to variation in religion, religion having been earlier identified as the primary mode of human socialization, the diversity of sects thus referring us to a larger diversity of culture.[16] If

---

12 Indeed, the apparently non-systematic structure of Machiavelli's work can be seen as representative of the non-systematic structure of reality. See, for example, Gennaro Sasso, *Niccolò Machiavelli: storia del suo pensiero politico* (Bologna: Società editrice il Mulino, 1980), 520; Joseph Anthony Mazzeo, "The Poetry of Power: Machiavelli's Literary Vision," *Review of National Literatures* 1, no. 1 (1970): 48; Filippo Del Lucchese, *Conflict, Power, and Multitude in Machiavelli and Spinoza* (London: Continuum, 2009), 47.

13 Negri, *Insurgencies*, 70. On the Heraclitean dimension of Machiavelli's thought see also Neal Wood, "Some Common Aspects of the Thought of Seneca and Machiavelli," *Renaissance Quarterly* 21, no. 1 (1968): 19.

14 Machiavelli, "Discorsi sopra la prima Deca di Tito Livio," bk. 2.5.

15 Ibid.

16 On the significance of religion as a comprehensive mode of socialization for Machiavelli, as opposed to a one-sided and instrumental compulsion to obey the law, see, for example, John M. Najemy, "Papirus and the Chickens, or Machiavelli on the Necessity of Intepreting Religion," *Journal of the History of Ideas* 60, no. 4 (1999):

knowledge of past cultures is inadequate – that is, if individuals do not adequately recognize the fact of social difference across time and space – it is because succeeding cultures undertake active war on them in the attempt to eliminate all memory of different modes of doing and being. Thus, for example, Christianity's war against the Gentiles: "It erased all its orders, all its ceremonies, and extinguished every memory of that ancient theology."[17] Machiavelli, however, goes on to note that it is not possible to completely eliminate remembrance of such prior modes, and hence the perpetuation through time of various cultural remnants, preserved, for example, through the continued use of Latin, and so on. Significantly, after detailing the contingency of human custom, Machiavelli proceeds to detail a seemingly analogous contingency of physical nature, suggesting the former is merely one element of a much more comprehensive philosophy of natural history. He writes that "as for the causes that come from heaven, they are those that extinguish the human race, and reduce to a few the inhabitants of part of the world, this coming through plague or through famine or through an inundation of water."[18] Machiavelli thus explicitly rejects belief in a regular and predictable movement of natural history, going so far as to partially locate cultural variation in the displacements that result from contingent natural events that interrupt the apparently static and regular being of the world.

Machiavelli can be seen to locate the chaotic structure of reality in a quasi-dialectical understanding of the objects of the world. This is certainly not a positive dialectical understanding that, in teleological fashion, assimilates historical events into a logical or causal time continuum culminating in the actualization of a synthetic end, but rather a negative dialectical understanding that emphasizes the internal non-identity of objects. Objects are subject to a play of different forces whose interaction and interpenetration generate a multitude of unique potentialities. Hence Machiavelli's characterization of the process of unpredictable objective movement in *Discourses* 3:37: "near the good there is always some evil, which arises so easily with that good that it seems impossible to be able to miss the one while wanting the other. And this is seen in all

---

659–81; Benedetto Fontana, "Love of Country and Love of God: The Political Uses of Religion in Machiavelli," *Journal of the History of Ideas* 60, no. 4 (1999): 639–58.

17 Machiavelli, "Discorsi sopra la prima Deca di Tito Livio," bk. 2.5.

18 Ibid.

the things that men work on. Therefore one acquires the good with difficulty, unless fortune aids you in such a way that it and its force defeat
this ordinary and natural inconvenience."[19] One must know not to put
all of one's force behind one mode, thus exposing oneself to ruin should
the form of the arrangement of those internal tendencies structuring the
being of the object shift. Even if we presume that the form of the object
will remain relatively stable over a period of time, the elements constituting it are so closely intertwined that human investigation will never
be sufficient to conceptually parse them one from the other, for things
"have bad so near to the good, and so much are they joined together,
that it is an easy thing to take the one, believing one has seized the
other."[20] And what is more, any human intervention will necessarily
upset the composition of elements, thus contributing to the emergence
of unforeseen and necessarily unconsidered permutations. Hence in 1:6
Machiavelli states that "in all human things he who will examine them
well sees this: that you can never remove one inconvenience without
another one emerging."[21] The world provides no opportunity for individuals to initiate modes which will produce assured ends: what is
"entirely clear, entirely without uncertainty, is never found."[22]

As will be elaborated on later, in the final instance it is the fact of
worldly contingency that makes impossible the thought of a political
project that looks to the instrumental mastery of human reality. No
virtue is compelling enough to provide a stable direction to the nondetermined movement of objects through the flux of time. Such is made
explicit in *Discourses* 2:29, where Machiavelli notes that this project of
mastery was impossible even for his largely fictional and idealized
Romans: "If you consider well how human affairs proceed, you will see
that many times things emerge and accidents take place that the heavens did not want to provide for at all. And if that which I say occurred
in Rome, where there was so much virtue, so much religion, and so
much order, it is not surprising that it occurs far more often in a city or
in a province that lacks the things said above."[23] Even the most virtuous

---

19 Ibid., bk. 3.37.
20 Ibid.
21 Ibid., bk. 1.6.
22 Ibid. See also Machiavelli, "L'Asino," in *Tutte le opere*, 967; "Istorie fiorentine," in
    Tutte le opere, bk. 5.1.
23 Machiavelli, "Discorsi sopra la prima Deca di Tito Livio," bk. 2.29.

of cities is thus incapable of definitively stabilizing the unstable and unpredictable temporality of the world. Obviously this is not to suggest, however, that human endeavour is wasted in the effort to negotiate the non-determinate, even if the latter cannot be shaped into the determinate. The possibility of such negotiation is revealed, for example, in *Discourses* 3:14, where the contingencies that perpetually arise in battles are presented as an element of the contingency of the world. Machiavelli writes: "Of how many times in conflicts and in battles a new accident arises because of a thing neither seen nor heard before is demonstrated in many places."[24]

As I showed in the previous chapter, given that the emergence of such accidents produces always new and unprecedented situations, the repetitions that prudent actors undertake in responding to them must refer not to actual patterns of behaviour, but to the imitation of a type of critical spirit or orientation that allows one to reflectively respond to contingency, and in some way neutralize the effects of necessity. Such a spirit, though, certainly does not look to overcome necessity, but actually depends upon a recognition and acceptance of its inevitability. Machiavelli states that "not so much are the orders of an army necessary to be able to fight in an orderly way, but so that every least accident not disorder you. For no other reason are multitudes of people not useful for war than that every noise, every voice, every uproar, alters them and makes them flee."[25] People must be socialized such that they are able to recognize the fact of unpredictability and act prudently in the face of it. They must, in other words, overcome the desire to stabilize and permanently fix the order of reality. In order to accustom his troops to the fact of contingency the prudent captain will thus deliberately introduce accidents to ill-prepared armies as a mode of disruption.[26] These new innovations have a double function, being used both to disrupt your opponents, but also to prepare your own soldiers to respond to the inevitable accidents that will arise and confront them. As Machiavelli says, "And so a good captain ought to do two things: one, to see, through some of these new inventions, to frightening the enemy; the other, to be prepared, so that if the enemy tries this against him, he can

---

24 Ibid., bk. 3.14.
25 Ibid.
26 Ibid.

uncover them and make them turn out in vain."[27] The recognition of the inevitability of unpredictability provides a condition for neutralizing the effects of unpredictability upon you.[28]

Although it is in the *Discourses* that Machiavelli most comprehensively articulates his understanding of the indetermination of worldly being, we can also point to several other passages throughout his work that seem to confirm the metaphysical instability reading. In *The Prince* 3, speaking of the Romans and the impossibility of deferring the moment of political decision in the hope that time will rectify one's problems, Machiavelli writes: "Nor did it ever please them, that which is in the mouth of all the wise of our day, to enjoy the benefit of time, but the good of their virtue and prudence; *for time drives all things forward*, and can lead him to good as well as bad, and bad as well as good."[29] In chapter 7 this process whereby time drives forward or alters the organization of the things of the world is once again referenced. Here Machiavelli argues that one who becomes a prince primarily through fortune acquires with ease but will maintain authority with great difficulty. This is due precisely to the inconstancy of the world, to the fact that the emergence of new objects and new relations perpetually upsets the stable order of things, the non-virtuous prince being ill-equipped to negotiate such fluctuations. The things of the world are constantly in motion, and the only means to keep what fortune has provided you is to act virtuously, to be able to recognize the opportunities presented in the displacements caused by the movement of time.[30] And just as in

---

27 Ibid.

28 Ibid.

29 Machiavelli, "Il Principe," in *Tutte le opere*, chap. 3. Emphasis added. On this subject Robert Orr argues that "Man, as Machiavelli sees him in society, inhabits a world ruled neither by fortune, nor by himself, but by time." Robert Orr, "The Time Motif in Machiavelli," in *Machiavelli and the Nature of Political Thought*, ed. Martin Fleisher (New York: Atheneum, 1972), 188. Michael McCanles, furthermore, writes that for Machiavelli "to conform oneself to the times really means to conform oneself to time itself." McCanles, *The Discourse of Il Principe*, 116. On the competing conceptions of time in Machiavelli's work see Antoine Chollet, *Les temps de la démocratie* (Paris: Dalloz, 2011), 87–135.

30 For an early recognition that Machiavellian thought grasps the political realm as being fundamentally one of movement, as opposed to one of static objects, see J. Condé, "La sagesse Machiavelique: politique et rhétorique," in *Umanesimo e scienza politica*, ed. E. Castelli (Milan: Marzorati, 1951), 84.

Discourses 2:5, here the instability of the political field simply reflects the instability of the natural one, Machiavelli again articulating a coextensive philosophy of natural history: "the states that come into being immediately, *like all the other things in nature* that are born and grow quickly, cannot have roots and corresponding elements, so that the first challenging time extinguishes them."[31] In chapter 10, speaking of the impossibility of attacking a prince who is not hated by his people without suffering embarrassing defeat, Machiavelli writes: "A prince, therefore, who has a strong city and does not make himself hated, cannot be attacked; and even if there is someone who would attack him, he would withdraw in disgrace, because *the things of the world are so variable* that it is almost impossible that one could stand with his armies idle for a year in a siege."[32] And in the penultimate chapter of the text this variability is considered in terms of the conceptual impossibility of generating a metaphysical schema capable of regulating and investing with a singular meaning the chaos of life, Machiavelli writing of "the great variability of things that have been seen and are seen now each day, beyond all human conjecture."[33]

Machiavelli and the Appearance of Human Wickedness

Despite some prominent exceptions, it is notable just how many commentators, despite their attempts to assimilate Machiavelli into highly distinct political positions – not just radical democratic ones, but proto-liberal,[34] civic humanist,[35] realist,[36] and even fascist[37] ones – agree on the question of his affirmation of the fact of worldly contingency.[38] Most of

---

31 Machiavelli, "Il Principe," chap. 7. Emphasis added.
32 Ibid., chap. 10. Emphasis added.
33 Ibid., chap. 25.
34 Isaiah Berlin, "The Originality of Machiavelli," in *Against the Current: Essays in the History of Ideas* (New York: Viking Press, 1980), 37.
35 Hanan Yoran, "Machiavelli's Critique of Humanism and the Ambivalences of Modernity," *History of Political Thought* 31, no. 2 (2010): 251.
36 Friedrich Meinecke, *Machiavellism: The Doctrine of Raison d'État and Its Place in Modern History* (New Haven: Yale University Press, 1957), 31.
37 Joseph Femia, "Machiavelli and Italian Fascism," *History of Political Thought* 25, no. 1 (2004): 5.
38 Besides the commentators already mentioned, see also, for example, Carl Roebuck, "A Search for Political Stability," *Phoenix* 6, no. 2 (1952): 55; Joseph Anthony Mazzeo,

these readers, however, despite recognizing that Machiavelli rejects all positive metaphysical frameworks that conceive being in terms of stability and rationally guided movement, abstract the human from the world, asserting a fixed Machiavellian human nature.[39] In general human essence is interpreted in terms of an acquisitive and invidious egoism that insatiably strives after possessions and honours, and which is moralized through the label of wickedness.[40] Quentin Skinner, for

---

"The Poetry of Power: Machiavelli's Literary Vision," *Review of National Literatures* 1, no. 1 (1970): 42; Gilbert, *Machiavelli and Guicciardini*, 198; Felix Gilbert, "The Humanist Concept of the Prince and *The Prince* of Machiavelli," in *History: Choice and Committment* (Cambridge: Belknap Press of Harvard University Press, 1977), 92; Klaus Held, "Civic Prudence in Machiavelli: Toward the Paradigm Transformation in Philosophy in the Transition to Modernity," in *The Ancients and the Moderns,* ed. Reginald Lilly, trans. Anthony Steinbeck (Bloomington: Indiana University Press, 1996), 119; Diego A. von Vacano, *The Art of Power: Machiavelli, Nietzsche, and the Making of Aesthetic Political Theory* (Lanham: Lexington Books, 2007), 78; Brook Montgomery Blair, "Post-Metaphysical and Radical Humanist Thought," *History of European Ideas* 27, no. 3 (2001): 200; Michael Dillon, "Lethal Freedom: Divine Violence and the Machiavellian Moment," *Theory and Event* 11, no. 2 (2008).

39 For explicit manifestations of this ambivalence with respect to the question of worldly vs. human nature see Berlin, "The Originality of Machiavelli," 172; Robert Kocis, *Machiavelli Redeemed: Retrieving His Humanist Perspectives on Equality, Power, and Glory* (Bethlehem: Lehigh University Press, 1998), 37, 60; Paul A. Rahe, "Situating Machiavelli," in *Renaissance Civic Humanism: Reappraisals and Reflections,* ed. James Hankins (Cambridge: Cambridge University Press, 2000), 270–308; Joseph V. Femia, *Machiavelli Revisited* (Cardiff: University of Wales Press, 2004), 13, 64. One of the few commentators to note the continuity between these two dimensions of Machiavelli's thought is Diego von Vacano. Von Vacano divides Machiavelli's metaphysics into two spheres: a cosmology that provides a model of the world and a philosophical anthropology that provides a model of the human being, both of which are subject to contingent dynamics to a degree that closes off the potential for systematic analysis. Von Vacano, *The Art of Power*, 78–9.

40 See, for example, Strauss, *Thoughts on Machiavelli*, 279; Olschki, *Machiavelli: The Scientist*, 18; Raymond Aron, *Machiavel et les tyrannies modernes*, ed. Rémy Freymond (Paris: Éditions de Fallois, 1993), 68; Mark Jurdjevic, "Machiavelli's Hybrid Republicanism," *English Historical Review* 122, no. 499 (2007): 1238; Hillay Zmora, "Love of Country and Love of Party: Patriotism and Human Nature in Machiavelli," *History of Political Thought* 25, no. 3 (2004): 425; Fischer, "Machiavelli's Rapacious Republicanism," xxxv; Gérald Sfez, "Deciding on Evil," in *Radical Evil*, ed. Joan Copjec, trans. James Swenson (London: Verso, 1996), 127–8. Oftentimes this anthropological assumption of human evil, furthermore, is seen to be a residual trace of the prevalence of Augustinian theology in Machiavelli's historical context. See, for example, Bjørn Qviller, "The Machiavellian Cosmos," *History of Political Thought* 27, no. 3 (1996): 328; Joseph Anthony Mazzeo, *Renaissance and Revolution: The Remaking of*

example, writes that Machiavelli has a "deeply pessimistic view of human nature," one that is reducible to the best-known characterizations of the people that we find in *The Prince*.[41] Machiavelli writes that "of men one can say this generally: that they are ungrateful, fickle, deceivers and dissimulators, avoiders of danger, covetous of profit."[42] Later in the same chapter, while discussing the prince's need to be feared in such a way that he is not hated, Machiavelli details the primary mode by which the possessive and acquisitive being of individuals is asserted. He maintains that the prince should above all else assure that he respects the property of his subjects, for individuals are so self-regarding as to privilege the security of their private possessions over the actual physical lives of, not only others, but close relations. He writes that the prince will succeed at his goal if he "refrains from the property of his citizens and his subjects, and from their women. And even if it is necessary to proceed against anyone's life, do it when there is reasonable justification and manifest cause; but, above all, refrain from the property of others, because men sooner forget the death of a father than the loss of a father's estate."[43] It thus seems difficult to imagine, given this apparently acquisitive and egoistic being, how a common political order grounded in mutual respect for the interests and needs of other citizens could be established. Indeed, Skinner will ultimately go so far as to claim that Machiavelli "is a consistent, an almost Hobbesian skeptic about the possibility of inducing men to behave well except by cajolery or force."[44] Hence even in the *Discourses* must the founder of the commonwealth presume that all men are wicked and that envy is a fundamental element of human nature. Neither education, inspiring leadership, nor religion are capable of transforming human nature to shape people such that they are able to privilege civic virtue over their private desire.[45]

European Thought (New York: Pantheon Books, 1965), 85; Giuseppe Prezzolini, "The Christian Roots of Machiavelli's Moral Pessimism," *Review of National Literatures* 1, no. 1 (1970): 33–7; Max Horkheimer, "Egoism and the Freedom Movement: On the Anthropology of the Bourgeois Era," trans. David Parent, *Telos*, no. 54 (1982): 13.

41 Quentin Skinner, *The Foundations of Modern Political Thought*, vol. 1: *The Renaissance* (Cambridge: Cambridge University Press, 1978), 137.

42 Machiavelli, "Il Principe," chap. 17.

43 Ibid.

44 Skinner, *The Foundations of Modern Political Thought*, vol. 1: *The Renaissance*, 185.

45 Quentin Skinner, "Machiavelli on *Virtù* and the Maintenance of Liberty," in *Visions of Politics*, vol. 2: *Renaissance Visions* (Cambridge: Cambridge University Press, 2002), 169–73.

The passage that Skinner is here referring to is the following, from *Discourses* 1:3: "it is necessary to one who provides a republic, and orders laws in it, to presuppose that all men are bad, and that they must always use the malignity of their spirit anytime they have a free occasion to."[46] There are, however, two issues that would seem to problematize the utilization of this statement as evidence for Machiavelli's belief in the universality of a human nature considered in terms of an orientation toward the invidious maximization of private good. The first, of course, is that Machiavelli does not state that all individuals *are* by their nature bad, but simply that the prudent orderer of the political regime must *presuppose* that they are so. The second issue, which provides us with an explanation as to why one seeking to order a republican way of life must presume this, is given an initial expression in this chapter, through one of Machiavelli's many accounts of the socializing power of custom and law. After the expulsion of the Tarquins the nobles of Rome were initially able to conceal their malevolence through feigning a popular spirit and a love for the plebs. Once the nobles perceived themselves as secure in their social position, however, their actual hatred of the plebs was allowed to externally manifest itself, there having not been established after the expulsion of the Tarquins a new political order that would have been able to successfully institutionalize the prior condition, that is, noble fear. Lacking a customary foundation for the preservation of the desired condition, law assumes responsibility for moral training: "it is said that hunger and poverty make men industrious, and the laws make them good. And where a thing works well itself without law, law is not necessary; but when that good custom is lacking, the law is immediately necessary."[47]

Although Machiavelli here uses the language of individuals being made good, one may nevertheless resist reading this lesson in terms of the potential to transform an apparent human nature, instead taking from it Machiavelli's understanding of the fundamental power of the law to compel good behaviour in spite of a perpetual human malevolence that always desires an external expression, regardless of whether or not a social space is available that would allow for such expression without fear. Such an interpretation, however, seems to be blocked by chapter 1:18. Here Machiavelli is speaking of a city that has been

---

46 Machiavelli, "Discorsi sopra la prima Deca di Tito Livio," bk. 1.3.
47 Ibid.

overcome by "universal corruption."[48] Under such conditions corruption is incapable of being overcome through legal means alone, but rather through a form of customary socialization that aims at a fundamental transformation of a deep substratum of human being. Machiavelli writes that "because, just as good customs need laws in order to be maintained, such laws need good customs in order to be observed."[49] Ultimately there is a co-determination between law and custom at play, good laws being respected where custom has moulded good people who voluntarily recognize the legitimacy of the legal order, and good custom being habitually preserved through the legal order that affirms the social values inculcated in individuals. And should a reader be unconvinced that Machiavelli is in this discussion not referring to an actual transformation of individual nature, he will go on to clearly differentiate between forms of society on the basis of a distinction between a generalized goodness and a generalized wickedness, through the account of the need to vary laws and orders through time in order to stay in accord with historical movement, writing that "the orders and the laws made in a republic at its birth, when men were good, are no longer appropriate later, when they have become bad."[50]

At this point we can return to Machiavelli's original formulation regarding the necessity of the republican founder to assume the wickedness of individuals, and how it can be read as simultaneously consistent with both Machiavelli's pessimistic characterization of individuals in *The Prince*, and his optimistic characterization of individuals later in Book One of the *Discourses*, which I will examine in more detail in the following section. Regarding the latter characterization let us consider, as just one example, *Discourses* 1:55, which is particularly notable given that Machiavelli here presents us with an example of a community of individuals who explicitly reject a mode of behaviour that is in *The Prince* taken to be the fundamental marker of invidious egoism. In 1:55 Machiavelli affirms that the establishment and preservation of a well-ordered republic depend upon a people in possession of what he calls goodness: "And truly, where there is not this goodness, one can expect nothing good, as nothing good can be hoped for in the provinces that in

---

48 Ibid., bk. 1.18.
49 Ibid.
50 Ibid.

these times are seen as corrupt, as in Italy above all others."[51] Crucially, the primary expression of this goodness is precisely the opposite of what had been taken to be the primary expression of human wickedness: against the egoistic drive to accumulate and secure private goods, we see instead individuals who, as a consequence of their positive integration into the life of the city, do not hesitate in contributing to it through the forfeit of their own property. This, for example, was seen in the Senate's trust that the plebs would fulfil Camillus's vow to contribute one-tenth of the booty of the Veientes to satisfy Apollo. Although this debt was ultimately not called in, "nevertheless one sees by this decision how much the Senate trusted in the goodness of [the plebs], and how they judged that nobody would not present precisely all that the edict had ordered. On the other hand, one sees how the plebs did not think of defrauding any part of the edict through giving less than they had to."[52]

Indeed, on Machiavelli's account we see many examples of the willingness of the people of Rome, as well as those of contemporary Germany, to financially contribute to the city, without being compelled and without the expectation of the benefits of recognition: "Those [German] republics, when they need to spend some quantity of money for the public account, have those magistrates or councils that have authority assess all the inhabitants of the city one percent, or two, of what each has of value. And after such decision, according to the order of the land, each presents himself before the collectors of the tax, and first having taken an oath to pay the proper sum, throws into a designated chest that which according to his conscience it appears he has to pay: of this payment there is no witness but the one paying. Hence one can conjecture how much goodness and how much religion is still in these men."[53]

---

51 Ibid., bk. 1.55.
52 Ibid.
53 Ibid. It is also worth bearing in mind at this point that even in *The Prince* Machiavelli suggests that individuals ultimately care about more than just the preservation of their own property, noting how the people may support the prince even if their goods are destroyed in the process of siege. Machiavelli, "Il Principe," chap. 10. See also the case of Spurius Cassius in *Discourses* 3:8 and the speech of a member of the Signori in the *Florentine Histories*, who, resisting the princely ambitions of Walter, duke of Athens, maintains that there is no amount of external goods sufficient to counter the desire for freedom. Machiavelli, "Discorsi sopra la prima Deca di Tito Livio," bk. 3.8; Machiavelli, "Istorie fiorentine," bk. 2.34.

There are two determining reasons for the appearance of such a willingness for civic financial contribution. The first is the external lack of invidious comparison and the resentful desire that it gives rise to. This lack is largely a consequence of the non-encounter with foreign goods, individuals "not having had major interactions with their neighbours; for the latter have not come to their home, nor have they to the home of others, because they have been content with those goods, to live from those foods, to dress with that wool, which their country provides."[54] The second, which I will examine in more detail later, is the internal lack of invidious comparison, a result of the establishment of a certain type of social equality, represented in the lack of an idle class of expropriating gentlemen: "those republics where a political and uncorrupt life is maintained do not allow that any of their citizens be or live in the way of a gentleman; indeed, they maintain among themselves a level equality, and to those lords and gentlemen in that province they are extremely hostile."[55] In the final instance what we see is that the establishment of certain social modes of existence provides the concrete conditions for overcoming that form of disposition that so many of Machiavelli's commentators take to be an ineradicable dimension of the human essence.

Almost all readers recognize the extent to which Machiavelli affirms the socializing power of law and custom. Such socialization, however, is generally interpreted in terms of a productive regulation or moderation of a basic set of essential human drives.[56] What the above example seems to demonstrate, however, is that there is nothing primary about appetitive acquisitiveness, which does not emerge in this situation as a consequence of the lack of those social conditions that stimulate its conventional development. What must be stressed is that for Machiavelli neither goodness nor badness in the sense of the properties or

---

54 Machiavelli, "Discorsi sopra la prima Deca di Tito Livio," bk. 1.56.

55 Ibid., bk. 1.55.

56 Such a reading most notably characterizes the neo-Roman interpretation of Machiavelli. For example, after identifying what he takes to be the vices "deeply rooted in human nature," Quentin Skinner goes on to note that Machiavelli believes "that the law can act to liberate us from our natural but self-destructive interests." Skinner, "Machiavelli on *Virtù* and the Maintenance of Liberty," 168, 177. Maurizio Viroli, meanwhile, interprets the law in terms of a necessary restriction of fundamental human appetites. Maurizio Viroli, *Machiavelli* (Oxford: Oxford University Press, 1998), 128.

dispositions described here can be reduced to constituent elements of human nature, but in both cases are contingent results of concrete social-historical conditions of life. This is why Machiavelli can simultaneously speak of human wickedness where individuals are socialized in an institutional context that does not value or stimulate communal sensibilities, and human goodness in an institutional context that does. As Claude Lefort writes, "The conduct of men is determined at once according to objective possibilities configured by circumstances, and rules or obligations imposed on them by institutions, and the latter are elaborated and modified according to the relations developed by the actors, engaged as they are in factual conduct."[57] What Lefort correctly perceives here is that Machiavelli's various and oftentimes seemingly contradictory declarations regarding the nature of individuals are analysable only within the context of the specific form of the political community under discussion at the moment of evaluation. Machiavelli assumes neither a natural human goodness nor a natural human badness, Lefort going so far as to claim that such questions are to Machiavelli ultimately irrelevant: "Are all men wicked or are they not? Is human nature in itself bad? Such questions hardly matter to Machiavelli. And if one insists on posing them, one will run up against contradictory statements that in fact acquire their meaning only once they are put back into context."[58]

If the majority of that human content that we take to be positive nature is just second nature, then in fact the defining human characteristic would be nothing other than the openness of nature to alteration and change. And if the primary factor stimulating alteration in nature is the form of social and political organization, then individuals themselves, to the extent that they are able to initiate common political projects and reflectively organize their lives according to certain principles of being, can themselves be seen as both the subjects and objects of such alteration. Human beings would thus be those who assume responsibility for creating their own nature; human essence would be negative as opposed to positive. In part three I will examine the mechanics by which individuals collectively perform such political operations through a study of the radically democratic

---

57 Claude Lefort, *Machiavelli in the Making*, trans. Michael B. Smith (Evanston: North-western University Press, 2012), 262.
58 Lefort, "Machiavelli and the *Verità Effetuale*," 129.

form of Machiavelli's republic. In the remainder of this chapter, though, I will highlight other key passages from Machiavelli's writings that suggest this open and negative understanding of the human essence.

Socialization and the Production of Human Nature

Machiavelli's critique of static and positive models of the human essence is revealed in two fundamentally related ways. The first has already been suggested: it is through Machiavelli's multiple assertions regarding the openness of human being to alteration via socialization. The second is revealed through Machiavelli's emphasis on the strong multiplicity that can be observed between different groups and individuals, a precise consequence of the potential for individual being to be developed in unique and myriad ways as a result of its openness to change. The potential for human being to change its form through exposure to unique socializing forces, often framed by commentators in terms of a distinction between first and second nature, is most clearly expressed in the *Discourses*.

One of Machiavelli's arguments that we see repeated over and over in the *Discourses* is that the institution of a republican form of life depends first of all on the creation of a collectivity whose individual members have been educated toward a particular type of civility. This civility is considered not simply in terms of a repression of an always-ineradicable wickedness, but rather in terms of an overcoming and abolition of it, possible to the extent that the latter is always contingent and socially grounded. As noted, individuals are by their nature neither good nor bad, which is not to say that they are incapable of being either good or bad. Indeed, a civil way of life depends upon a social mutuality that is grounded in a certain human goodness, that is to say, a human form of being that eschews as primary the instrumental and egoistic pursuit of private goods. Hence Machiavelli's distinction between shackled and unshackled populations, and how the people's relation to the law fundamentally informs its "nature."[59] The key chapter here is 1:58, which will be analysed in more detail below in part three. The lesson, though, is repeated in various places. It appears, for example, in 1:11, during a discussion of Roman religion and the extent to which it

---

59 Machiavelli, "Discorsi sopra la prima Deca di Tito Livio," bk. 1.58.

was necessary for Numa to institute religious rites in order for him to engage with a "ferocious people" in need of pacification.[60]

This discussion of the necessity of religion to political foundation takes place in the context of Machiavelli's recognition of the present corruption of Italy, suggesting that the utilization of religious techniques is not universally necessary for foundation, but rather only in certain social-historical situations, including Machiavelli's and Numa's, situations in which individuals are defined in terms of particular asocial yet transcendable forms of being. Hence Machiavelli writes that "without doubt, those who would wish to found a republic in the present time would find it easier among mountain men, where there is no civilization, than among those who are used to living in cities, where civilization is corrupt: and a sculptor will get more easily a beautiful statue from rough marble than from one poorly shaped by others."[61] That the utilization of religion as a political technique is only required as a mode of socialization where individual nature is deficient from the standpoint of republican life is confirmed in 1:13. Here Machiavelli shows how the use of religion is oriented toward the establishment of an internal social homogeneity that minimizes the potential for social conflict. What is crucial to recognize, and what again refers us to the always present need for contextual sensitivity to social-historical facts of existence when interpreting Machiavelli, is that he is thus not yet discussing his normative ideal – a well-ordered political regime in which disunion is productive – but rather a corrupt state where all forms of heterogeneity have the potential to immediately dissolve into sectarianism. The chapter speaks of the various noble uses of religion that were designed to break the instituted power of the plebs. Since we know, however, that Machiavelli does not ultimately think the plebs should be subordinated to the will of the nobles, it follows to assume that Machiavelli only thinks the utilization of religion as a mode of pacification is justified when the popular matter is ferocious and corrupt, that is, wicked.

---

60 Ibid., bk. 1.11.
61 Ibid. Daniel Waley takes this observation to be one element of what he calls Machiavelli's primitivism, people who are rough and coarse being seen as more malleable and open to change. Daniel Waley, "The Primitivist Element in Machiavelli's Thought," *Journal of the History of Ideas* 31, no. 1 (1970): 92.

This theme is returned to in a new context three chapters later in 1:16, where Machiavelli maintains that it is extremely difficult for people living under a prince to maintain their freedom after being liberated, for they have not been educated to that civic mode of life necessary for the perpetual reproduction of free political self-activity. Machiavelli notes that "such difficulty is reasonable, because that people is not otherwise than a brute animal, which, although of a fierce and savage nature, has always been nourished in prison and in servitude. Afterwards, left free to its fate in the countryside, not being used to feeding itself nor knowing the places where it must take refuge, it becomes the prey of the first who seeks to rechain it."[62] Needless to say, though, human beings are not mere beasts, even if they might appear so under such conditions. Indeed, what precisely differentiates the human being from other animal beings, what marks its specificity, is the openness of its nature to change through the confrontation with educating modes and orders. Machiavelli's most detailed differentiation of human from animal nature occurs in *The Ass*, specifically as it is articulated in the speech of the boar. In particular, the boar revels in the regular and constant nature of its life, a life unsubjected to the desires and ambitions of humans: "Our species does not care for other food than the product of heaven without art, and you want that which nature cannot bring. / You are not content with a single food, like us, but, to satisfy better your greedy desires, journey for these unto the kingdoms of the East. / It is not enough that which you collect on earth, so you enter the Ocean's breast to satiate yourself with its spoils."[63] The boar will go on to locate the insatiability of desire in the human capacity to produce and speak, and through the exercise of these capacities cancel out the immediacy of nature, simultaneously transforming the structure of the world and also the structure of the self. Unlike the animal, the human being can through its life activity transcend its nature.[64] The question at this point

---

62 Machiavelli, "Discorsi sopra la prima Deca di Tito Livio," bk. 1.16.

63 Machiavelli, "L'Asino," 975.

64 Here there would seem to be a parallel between Machiavelli and Marx, a fact recognized by various Marxian inspired readers of Machiavelli. See, for example, Benedetto Fontana, *Hegemony and Power: On the Relation between Gramsci and Machiavelli* (Minneapolis: University of Minnesota Press, 1993), 127; Antonio Gramsci, "The Modern Prince," in *Selections from the Prison Notebooks*, ed. and trans. Quintin Hoare and Geoffrey Nowell Smith (New York: International Publishers, 1971), 133.

is not whether Machiavelli thinks it is a more genuine or truer happiness to be self-identical and constant like the sated pig.[65] It is essential to note simply that the specificity of human nature is articulated in terms of the human ability to subvert its immediate forms.

If human beings are habituated to living like animals, then it makes little sense to expect them to immediately possess the ability to enjoy a free way of life, to the extent that freedom is largely thought in terms of a certain reflective self-questioning. A liberated people lacking such a nature, since it is "used to living under the governments of others, not knowing how to reason about any public offence or defence, not knowing of princes nor being known by them, soon returns under a yoke that most of the time is more severe than the one that, a little earlier, it had threw off its neck; and it finds itself in these difficulties although its matter is not corrupt. Because a people where everything has entered into corruption cannot live free."[66] Whenever referring to human capacity then, often framed in terms of the form of appearance of human nature, we must begin our analysis with a consideration of the distinction between forms of social being, between a people socialized to concern for civic life in common and a people socialized to concern for merely private advantage. Such contextual need is suggested by Machiavelli's specification in 1:16 that "our reasonings are of those peoples where corruption is not very extended, and where there is more of the good than of the spoiled."[67] Once again, though, despite Machiavelli's utilization of the language of corruption, it is not a matter of isolating either a primary goodness or a primary badness, locating apparent badness in the mere corruption of fundamental goodness, or apparent goodness in the repression of fundamental badness. The existence of an essentially bad substratum is explicitly rejected in 3:29, where Machiavelli writes that "princes should not complain of any sin committed by the people they rule, because these sins necessarily arise either from his negligence, or from him being guilty of similar errors. And whoever discourses on the people who in our times have been held full of

---

65 In *The Ass* this ability for self-transcendence is identified as the source of human misery, as seen for example in the violent attempts of individuals to realize their private ambition. As I will argue later, though, the actualization of ambition need not proceed in these terms, that is violently, privately, and against others, but can be realized through a form of non-antagonistic democratic practice.
66 Machiavelli, "Discorsi sopra la prima Deca di Tito Livio," bk. 1.16.
67 Ibid.

robberies and similar sins, will see that it is *entirely created* by those who ruled, who were of a similar nature."[68] Once again, the nature of individuals is a productive result of processes of political socialization.

Just as it would be a mistake to read Machiavelli's account of socialization as mere mediation of an essential human disposition toward a positive mode of doing or being, so too it would be a mistake to interpret it as mere habituation that produces a second nature that is as static as our "first" nature.[69] Against such readings that emphasize the rigid form of habitual character, I would argue that Machiavelli provides us with many examples of cases in which second nature reveals its perpetually open character through non-protracted socialization. Such seems to be clearly disclosed in *Discourses* 1:42, significantly entitled "How easily men can be corrupted." This ease is a consequence precisely of the instability of human nature, revealed here through the example of life under the Decemvirate. Machiavelli writes: "We note also, in this Decemvirate matter, how easily men are corrupted, and made to assume a contrary nature, despite how good and well-trained."[70] It took very little indeed for the youth attracted by Appius to abandon or lose their prior disposition and throw their support behind the Ten, for instance. The most specific examples Machiavelli provides of short-term alteration in preformed nature occur in the military context; hence the chapter immediately following 1:42, again on the destructive influence of the Decemvirate, in the context of a discussion of the uselessness of mercenaries and their orientation toward the

---

68 Ibid., bk. 3.29. Emphasis added. Mark Jurdjevic reminds us that Machiavelli never shied away from placing all of the blame for Italy's woes on rulers. Mark Jurdjevic, "Virtue, Fortune, and Blame in Machiavelli's Life and *The Prince*," *Social Research* 81, no. 1 (2014): 40.

69 See, for example, Janet Coleman, *A History of Political Thought: From the Middle Ages to the Renaissance* (Oxford: Blackwell, 2000), 255; Cary J. Nederman, "Rhetoric, Reason, and Republic: Republicanisms – Ancient, Medieval, and Modern," in *Renaissance Civic Humanism: Reappraisals and Reflections*, ed. James Hankins (Cambridge: Cambridge University Press, 2000), 363. Compare such readings with that of someone like Pierre Manent. For Manent what defines the new prince is the ability to live without a habitus, this being just one manifestation of Machiavelli's affirmation of the capacity for self-variability that is at the heart of his anthropology: "If Machiavelli asks the Prince of enough freedom of mind to exit the path of the good, it is as test and guarantee of the indefinite plasticity of his soul." Pierre Manent, *Naissances de la politique moderne* (Paris: Gallimard, 2007), 22.

70 Machiavelli, "Discorsi sopra la prima Deca di Tito Livio," bk. 1.42.

achievement of their own glory. Machiavelli notes that Roman soldiers were in possession of exactly the same set of technical skills in the interim as before and after the rule of the Ten yet nevertheless lacked the spiritual disposition to function as good soldiers, and this precisely because they lacked an orientation toward a free way of life. Nevertheless, a change in the customary mode was sufficient to reinstall this orientation and correct the lack that the Decemvirate arbitrarily produced: "But as soon as the magistracy of the Ten was eliminated, and they began a free military life, the same spirit returned to them; and in consequence their enterprises had the same happy end as before, in accordance with their old custom."[71] The new situation produced not only a new character, but a new character defined in terms of a capacity for free action. Overall, it seems as if Machiavelli believes that once an individual's character or nature becomes generated there nevertheless always remains the potential for further alteration through exposure to new forces. Individuals and armies can transform from bad to good and back again as a result of subjection to new customs, orders, and institutions. As Machiavelli puts it in the "Discourse on Florentine Affairs," "men mutate easily and turn from good to miserable."[72]

The Multiplicity of Human Being

The non-determination of human nature for Machiavelli is second revealed through the strong multiplicity of forms of human doing and being that we can observe in the world. This multiplicity is the social consequence of the openness of internal nature to alteration via engagement with specific processes of socio-cultural and political socialization. Readers of Machiavelli most often interpret the latter's understanding of social difference as exhausted by the seemingly primary differentiation of humours that Machiavelli associates with the plebs and the grandees respectively. Whereas the latter are defined in terms of their desire to oppress and dominate, the former are defined in terms of their desire to not be oppressed or dominated. In chapter 4 I will argue that this distinction of humours is not only not originary, but simply the form of appearance of a fundamental

---

71 Ibid., bk. 1.43.
72 Machiavelli, "Discursus florentinarum rerum post mortem iunioris Laurentii Medices," in *Tutte le opere*, 24.

human desire for self-creation. In this section, though, I will point to several passages in Machiavelli's work that reveal the fact that social difference is actually much more complex and variegated than normally thought, and ultimately irreducible to the binary division of noble and plebeian humours.

The link between the two manifestations of the contingency of human nature is established by Machiavelli in *Discourses* 3:22, in the discussion of the differing modes of Manlius Torquatus and Valerius Corvinus. As in the case of Quintius and Appius Claudius presented three chapters earlier, the modes of Manlius and Valerius are seen as providing us with contrasting examples of potential means of command: "Manlius, with every severity, without intervening in his soldiers' fatigue or pain, commanded them; Valerius, on the other hand, with every human mode and way, and full of familiar attachment, delighted them."[73] Despite the opposite modes, however, both actors achieved the same success. This raises several questions, the most significant for our purposes being, how could two individuals raised in the same place proceed so differently? The answer to this question lay in the internally differentiated modes of education that mark all cities, and republican ones in particular. The specificity of Manlius's upbringing produced a strong nature that inclined him to extraordinary command. One not socialized in this way, and hence not in possession of this nature, would not be able to act by such extraordinary modes. As Machiavelli says, "whoever is not of this strength of spirit ought to guard himself from extraordinary controls, and in the ordinary ones use his humanity; for ordinary punishments are not imputed to the prince, but to the laws and to those orders."[74] There is thus a co-determination between the multiplicity of being and the openness of being to change, the form of internal nature and the modes of action that this nature allows for being delimited by embeddedness in a part of this multiplicity. Ultimately the question of education and upbringing speaks to the social difference of the polity, to the fact that there will never exist in the city a form of homogeneous socialization that is capable of levelling human being, producing an exact identity among citizens.

I have suggested in this chapter that Machiavelli's theorization of the variability of internal nature is a constituent element of his recognition

---

73 Machiavelli, "Discorsi sopra la prima Deca di Tito Livio," bk. 3.22.
74 Ibid.

of the variability of external nature, as represented in his account of the world as chaotic and subject to historical flux. This relationship is nowhere articulated with more precision than in certain of Machiavelli's private letters. In the *Ghiribizzi*, for example, Machiavelli writes to Giovan Battista Soderini that "my luck has exhibited to me so many things, and so varied, that I am rarely compelled to be surprised or confess that I have not savoured, either through reading or through practice, the actions of men and their modes of proceeding."[75] Such a diversity of individuals and modes is for Machiavelli taken to be simply a reflection of the natural diversity that he sees all around him in the temporal world, nature having bestowed on individuals, even prior to their socialization, unique forms and tendencies: "I believe that, as Nature has created men with different faces, so it has created them with different temperaments and imaginations. From this emerges that each one governs himself according to his own temperament and imagination."[76] It is precisely because the world is in a perpetual state of movement that the modes of one individual may at one point in time lead to success while at another lead to ruin.

Machiavelli's apparent belief in the stability of individual beings, themselves fixed manifestations of the diversity of human being, might seem to suggest that individuals are thus at the mercy of time. Indeed, he goes on to write that "because times and things in general and in particular mutate frequently, and men change neither their imaginations nor their modes of proceeding, it results that one has good fortune at one time and miserable at another."[77] Yet of course we know given the discussion above this cannot be the case. As will be argued in the following chapter, Machiavelli is here referring only to the impossibility of individuals completely mastering reality, simultaneously achieving complete rational dominance over their psyches and their world. Hence when the theme of the relationship between one's temperament

---

75 Machiavelli, "Lettere, 116, Niccolò Machiavelli a Giovan Battista Soderini," in *Tutte le opere*, 1082. For an account of Machiavelli's theory of imagination such as it is elaborated in this letter, see K.R. Minogue, "Theatricality and Politics: Machiavelli's Concept of *Fantasia*," in *The Morality of Politics*, ed. Bhikhu Parekh and R.N. Berki (London: George Allen and Unwin, 1972), 148–62.

76 Machiavelli, "Lettere, 116, Niccolò Machiavelli a Giovan Battista Soderini," in *Tutte le opere*, 1083.

77 Ibid.

and the times is returned to in *Discourses* 3:9, Machiavelli highlights the actor's ability to autonomously match his or her mode with the worldly reality.[78] Indeed, here it is precisely the diversity of republics that is identified as that which allows them to vary with the times more adequately than republics, the people being, if slower as a consequence of their number, equally able to reorient their mode of being in light of their perception of the shifting nature of the historical conjuncture.[79]

It is not true that the unique internal nature bestowed on the individual by external nature is incapable of being altered. On the contrary, Machiavelli theorizes virtuous action precisely in terms of such reflective alteration, the successful political actor being he or she who is most able to imitate the diversity of the world through the adoption of a diversity of natures or personas. For Machiavelli the multiplicity of human life is a moment or element of the multiplicity of nature, one which individuals must seek to imitate for the sake of environmental orientation.[80] This multiplicity of internal and external nature is explicitly affirmed by Machiavelli in a letter to Francesco Vettori, Machiavelli using the experiences of himself and his friend as examples of the dynamics here at play: "Whoever would see our letters, honourable comrade, would see the diversity of them, and would greatly marvel, because it would immediately seem that we were serious men, entirely directed toward great things, and that no thought could pass through our heads that did not have integrity and grandeur. But afterwards, turning the page, it would seem to them that we ourselves be frivolous, inconstant, lascivious, and directed toward useless things. This mode of proceeding, if for someone it appears to be shameful, to me it appears laudable, because we are imitating nature, which is changeable; and whoever imitates that cannot be reprimanded."[81]

Overall, Machiavelli's letters reveal his belief that to imitate nature is to be receptive to adaptation, to the need to shift one's mode of doing and being in order to actualize the human potential to create one's nature. In Arlene Saxonhouse's words, "Unlike the Nature of the

---

78 Machiavelli, "Discorsi sopra la prima Deca di Tito Livio," bk. 3.9.
79 Ibid.
80 On this point see Del Lucchese, *Conflict, Power, and Multitude in Machiavelli and Spinoza*, 145.
81 Machiavelli, "Lettere, 239, Niccolò Machiavelli a Francesco Vettori," in *Tutte le opere*, 1191.

ancients and medieval philosophers, Machiavelli's Nature demands that we not affirm a fixed form to ourselves lest we be broken by the rigidity of our characters, that we not mire ourselves in the moralistic pieties of those who lose in the comic stories of Italian literature."[82] Indeed, Saxonhouse argues that tracing the comedic elements in Machiavelli's letters allows us to reconstruct his strong emphasis on the human potential to create, refound, and redefine being. Machiavelli's letters "become an explicit arena for the exercise of his imagination, for the creation of stories and drama – for the leap from what is to what might be, from what we observe to what we suspect based on observation."[83] The emphasis is on the ability of the actor to become other than what he or she is prior to imaginative creation. Hence in the most famous letter to Vettori, Machiavelli's personal adaptability, his everyday imitation of the diversity of nature, is expressed through his constant oscillation between various social roles, such as a writer on principalities, a student of the ancients, a hunter, a gamesman, and so on.[84] This diversity of being was stimulated by Machiavelli's engagements with the locals, who compelled him to an even greater degree to recognize and appreciate the diversity of humankind: "moving then up the road toward the inn, I talk to those who pass by, I ask news of their countries, I come to understand various things, and I note the manifold tastes and different patterns of men."[85]

Machiavelli's letters thus reveal that human multiplicity has a double form: individuals are non-identical both with respect to others, and

---

82 Arlene W. Saxonhouse, "Comedy, Machiavelli's Letters, and His Imaginary Republics," in *The Comedy and Tragedy of Machiavelli: Essays on the Literary Works*, ed. Vickie B. Sullivan (New Haven: Yale University Press, 2000), 61. See also Arlene W. Saxonhouse, "Machiavelli's Women," in *Machiavelli's Legacy: The Prince after Five Hundred Years*, ed. Timothy Fuller (Philadelphia: University of Pennsylvania Press, 2016), 70–86.

83 Saxonhouse, "Comedy, Machiavelli's Letters, and His Imaginary Republics," 63. Maurizio Viroli also observes that in his letters Machiavelli "asserted as clearly as possible that the right way of living and thinking is to intelligently accommodate different and even contradictory aspects of human life, like passions and reason, gravity and lightness, civic integrity and playful transgression." Viroli, *Redeeming The Prince*, 67.

84 Saxonhouse, "Comedy, Machiavelli's Letters, and His Imaginary Republics," 75.

85 Machiavelli, "Lettere, 216, Niccolò Machiavelli a Francesco Vettori," in *Tutte le opere*, 1159.

with respect to themselves. This double form is further revealed in the *Discourses*, where it will ultimately influence Machiavelli's theorization of the ideal form of his republican regime, a regime that is able to harness this double difference for the sake of political generation. Both the external and internal non-identity of individuals are clearly and simultaneously articulated in the preface to Book Two during one of Machiavelli's discussions of the misappropriation of past historical objects. Machiavelli here asks the following question: if individuals misjudge ancient things because of a lack of direct experience with them, should they then not be able to properly judge those events that they have lived through themselves and that they have experienced directly? Machiavelli determines that it is ultimately impossible to establish a universality of perception grounded in an equivalent experience of all subjects. This is because individuals are different from one another, appropriating and judging the world in unique ways, and also because individual forms of being themselves change over time, such that objects are experienced and perceived in different ways at different points in the subject's life. On the one hand we see a general "variation of customs."[86] On the other hand, even if this were not the case, there would still not be a ground for assuming consistent judgment: "This thing would be true if men through all the times of their lives were of the same opinion, and had the same appetites; but since these vary even if the times do not vary, they cannot appear the same to men who have other appetites, other delights, other considerations in old age than in youth."[87] In short, people are capable of occupying a variety of seemingly incompatible subject positions. As will be detailed in the following chapter, Machiavelli associates the ability of individuals to shift such positions with virtuous political action, as revealed for example through the figure of the centaur Chiron in *The Prince*, who is able to exploit the diverse modes of both beast and human.

In other places throughout the *Discourses* the general fact of human difference is expressed in various contexts and in various ways. For example: in 1:9, during a discussion of the many versus the one with respect to the efficiency of foundation and preservation, Machiavelli speaks of the "diverse opinions" naturally held by people;[88] in 3:6,

---

86 Machiavelli, "Discorsi sopra la prima Deca di Tito Livio," bk. 2, preface.
87 Ibid.
88 Ibid., bk. 1.9.

during his discussion of the causes of the failures of conspiracies, and in particular of the inability to control or map the motivations of others, Machiavelli again affirms the fact of differential rationality, writing that "two cannot be agreed together in all of their reasonings";[89] and in 3:9, the intensification of difference in republican contexts is pointed out, an essential feature of republics being the existence of "diverse citizens and diverse humours."[90] Machiavelli's affirmation of social difference, however, at least inasmuch as it is articulated within his major political writings, is most clearly revealed in 3:46. Here Machiavelli makes clear that human division manifests itself not only between unique political communities, between cities that are considered internally homogeneous though distinguished from one another via cultural or social-political variation. There is also a division internal to cities, and not just republican ones: "It appears that not only one city has certain modes and institutions different from another, and produces men more hard or more effeminate, but in the same city one sees such difference existent in families, one from the other. This is found to be true in every city."[91] Machiavelli gives as evidence for this claim certain distinguishable tendencies found within Rome, such as the particular toughness of the Manlii, the kindness of the Publicoli, the ambition of the Appii, and so on, for "many other families had each of its qualities distinct from the others."[92]

Machiavelli's framing of difference in terms of familial singularity might mislead us into reading division in simply genetic terms, as a manifestation of an intrinsic and ineradicable biological logic that operates independently of human intervention. Machiavelli, though, will immediately go on to close off such potential readings, locating difference in a variety of contingent social relations and determinations. Machiavelli thus explicitly posits here, again, a co-relationality between the two markers of the contingency of human nature that I have

---

89 Ibid., bk. 3.6.
90 Ibid., bk. 3.9. As Pocock notes, and as will be investigated later, one of the key reasons the republic is a more adaptable regime than the principality is because it has "a diversity of personality types at its disposal." J.G.A. Pocock, "Machiavelli and Rome: The Republic as Ideal and as History," in *Machiavelli and Republicanism*, ed. John M. Najemy (Cambridge: Cambridge University Press, 2010), 153.
91 Machiavelli, "Discorsi sopra la prima Deca di Tito Livio," bk. 3.46.
92 Ibid.

identified, the openness to alteration and the fact of difference. He writes: "These things cannot arise only from the blood, because that should vary by means of the diversity of marriages, but must necessarily come from the diverse education of one family from another. So it is very important that a youth of tender years begin to hear good or bad said of a thing, because it should make an impression, and from then on regulate the mode of proceeding in all the times of his life."[93] The latter contention, furthermore, that socialization produces an impression that the subject will bear with him or herself throughout his or her life, should not be interpreted as Machiavelli's concession that once one's character becomes fixed it assumes an essential form that closes the potential for future alteration. On the contrary, it is simply Machiavelli's recognition that individuals are always historical beings, beings from some time and some place, with a particular past, and whose existence always leans upon and is delimited by their social location and experience. As noted by many commentators, it is precisely such social difference that any political project must seek to negotiate, each of Machiavelli's major political works being largely oriented toward a consideration of the potential nature of such negotiations.[94] Part three of this study will be concerned with articulating how difference is negotiated in Machiavelli's republican writings, as I will argue that Machiavelli's defence of the republic is grounded in an ethical imperative to affirm human difference through a form of agonistic democratic institutionalization.

Once again, it must be stressed that Machiavelli's theorization of the indetermination of human being is a correlate of his theorization of the indetermination of the world. Readers of Machiavelli are generally far too quick to attribute to him belief in a positive human nature, that is,

---

93 Ibid.
94 See, for example, Jane S. Jacquette, "Rethinking Machiavelli: Feminism and Citizenship," in *Feminist Interpretations of Machiavelli*, ed. Maria J. Falco (University Park: Pennsylvania State University Press, 2004), 339–40; Maurizio Viroli, *From Politics to Reasons of State: The Acquisition and Transformation of the Language of Politics, 1250–1600* (Cambridge: Cambridge University Press, 1992), 173; S.M. Shumer, "Machiavelli: Republican Politics and Its Corruption," *Political Theory* 7, no. 1 (1979): 15; Terray, "An Encounter: Althusser and Machiavelli," 273.

a determinate human orientation toward certain universal modes of doing and being, closing off or denying the potential for the human being to create its own nature, thus transcending human nature's immediate form of appearance. Recognition of the co-implication of worldly and human being has important consequences for how we interpret Machiavelli's political theory. Machiavelli's rejection of natural teleology certainly does not necessitate an equivalent rejection of all normative political ethics.[95] On the contrary, the former fundamentally structures the latter. For Machiavelli the lack of a human telos is not coextensive with the lack of political essence because essence is negative, speaking only to the human potential for creative self-alteration. Machiavelli will thus think the being of the political in precisely such creative terms: politics is not oriented, for example, toward deliberation aimed at the mutual recognition of common human goods, but toward agonistic debate over the always highly contentious direction of the form of the political community, which is never capable of being fixed due to the fact of human multiplicity and the capacity for self-alteration. For Machiavelli the human being is indeed a political animal, just not an Aristotelian political animal. Specifically, the human being is a political animal to the extent that politics is considered by Machiavelli as the mode by which individuals are capable of expressing their fundamental capacity for creative self-overcoming. Before examining the outlines of such a mode of politics, however, we must first investigate in more detail Machiavelli's theorization of this creativity that is suggested by the account of the indetermination of human being. In this chapter I have detailed the extent to which Machiavelli rejects all positive philosophical anthropologies. In the next chapter I will go on to attempt, primarily through a study of the form of subjectivity that Machiavelli presents us with in *The Prince*, to reconstruct an alternative philosophical anthropology that more comprehensively highlights the ethos of creativity that I have been referring to throughout this study.

---

95 For manifestations of this position see Paul A. Rahe, *Against Throne and Altar: Machiavelli and Political Theory under the English Republic* (Cambridge: Cambridge University Press, 2008), 55; Rahe, "Situating Machiavelli," 305; Leo Strauss, "Machiavelli and Classical Literature," *Review of National Literatures* 1, no. 1 (1970): 10.

Chapter Three

Politics and the Human Essence: *The Prince* as a Model of Human Subjectivity

In this chapter I provide a first element of my proposal for a new mode of reading Machiavelli's *Prince* in relation to the *Discourses on Livy*. I argue that in *The Prince* Machiavelli is assembling a theoretical constellation aimed at the articulation of the ideal mode of political subjectivity, the form of being of the virtuous political actor. In the *Discourses*, meanwhile, Machiavelli develops a different constellation of thought, this one looking toward the figure of a political regime that is capable of generalizing this form of subjectivity, and providing the institutional conditions for a popular actualization of political virtue. In this chapter I will concentrate on the first of these two constellations. I will argue that through extracting and juxtaposing certain conceptual elements from the text, and through presenting them in light of Machiavelli's critique of positive models of essence as detailed in the last chapter, we can reread *The Prince* as a treatise on the nature of the human capacity for creative self-expression.

The form of subjectivity that Machiavelli develops in *The Prince* is the foundation of his reorientation of human ethics, a reorientation that is only fully articulated in the normative defence of democratic republican life in the *Discourses on Livy*. With respect to *The Prince*, although commentators are correct to point out the extent to which Machiavelli here rejects all totalizing moralities that delimit in advance the legitimate scope of political behaviour, often they are far too quick to interpret such a rejection in terms of a refusal of any ethical principle as such.[1]

---

1 See, for example, Yoran, "Machiavelli's Critique of Humanism," 256; Plamenatz, *Machiavelli, Hobbes, and Rousseau*, 20.

Contrary to such interpretations, in this chapter I argue that Machiavelli's text articulates a new ethical paradigm grounded in a consideration of the fundamental creative power of the individual. The Machiavellian concept of *virtù* will ultimately refer us to a particular form of reflective judgment that looks toward – through the critical interrogation of the being of the world and the opportunities for action this being opens up to the actor – the energetic expulsion of a fundamental human ambition, an expulsion that actualizes itself in the generation of new political modes and orders.[2] Machiavelli's ethics is thus one of self-creation. He attempts to think the conditions for the realization of a particular type of negative human essence considered in terms of the transgressive ability to perpetually overcome existent forms through the institution of new political realities.

The Affirmation of Creativity and the Constellative Form of *The Prince*

What immediately strikes one as consistent across the wide range of Machiavelli's writings is the strong emphasis placed on the value of novelty or innovation. Machiavelli's valorization of the new and of beginnings is well known. The principle of creativity affirmed by Machiavelli can be seen as operative in a diversity of human fields, Machiavelli constructing a hierarchy of foundation that moves from founders of religions, to founders of states, to expanders of states, to literary creators.[3] In this construction Machiavelli establishes a strong link between political creation, artistic creation, and productive creation, seeing each as moments of a larger general orientation toward innovative institution. The potential range of such institution, furthermore, extends outwards indefinitely: "To any other man, the number of

---

2 Inversely, in the *Mandragola* Machiavelli explicitly associates stupidity with the incapacity to interrogate the legitimacy of existing realities. Machiavelli, "Mandragola," in *Tutte le opere*, 877. This incapacity defines the being of Messer Nicia, whose uncritical nature is revealed through his subservience to established authority, most notably in his naive belief in kings' and nobles' manipulation of the sexual power of the mandrake. For example, after being told of the practice of consuming the mandrake for pregnancy, and having another sleep with the woman in question first in order to draw out the poison, Nicia states: "I am content, because you say that kings and princes and lords have held to this mode." Ibid., 876.

3 Machiavelli, "Discorsi sopra la prima Deca di Tito Livio," in *Tutte le opere*, bk. 1.10.

which is infinite, is credited with some part of the praise that his art or practice brings him."[4] Those actors deserving of praise, in whatever sphere they operate in, are creators. Hence in *The Art of War*, for example, Machiavelli is explicit that one cannot determine in advance a set of qualities that mark one as a good commander, for such is revealed only in concrete creative practice, which is largely identified with the ability to reflectively self-generate modes of action. Fabrizio states that "I would not know how to choose any other man than he who knew how to do all those things that we have reasoned about today; yet these would not be enough, if he did not know how to find them himself. Because no one without invention was ever a great man in his art; and if invention brings honour in other things, in this above all it honours you. And one sees every invention, however slight, is celebrated by the writers."[5] All human beings, regardless of the mode of activity that they are engaged in, deserve praise to the extent that they move to actualize this potential for creative invention. Needless to say, however, what most interests Machiavelli is the specifically political form of this actualization. Hence in *The Prince* the founding of new political orders, the creative reinstitutionalization of the social field, is considered as the greatest of acts: "nothing does so much honour to a newly emerging man as do the new laws and new orders he founds. These things, when they are well founded and have greatness in them, make him revered and admirable."[6] As I will attempt to show, Machiavelli's entire theoretical project can be considered in terms of his fundamental affirmation of the human capacity for creation.

Machiavelli to this degree can be seen as participating in a more general philosophical trajectory of which he is an exceptional contributor. Indeed, Skinner notes that the "emphasis on man's creative powers came to be one of the most influential as well as characteristic doctrines of Renaissance humanism."[7] The early Renaissance civic humanist claim that individuals were capable of achieving excellence required a certain model of human creation: "To assert that men are capable of reaching the highest excellence is to imply that they must be capable of

---

4 Ibid.
5 Machiavelli, "Dell'Arte della guerra," in *Tutte le opere*, 386.
6 Machiavelli, "Il Principe," in *Tutte le opere*, chap. 26.
7 Skinner, *The Foundations of Modern Political Thought*, vol. 1: *The Renaissance*, 98.

overcoming any obstacles to the attainment of this goal. The humanists willingly recognize that their view of human nature commits them to just such an optimistic analysis of man's freedoms and powers, and in consequence go on to offer an exhilarating account of the *vir virtutis* as a creative social force, able to shape his own destiny and remake his social world to fit his own desires."[8] Roberto Esposito, meanwhile, highlights how the Italian humanist emphasis on creation was often explicitly anti-essentialist in orientation, this anti-essentialism being characterized in particular by a substitution of becoming for being, in a recognition of the specifically innovative capacities of the human being, and the openness of this being to change and self-alteration. This orientation is given a characteristic expression, for example, in the work of Giovanni Pico della Mirandola, who represents "the breaking of the classical scheme in favor of a new dynamic that has at its center the transition from being to becoming: human beings are nothing other than what they become, or better, what they intend to 'make' of themselves."[9]

On those few occasions when Machiavelli speaks of the fixity of human nature, the most we can attribute to this statement given his account of the indeterminacy of the human being such as was detailed in the previous chapter, is the universal orientation toward creativity, an expression of the perpetual human ability to constantly overcome the form of its existence and reshape its being.[10] My suggestion is that it is possible to read *The Prince* not only as a text detailing the mechanics of a certain type of political regime, the new principality, but also as one detailing Machiavelli's understanding of the form of being of this creative human practice. *The Prince* is a text that operates on multiple registers. Just as it is possible to interpret it as a political treatise articulating the mode of functioning of a civil principality, or as an initial

---

8 Ibid., 94.

9 Roberto Esposito, *Living Thought: The Origins and Actuality of Italian Philosophy* (Stanford: Stanford University Press, 2012), 41 See also Michelle Zerba, "The Frauds of Humanism: Cicero, Machiavelli, and the Rhetoric of Imposture," *Rhetorica: A Journal of the History of Rhetoric* 22, no. 3 (2004): 222. On the human being's capacity to voluntarily create its own nature and perpetually reinvent itself see especially Giovanni Pico della Mirandola, *On the Dignity of Man*, trans. Glenn Wallis (Indianapolis: Hackett, 1965), 4–5.

10 Such is recognized, for example, by Diego von Vacano, who understands Machiavelli as interpreting the individual in terms of an innate tendency for creative self-actualization. Von Vacano, *The Art of Power*, 16.

programmatic statement regarding the process of republican institutionalization, it is also possible to read it as an account of the nature of
the human actor considered as a virtuous subject. The foregrounding
of any particular interpretative reading – that is, the generation of any
particular textual constellation – depends upon the precise set of elements that are highlighted, and the nature of their arrangement or
juxtaposition.

On my reading *The Prince*'s surplus, which is not to say non-political
nature, lay in its articulation of the general characteristics of human subjectivity.[11] It is significant that these characteristics are not drawn from
any one historical source. We must remember our discussion from chapter 1 on the significance of Machiavelli's perspectivism, on the necessity
of the virtuous subject's capacity for perspectival representation. What
the new prince understands above all is that his understanding is structured by his particular location in a shifting historical field, each loca-
tional movement affecting the form and object of his perception. Even if
we believe it is justified to ascribe to the object a stable and determinate
being – and we know from chapter 2 that such a belief is highly prob-
lematic given Machiavelli's theorization of the world in terms of perpetual movement and flux – human beings are not epistemologically
capable of singularly subsuming this being under the sign of the concept. There is no Archimedean point that would allow for a complete
schematization of the contours of objective being, hence Machiavelli's
occupation with the necessity of engaging with, not the essence of
things, but the appearance of things: "And men universally judge more
with their eyes than with their hands, because seeing moves everyone,
feeling a few. Everyone sees what you appear to be, few perceive what
you really are."[12] One can read Machiavelli here as positing an inequality of intelligences whereby a certain minority of individuals is endowed
with the capacity to grasp genuine being. As is suggested, though, by
his claim that it is a universal feature of humans that they are incapable

---

11 Giulio Ferroni is one of the rare readers who perceives that in *The Prince* Machiavelli
    is developing a specific anthropology, it being "not only a political treatise but also
    the construction of a model of human behavior." Giulio Ferroni, "'Transformation'
    and 'Adaptation' in Machiavelli's Mandragola," in *Machiavelli and the Discourse of
    Literature*, ed. Albert Russell Ascoli and Victoria Kahn, trans. Ronald L. Martinez
    (Ithaca: Cornell University Press, 1993), 84.
12 Machiavelli, "Il Principe," chap. 18.

of touching the essence of being, we could also read Machiavelli as maintaining that there exists no privileged spectator who escapes the field of appearance, or at least no spectator whose privilege allows him or her such an escape. There are no exalted viewers, only vulgar ones: "for the vulgar are always taken in by what appears, and with the outcome of the thing, and in the world there are none but the vulgar; and the few have no place there when the many have somewhere to lean on."[13] What in any case seems clear is that in a world in which at least the vast majority of people are incapable of comprehending the essence of things, a political project grounded in the consideration of this essence, as opposed to the manipulation of appearances, is impossible. Even if there are those few who can touch the essence of the object (and in chapter 4 I will argue that there are not), the transmission of such perception cannot be the basis for political determination in a world dominated by those who can only see. Hence in the final instance there is no possibility for the transcendence of the stratified field of appearance, either through the subjective possession of unique properties or capacities, or through the occupation of a certain objective social position.

Given the impossibility of a political actor acquiring a complete knowledge of the essence of things, of mastering political reality, it should not surprise us that Machiavelli is unwilling to give the reader an archetypal model of the new prince who completely actualizes his political ethic.[14] Peter Breiner notes the significance of the fact that Machiavelli does not provide his reader with any single example of a particular historical prince who embodies the ethic of virtue that the text is intended to reveal. On the contrary, Machiavelli selectively extracts traits and qualities from a multiplicity of sources, constructing a mental image of the new prince through the arrangement of these elements in a specific figure of thought: "To be sure, Machiavelli presents

---

13 Ibid. That the political world is constituted only by the vulgar is noted in Smith, *Politics and Remembrance*, 94; Erica Benner, *Machiavelli's Ethics* (Princeton: Princeton University Press, 2009), 62.

14 Indeed, there is very little reason to believe Machiavelli thought that such a prince ever existed. It would thus be a mistake to read the text as a form of historical investigation meant to identify virtuous precedents. See, for example, Federico Chabod, "*The Prince*: Myth and Reality," in *Machiavelli and the Renaissance*, trans. David Moore (London: Bowes and Bowes, 1960), 61; Charles D. Tarlton, "Machiavelli's Burden: *The Prince* as Literary Text," in *Seeking Real Truths: Multidisciplinary Perspectives on Machiavelli*, ed. Patricia Vilches and Gerald Seaman (Leiden: Brill, 2007), 66.

numerous candidates for such a role: Louis XII of France, Cesare Borgia, Francesco Sforza, Ferdinand of Aragon, and Pope Julius II, but none of these figures represent 'the new prince' as such but only fragments of what a new prince might do or have to do."[15] Breiner will go so far as to recognize that this constellative form of arrangement has a major significance for the reader of the political text, who is encouraged to selectively appropriate Machiavelli's conceptual content in light of his or her own concrete historical situation, for "who that reader is specifically depends on the way s/he cobbles together that political advice and examples for his/her own constellation of governments, territory, and conflicting groups. In short, Machiavelli leaves open who that reader might be and where s/he is located in the matrix of political forces."[16] The act of interpreting Machiavelli's constellation is thus seen as a constellative act in itself. In the final instance, "it is, thus, the reader as potential political actor who must put the text together relative to his/her (political) situation which fortune always serves up in unpredictable and unique ways."[17] The political significance of such constellative reading is highlighted in the concluding chapter of the text, where Machiavelli maintains that it is possible for a contemporary actor to seize the historical moment and work toward the political task at hand, the unification and liberation of the peninsula, provided he or she is able to properly synthesize the relevant concepts that are articulated through the juxtaposition of examples provided. In Machiavelli's words, to learn the lessons of the text "is not very difficult if you take before you the actions and lives of those named above."[18]

Machiavelli himself notes that the prudent actor's political success is largely grounded in his or her ability to selectively appropriate princely

---

15 Peter Breiner, "Machiavelli's 'New Prince' and the Primordial Moment of Acquisition," *Political Theory* 36, no. 1 (2008): 66–7. Agnès Cugno also recognizes the non-empirical being of the new prince, writing that "the Machiavellian prince has no reality, neither empirical nor logical. It is a pure idea." Agnès Cugno, "Machiavel et le problème de l'être en politique," *Revue philosophique de la France et de l'étranger* 189, no. 1 (1999): 23. And Diego von Vacano writes that "*The Prince*, ostensibly written about principalities, is also a *representation* of the ethic of the great man in terms of the human condition … It is the *imaginary* portrayal of the quintessentially political man." Von Vacano, *The Art of Power*, 44.

16 Breiner, "Machiavelli's 'New Prince,'" 84.

17 Ibid., 86.

18 Machiavelli, "Il Principe," chap. 26.

traits in response to the necessity of the situation. This, for example, is the lesson of the presentation of the examples of Marcus Aurelius and Severus in chapter 19. It is within the context of a discussion of whether a prince should privilege the satisfaction of the people or the satisfaction of the soldiers that Machiavelli introduces these contrasting examples. From whom should the contemporary actor take his or her lead? Should he or she aim to replicate the brutality and ferocity of Severus or the humaneness and constancy of Marcus? For Machiavelli the opposition is a false one, for imitation is not a matter of deliberating and choosing between antithetical and self-contained positions that are seen to exhaust all possible options. It is not at all a matter of choosing between pre-existing forms of proceeding: "a new prince in a new principality cannot imitate the actions of Marcus, nor yet is it necessary to follow those of Severus; but he ought to take from Severus those parts that are necessary to found his state, and from Marcus those that are appropriate and glorious to conserve a state that is already established and firm."[19] It is not sufficient for the actor to simply aim to replicate in an immediate way past patterns, and in fact such non-reflective and one-sided imitation is identified as being that fundamental error that caused the downfall of Pertinax and Alexander, as well as Caracalla, Commodus, and Maximus. Whereas the former group attempted to imitate the modesty of Marcus without possessing a hereditary right to their state, and hence with a need to satisfy the soldiers and the people, the latter attempted to imitate the cruelty of Severus without possessing the virtue that allowed him to appear "so admirable in the sight of the soldiers and the people that the latter remained in a certain way astonished and stupefied, and the former reverent and satisfied."[20] It is by no means insignificant, furthermore, that in the *Discourses* Machiavelli identifies the same Severus as a criminal, from which there seems not to be any precise lessons to be drawn.[21] This results exactly from the fact that in the *Discourses* we are dealing with a fundamentally different constellation of thought, the unique organization of concepts generating unique figures of meaning and hence unique imperatives.

---

19 Ibid., chap. 19.
20 Ibid.
21 Machiavelli, "Discorsi sopra la prima Deca di Tito Livio," bk. 1.10.

Ambition and the Function of the New Prince

What the constellative presentation of examples is meant to reveal is the creative human faculty, the ability of the human actor to institute the new through exercising the capacity for innovation. This concern with the new is first of all revealed in the very specificity of the topic discussed, that is, in Machiavelli's clear differentiation of the new principality from the hereditary and the ecclesiastical principalities.[22] Machiavelli's refusal to discuss these latter two forms in any detail is grounded in his perception of their ahistorical existence, in his recognition that each is governed by a logic of development that closes off the potential for human intervention and fixes the trajectory of each. The new principality's situation in a historical continuum that structures activity but does not determine it is represented in his characterization of the instability that always haunts the new principality, in chapter 3 represented by the non-security of political leaders and the fickleness of political subjects.[23] The new prince will ultimately be seen as one who can insert himself into time in order to create new modes and orders, thus altering the constitution of the historically variable and unstable political world.

Although it is not unusual for readers of Machiavelli to note his valorization of an ethic of *virtù* that is identified with novelty and political innovation, it is rare for commentators to attempt to ground this valorization in what I take to be Machiavelli's negative philosophical anthropology.[24] The central element of this anthropology is a dynamic human desire emanating from the psychic flux of the mind. Martin Fleisher notes that for Machiavelli, as is often pointed out, "politics is the very life of the soul."[25] Very few readers, however, have attempted to reflect

---

22 On the significance of this differentiation see, for example, Sheldon Wolin, *Politics and Vision: Continuity and Innovation in Western Political Thought* (Princeton: Princeton University Press, 2004), 180; J.G.A. Pocock, *The Machiavellian Moment: Florentine Political Thought and the Atlantic Republican Tradition* (Princeton: Princeton University Press, 1975), 158; Gaille-Nikodimov, "An Introduction to *The Prince*," 34; Negri, *Insurgencies*, 50.

23 Machiavelli, "Il Principe," chap. 3.

24 Although not clarifying its content in detail, Filippo Del Lucchese does specify that Machiavelli's anthropology is a specifically negative one. Filippo Del Lucchese, "On the Emptiness of an Encounter: Althusser's Reading of Machiavelli," trans. Warren Montag, *Décalages* 1, no. 1 (2010): 2.

25 Martin Fleisher, "A Passion for Politics: The Vital Core of the World of Machiavelli," in *Machiavelli and the Nature of Political Thought*, ed. Martin Fleisher (New York: Atheneum, 1972), 119.

more literally on this image. Doing so leads us to recognize that Machiavelli's concept of *animo* refers us very specifically to politics as an essential mode of human being. Machiavelli's concept of the soul is not static; it does not refer us to a set of fixed parts that may be arranged into a harmonious whole or architechtonic psychological system. On the contrary, the soul "is, rather, in continual motion."[26] This motion, furthermore, is not uniform or subject to a transcendentally or rationally guided movement, but is irregular and stratified, the soul being a vital force of expression whose trajectory is continually being redirected. In Dante Germino's words, "the psyche is a field of perpetually shifting and contending passions, one or more of which may temporarily gain control, only later to be replaced by a contradictory passion or set of passions."[27] As constant motion and variation, the soul is a field for the "agonistic" play of passion.[28] All that we can say is that the soul is perpetually oriented toward creation: "The *animo* continually and changeably desires or values things. It is truly vital – the genuine source of human values. And what it desires or values most is the ability to command any desire or bestow any value it wishes."[29] Hence the "supreme value" is "*the power to designate and appropriate values.*"[30]

The vitality of the psyche, the perpetual desire of the *animo*, is most significantly expressed through the concept of ambition. As Yves Winter writes, "if *ambizione* is what distinguishes the human among other animals, then the definitional attribute of being human is the capacity to be or become unnatural," the human thus being "that animal whose nature is to undo nature."[31] The key text detailing Machiavelli's

---

26 Ibid.
27 Dante Germino, "Machiavelli's Political Anthropology," in *Theorie und Politik: Festschrift zum 70. Geburstag für Carl Joachim Friedrich*, ed. Klaus von Beyme (Haag: Martinus Nijhoff, 1971), 39.
28 Ibid. On the dynamism of desire and its implications for political theory see also Nicole Hochner, "Machiavelli: Love and the Economy of the Emotions," *Italian Culture* 32, no. 2 (2014): 85–97; Bonnie Honig, *Political Theory and the Displacement of Politics* (Ithaca: Cornell University Press, 1993), 70.
29 Fleisher, "A Passion for Politics: The Vital Core of the World of Machiavelli," 124.
30 Ibid. Original emphasis.
31 Yves Winter, "Necessity and Fortune: Machiavelli's Politics of Nature," in *Second Nature: Rethinking the Natural through Politics*, ed. Crina Archer, Laura Ephraim, and Lida Maxwell (New York: Fordham University Press, 2013), 27. On the specifically human nature of ambition see also Wendy Brown, *Manhood and Politics: A Feminist Reading of Political Theory* (Totowa: Rowman and Littlefield, 1988), 77; Haig Patapan,

thinking on the nature of human ambition is his poem "Of Ambition." The significance of the poem lies in Machiavelli's explicit identification of ambition, which throughout *The Prince* and the *Discourses* is conceptually deployed in order to articulate the direction and insatiability of human desire, with objective alteration. Here Machiavelli presents most concisely the fundamental psychic element that structures his philosophical anthropology, reading the essence of the human being (and crucially, there is here no bifurcation of desire into popular and noble humours, the significance of which will be elaborated on in chapter 4) in terms of a vital creative energy that is fundamentally transgressive, looking to perpetually interrogate and potentially overcome existing forms: "meditate a little better on human desire. / For from the sun of Scythia to that of Egypt, from England to the opposite shore, one sees the germination of this offence. / What country or what city is devoid of it? What village, what hovel? In all places Ambition and Avarice reach."[32] Machiavelli in "Of Ambition" is explicit: wherever you find human beings you find this transgressive and limitless energy looking to overcome the being of the merely existent, the birth of it necessarily accompanying the birth of humanity.[33]

In "Of Ambition," however, the linking of ambition and avarice reveals the degree to which the expression of value creation takes place through violence, through the external deployment of psychic energy against others: "Oh human mind insatiable, proud, sly, and changeable, and above everything malignant, iniquitous, impetuous, and wild, / for through your ambitious desire was seen the first violent death in the world, and the first bloody grass!"[34] The externalization of ambitious energy thus has a double consequence: the satisfaction of the desire of the one is paid for with the denial of the other ("you will see from Ambition one or the other art: as the one robs the other weeps for its tattered and scattered fortune").[35] Machiavelli's sympathy for those

---

Machiavelli in Love: The Modern Politics of Love and Fear (Lanham: Rowman and Littlefield, 2006), 52.

32 Machiavelli, "Dell'Ambizione," in *Tutte le opere*, 983.

33 Ibid., 984.

34 Ibid. On what Machiavelli takes to be the inhumanity of violence in itself (as opposed to the utilization of violence as a performative modality of human virtue) see Machiavelli, "Discorsi sopra la prima Deca di Tito Livio," bk. 1.26.

35 Machiavelli, "Dell'Ambizione," 986.

who are the victims of ambition, along with his recognition that ambition cannot simply be willed away, since "man by himself cannot expel it,"[36] leads him to attempt to find a solution to the problem of energetic discharge, which if ignored will bring a city to ruin.[37] Here that solution is identified with the outward projection of passion against external cities through war making. The violence that accompanies transgressive creation is simply displaced onto other peoples and cities, the non-possibility of an internal expression being suggested by the purely negative characterization of the function of law in terms of restraint, in terms of the repression of human desire: "To this our natural instinct leads us by our own motion and our own passion, if law or greater force do not restrain us."[38] The internal expression of desire would result in the ruin of the city, hence the need for law to place limits on such expression, while at the same time providing a field for outward projection: "When a country lives unbridled by its nature, and then, by accident, is established and ordered by good laws, / Ambition uses against foreign people the furore that neither the law nor the king grants it to use at home."[39] Clearly the simple displacement of violence onto another register, from the citizens of one city to the citizens of another city, is from an ethical standpoint no meaningful solution to what Machiavelli identifies as the problem of ambitious expression. In *The Prince*, however, although Machiavelli will continue to think about the essentiality of ambition to human being – viewing it as the source of the innovation of the virtuous actor – he will fundamentally reconceptualize its mode of expression, specifically through a rearticulation of the relationship between desire and law.

In *The Prince* law is not considered as the means for the one-sided repression of ambitious desire, but rather as a medium that is able to productively channel this desire in socially beneficial ways. Although in the *Discourses on Livy* Machiavelli will attempt to think the institutional conditions for a universal expulsion of desire mediated by law, a situation in which all citizens are able to legally vent their ambitious energy, in *The Prince* it is the new prince alone who is able to actualize ambition. This results from the specific social situation that Machiavelli

---

36 Ibid.
37 Ibid., 985. On the mechanics of this ruin see also Machiavelli, "L'Asino," 966.
38 Machiavelli, "Dell'Ambizione," 985.
39 Ibid.

is detailing. We must recall the double variability of people: not only are individuals distinct from each other, but they are also distinct from themselves, their desires and wants changing form over time as a consequence of their experiences in a historically fluctuating world. This double variability is summed up in *The Prince* when Machiavelli writes that "the nature of peoples is variable, and it is easy to persuade them of a thing, but difficult to hold them in that persuasion."[40] The function of the prince is comprehensible only in the context of the recognition of this primary fact of human difference. In the previous chapter I made an initial bifurcation between two social contexts, one that produced human badness – that is, an orientation in individuals toward the egoistic self-maximization of private good – and one that produced human goodness, considered in terms of the renunciation of such an orientation and a willingness to affirm civic mutuality. I also suggested that *The Prince* corresponds to the former situation. The political imperative in *The Prince* is thus structured by the objective reality of this form of social existence. We can consider the totality of Machiavelli's political project as responding to the question of the problem of social difference. *The Prince* and the *Discourses* give two fundamentally different answers to this question, to the extent that they speak to two fundamentally different social realities. As I will detail later, in the *Discourses* Machiavelli demonstrates how difference can be given a positive institutional expression in a political context in which all citizens recognize the claim of other citizens to expel their ambition in order to satisfy their desire for value formation. In *The Prince*, however, individuals are not capable of making such a recognition to the extent that they are invidiously motivated, seeking to actualize their own desire at the expense of the actualization of others. In such a context the universal expulsion of difference must result only in violence and destruction, such as the kind detailed in the *Florentine Histories*.

Hence the function of the new prince is not to provide the institutional conditions for the affirmation of social difference, but rather to cover up this difference through a project of social unification. Machiavelli would make this explicit in a letter to Francesco Vettori, where he maintains that a new prince of a corrupt city must look to homogenize the social field through imposing unity on the diverse elements that

---

40 Machiavelli, "Il Principe," chap. 6.

compose it: "One who becomes a prince ought, therefore, think of making it a unified body, and accustom [the diverse members] to recognize it as one as soon as possible. This can be done in two modes: either by staying there in person, or by appointing one of his lieutenants to command everyone, so that those subjects, even if from diverse towns and moved by different opinions, begin to observe one alone, and know him as prince."[41] To the extent that individuals are multiple, it is unrealistic to expect to be able to achieve universal agreement on the legitimacy of the form of princely constitution independent of the potential to deploy force as a means of coercion. It is for this reason that unarmed prophets invariably come to ruin: "Moses, Cyrus, Theseus, and Romulus would not have been able to ensure respect for their constitutions for long if they had been unarmed, such as happened in our time with Brother Girolamo Savonarola, who was destroyed in his new orders as the multitude began to not believe in them; and he had no way to keep firm those who believed, nor to make believe the unbelieving."[42] The prudent political orderer is thus identified as one who not only recognizes social variability and its potentially destructive consequences, but also is willing and able to deploy force in order to bring that variability under control, uniting the diverse elements that constitute the social body under the image of the prince. The prince is thus an external mediator who imposes an artificial unity on the fragmented social field.

This movement, which does constitute one dimension of the text, is captured by what might be called the transitional reading of the relationship between *The Prince* and the *Discourses*. According to this now-standard interpretation, the political function of the prince is the production, within the context of a general corruption of the body politic, of the institutional conditions for the re-education of a group of citizens fit for republican life.[43] If the social field upon which the

---

41 Machiavelli, "Lettere, 239, Niccolò Machiavelli a Francesco Vettori," in *Tutte le opere*, 1191.

42 Machiavelli, "Il Principe," chap. 6.

43 In the words of Maurizio Viroli in his recent reading of the prince as redeemer, this political founder is specifically "one who acts as a monarch but then opens the path for a republic." Viroli, *Redeeming The Prince*, 18. See also G.H.R. Parkinson, "Ethics and Politics in Machiavelli," *Philosophical Quarterly* 5, no. 18 (1955): 41; Norman Jacobson, *Pride and Solace: The Functions and Limits of Political Theory* (Berkeley: University of California Press, 1978), 44; Sebastian de Grazia, *Machiavelli in Hell* (Princeton: Princeton University Press, 1989), 236; Robert Kocis, *Machiavelli*

new principality is instituted is considered largely in terms of the chaotic distribution of matter lacking a form that integrates diverse and self-referring elements, the new prince is that actor who introduces those modes and orders that look toward a positive socialization capable of generating civic-minded citizens, citizens able to orient themselves away from a quest for the realization of their private interest and toward a quest for the realization of a common interest of which their private interest is a non-abstractable part.[44] This suggests that the goal of the prince is not the simple and immediate unification of the social, but the institution of a precise form of social unity, one that integrates the singular elements in a specific pattern. This pattern is revealed through Machiavelli's consideration of whether the prince should rely on the people or the great in his effort at stabilization. In chapter 9 Machiavelli is clear that the civil principality requires a form of social approval in order to be established. It is instituted "when a private citizen, not through wickedness or other intolerable violence but through the support of his fellow citizens, becomes prince of his country."[45] This support will take one of two forms, being grounded in the backing of one of the two poles constituting society's fundamental social division, that between the people and the great. This division is relationally defined

---

Redeemed: Retrieving His Humanist Perspectives on Equality, Power, and Glory (Bethlehem: Lehigh University Press, 1998), 149; Alissa M. Ardito, *Machiavelli and the Modern State: The Prince, the Discourses on Livy, and the Extended Territorial Republic* (Cambridge: Cambridge University Press, 2015), 13. For examples of scepticism that Machiavelli could have intended single-person foundation to be a plausible solution to the problem of political rejuvenation see, for example, Mary G. Dietz, "Trapping the Prince: Machiavelli and the Politics of Deception," *American Political Science Review* 80, no. 3 (1986): 780; Hanna Fenichel Pitkin, *Fortune Is a Woman: Gender and Politics in the Thought of Niccolò Machiavelli* (Berkeley: University of California Press, 1984), 295; John M. Najemy, "Society, Class, and State in Machiavelli's *Discourses on Livy*," in *The Cambridge Companion to Machiavelli*, ed. John M. Najemy (Cambridge: Cambridge University Press, 2010), 101–2; John M. Najemy, "The 2013 Josephine Waters Bennett Lecture: Machiavelli and History," *Renaissance Quarterly* 67, no. 4 (2014): 1147.

44 Needless to say, such an integration is achieved at the level of appearance alone, it not being possible to objectively unify the disparate constituents of the social field. See, for example, Farhang Erfani, "Fixing Marx with Machiavelli: Claude Lefort's Democratic Turn," *Journal of the British Society for Phenomenology* 39, no. 2 (2008): 204.

45 Machiavelli, "Il Principe," chap. 9.

according to the form of appearance of human desire. As will be elaborated on later, whereas the great seek to satisfy their ambition through the desire to oppress and dominate other citizens, the people seek to simply not be oppressed and dominated.[46] The prince must thus decide which of these two social groups he will rely on in order to institute the civil principality.

A principality is supported by the great when it is instituted so as to overcome the noble fear of being overwhelmed by the people, providing a space for the satisfaction of the noble desire for oppression. The great agree to invest all legitimate civil authority in a single figure, "so that they can, under his shadow, vent their appetite."[47] Ultimately, however, Machiavelli advises the prince against attempting to stabilize his authority through the construction of a space upon which the *grandi* are able to express their desire to dominate. On the one hand, such an organization is a threat to the stable being of the prince, who is able to secure himself with more ease when aligned against few as opposed to many.[48] What is more, this few that constitutes the *grandi* is differentiated from the people precisely in its desire to command, and thus constitutes a continual threat to the authority of the prince, whom they might seek to overwhelm or resist at any point through the redirection of their hostility. Machiavelli thus writes that "he who comes to the principality with the aid of the great maintains himself with more difficulty than he who does so with the aid of the people, because he finds himself with many around him who think themselves equal to him, and because of this he cannot command them nor manage them in his own way."[49] It thus seems that it is the potential confrontation with the power of the *grandi* that motivates the prince to recruit the people.[50] Crucially, however, beyond these two apparently instrumental considerations we also see in this chapter the introduction of the germ of an ethical imperative to limit human suffering, Machiavelli noting that

---

46 It is important to note, however, that the people's desire not to be oppressed does not preclude on their part a desire for ambitious expression, as I will demonstrate in chapter 4.
47 Machiavelli, "Il Principe," chap. 9.
48 Ibid.
49 Ibid.
50 Alfredo Bonadeo, "The Role of the 'Grandi' in the Political World of Machiavelli," *Studies in the Renaissance* 16 (1969): 17.

"no one can with decency satisfy the great without injury to others, but one can the people, because the end of the people is more upright than that of the great."[51]

A principality supported by the people is created when the latter grant authority to an individual who it is hoped will defend them from the insolence and oppression of the great. The people in this institution are no mere passive components, but an active force that consciously assents to the establishment of the regime. And unlike the great, the problem of popular assent cannot simply be evaded through the elimination of the discontented party, for unlike members of the *grandi* the people cannot be purged from the city: "It is necessary still that the prince live always with the same people, but he can do well without the same nobles, being able to make and unmake them every day, and take away and give them their reputation as he pleases."[52] Even under a non-ideal condition where authority is established through the support of the great, the new prince should immediately move to ally himself with the people at the first opportunity: "one who, against the people, becomes prince through the support of the great must above all seek to win the people, which is easy to do if he takes them under his protection."[53] In the final instance Machiavelli will reject the maxim that the ruler who founds on the people does so on shaky ground, arguing on the contrary that such a foundation is in fact the necessary condition for the establishment of a relatively stable civil principality. The ultimate lesson of chapter 9 is that the historical function of the new prince, the neutralization of human difference so as to homogenize the social field

---

51 Machiavelli, "Il Principe," chap. 9. See also Erica Benner, "The Necessity to Be Not-Good: Machiavelli's Two Realisms," in *Machiavelli on Liberty and Conflict*, ed. David Johnston, Nadia Urbinati, and Camila Vergara (Chicago: University of Chicago Press, 2017), 167. For an account of what is to be taken to be Machiavelli's self-declared philanthropy see Patrick Coby, "Machiavelli's Philanthropy," *History of Political Thought* 20, no. 4 (1999): 604–26. Fredi Chiappelli also emphasizes what he takes to be Machiavelli's empathy, which he sees as expressed not only in the theoretical writings, but the diplomatic ones as well. Fredi Chiappelli, "Machiavelli as Secretary," *Italian Quarterly* 14, no. 3 (1970): 27–44.

52 Machiavelli, "Il Principe," 9. Erica Benner, for example, calls attention to the fact that Machiavelli always advises those in power to establish authority via consent, respecting the potential capacity for the self-legislation of the people. Benner, *Machiavelli's Ethics*, 259.

53 Machiavelli, "Il Principe," chap. 9.

and mitigate the expression of civic violence, is not an immediate one, but rather one that must proceed according to a specific logic, that is, a popular logic looking toward the good of the people.

Although the above discussion reveals the extent to which *The Prince* can be seen to be governed by a popular logic, it can nevertheless not be interpreted as a specifically democratic text.[54] In *The Prince* it is the new prince alone who is able to realize his creative desire for value formation, such a realization being achieved through the denial of a similar realization to all other citizens. The fact of princely desire, though, that the prince himself is in possession of ambitious energy seeking externalization, must not be forgotten. The prince's desire for rule is achieved through his support for the people, through his placing definite limits on the ability of other nobles to pursue their desire to dominate via the subjection of the people. It is precisely in this limitation, though, that we can begin to see the reconfiguration of the means by which desire is realized. The prince, if he is to separate himself from the nobles, must do so via the support of the people, which is achieved through the institution of laws that limit the ability of some to dominate many. It is in this initial movement that we begin to see come into focus the function of the law in the mediation of the discharge of desire. The prince, of course, to the extent that he projects an image of himself that exists above society, is not subject to the limitations of the law in the same manner that his subjects are. Nevertheless, already in *The Prince* Machiavelli is beginning to anticipate that relation between desire and law that will be fully articulated in the contrast between the modes of energetic expulsion that we see contrasted in the *Discourses* and the *Florentine Histories*. Consider again a passage I have already cited, his advice to the prince, in the context of the recognition of the impossibility of being simultaneously loved and feared, on how to avoid being feared in such a way so as not to be hated: "this he will always do if he refrains from the property of his citizens and his subjects, and from their women. And even if it is necessary to proceed against anyone's life, do it when there is reasonable justification and manifest cause."[55] In short, Machiavelli is conceding that the self-affirmation of the prince cannot be

---

54 In this sense I disagree with the conclusion drawn by Vatter, for whom "*The Prince* is the first philosophical grounding of a democratic project of modernity." Miguel Vatter, *Machiavelli's The Prince* (London: Bloomsbury, 2013), 29.

55 Machiavelli, "Il Principe," chap. 17.

achieved through an arbitrary exercise of will. After all, one of the fundamental foundations of all states is "good laws,"[56] and princes "begin to lose their state at the hour they begin to break the laws."[57] As will be elaborated on in more detail in part three, in Machiavelli's political writings the relationship between law and desire is articulated in a fundamentally different way than in "Of Ambition," law existing not in order to one-sidedly repress desire, but rather as a means for the productive channelling or sublimation of it.[58]

The Dialectic of *Virtù* and *Fortuna*

In detailing the activity of the virtuous prince Machiavelli articulates a form of energetic expulsion that looks toward the productive creation of new political objects. It is of the utmost significance that the possibility of such controlled or mediated creation is seen as dependent on the openness or contingency of the being of the world, such as was detailed in the previous chapter. What is essential to recognize is the extent to which early in *The Prince* Machiavelli establishes a conjunction between the actor's ability to create the new and the instability of existent forms. It is the latter, a consequence of the indetermination and inconstancy of life in a historical world, which makes possible the former. To the extent that the temporal world is thought of in terms of a radical indetermination in which human objects are perpetually unstable and subject to unpredictable movement, the Machiavellian concept of creation that is given an initial expression in the generative activity of the prince must not be reduced to a production of the new that might result from the simple recombination or reorganization of already existing elements.[59]

---

56 Ibid., chap. 12.

57 Machiavelli, "Discorsi sopra la prima Deca di Tito Livio," bk. 3.5.

58 On the linking of institutionalization with sublimation in Machiavelli see Christopher Holman, "Machiavelli and the Concept of Political Sublimation," *Italian Culture* 35, no. 1 (2017): 1–20; Pitkin, *Fortune Is a Woman*, 316–20; Dante Germino, *Machiavelli to Marx: Modern Western Political Thought* (Chicago: University of Chicago Press, 1979), 53. For an example of a reader who claims that Machiavelli ultimately does not believe it possible to channel "superlative ambition" toward socially beneficial ends see Alexander F. Duff, "Republicanism and the Problem of Ambition: The Critique of Cicero in Machiavelli's *Discourses*," *Journal of Politics* 73, no. 4 (2011): 980–92.

59 This, for example, characterizes certain Marxist or Gramscian readings that, although identifying a principle of creation in Machiavelli's thought, reduce it to

As Althusser notes, Machiavellian creation is creation *ex nihilo*, as it does "*not rely on anything*, neither on an existing State nor on an existing Prince, but on the non-existent impossibility: a new Prince in a new Principality."[60] As pointed out by Cornelius Castoriadis, however, it is clear that to posit the possibility of creation from nothing is not to posit creation as in nothing (*in nihilo*) or as with nothing (*cum nihilo*).[61] As I have suggested above, the prince as a historical construction always emerges at some time and in some place, his actions leaning on already instituted forms and determinations. It is simply that the political orders that he institutes cannot be reduced to these prior forms and determinations, as if the latter were merely sequential moments in a causal sequence culminating in the positive creations of the prince.[62]

---

the productive consequence of a necessary or deterministic logic. See, for example, Gramsci, "The Modern Prince," 130; Fontana, *Hegemony and Power*, 6. For a contrary interpretation arguing that Gramsci, along with Althusser, is using Machiavelli in order to aid in "the development of a non-determinate Marxism," see Ross Speer, "The Machiavellian Marxism of Althusser and Gramsci," *Décalages* 2, no. 1 (2016): 1.

60 Althusser, "Is It Simple to Be a Marxist in Philosophy?," 171. Original emphasis. For elaboration on the significance of the ideas of beginning and creativity in Althusser's reading of Machiavelli see Mohamed Moulfi, "Lectures machiavéliennes d'Althusser," in *The Radical Machiavelli: Politics, Philosophy, and Language*, ed. Filippo Del Lucchese, Fabio Frosini, and Vittorio Morfino (Leiden: Brill, 2015), 406–19. On Machiavelli and creation *ex nihilo* see also Negri, *Insurgencies*, 52; Terrence Ball, "The Picaresque Prince: Reflections on Machiavelli and Moral Change," *Political Theory* 12, no. 4 (1984): 531; Terray, "An Encounter: Althusser and Machiavelli," 264–5.

61 See, for example, Cornelius Castoriadis, "Time and Creation," in *World in Fragments*, ed. and trans. David Ames Curtis (Stanford: Stanford University Press, 1997), 392.

62 It is the non-recognition of the historical being of creation *ex nihilo* which I think has led certain commentators to reject the idea of creation as being a normative ideal in Machiavelli's thinking. Erica Benner sees the reading that associates *virtù* with the capacity for self-creation as "grounded in an unrealistic view of human capabilities. It reflects a longing for total control of circumstances that cannot be completely controlled – though they can be 'managed' or 'governed' by self-ordering *virtù*." Benner, *Machiavelli's Ethics*, 68. As I will argue below, however, to affirm the human capacity for self-creation is certainly not to affirm the human capacity for rational mastery, the creative potential indeed always being limited by the constraints of life in a historical world. For Dante Germino, as well, Machiavelli's recognition that individuals are incapable of completely mastering fortune is a concession regarding the incapacity for human self-creation. Machiavelli's alleged realism – that is, his non-belief that individuals are capable of creating the conditions of their own existence – is counterposed to what Germino labels the "fantasies of Marx." Germino, "Second Thoughts on Leo Strauss's Machiavelli," 814. In fact, however, Machiavelli

This relationship between the already instituted and the process of creative institution is articulated in Machiavelli's establishment of a relational proximity between the concepts of *virtù* and *fortuna*, a proximity that closes off the possibility of an independent evaluation of either category.

In *The Prince* the relation between the form-giving activity of the political actor and the field of action which conditions and facilitates creation is expressed through Machiavelli's positing of a dialectical relationship between the concepts *virtù* and *fortuna*.[63] To understand the meaning of these categories we must first resist the urge to reduce or subsume them to concepts already established in the tradition of

and Marx appear to be quite close in this respect, Machiavelli's dialectic of creation as revealed in the interpenetration of virtue and fortune anticipating Marx's contention that "men make their own history, but they do not make it just as they please; they do not make it under circumstances chosen by themselves, but under circumstances directly encountered, given and transmitted from the past." Karl Marx, *The Eighteenth Brumaire of Louis Bonaparte* (Moscow: Progress Publishers, 1934), 10. For an alternative interpretation of Machiavelli's realism, one that emphasizes the imaginative powers of human actors, see Maurizio Viroli, "Machiavelli's Realism," *Constellations* 14, no. 4 (2007): 466–82. For a study of the relationship between Marx and Machiavelli with respect to the idea of the real see Claude Lefort, "Réflexions sociologiques sur Machiavel et Marx: la politique et le réel," in *Les formes de l'histoire: essais d'anthropologie politique* (Paris: Gallimard, 1978), 169–94.

63 The specifically dialectical form of this relationship has been pointed out by several readers. See, for example, Leonardo Olschki, *Machiavelli: The Scientist* (Berkeley: Gillick Press, 1945), 40; André Rélang, "La dialectique de la fortune et de la *virtù* chez Machiavel," *Archives de philosophie* 66, no. 4 (2003): 649–62; Angus Fletcher, "The Comic Ethos of *Il Principe*," *Comparative Drama* 43, no. 3 (2009): 293–315; Dick Howard, *The Primacy of the Political: A History of Political Thought from the Greeks to the French and American Revolutions* (New York: Columbia University Press, 2010), 195; Virginia Cox, "Rhetoric and Ethics in Machiavelli," in *The Cambridge Companion to Machiavelli*, ed. John M. Najemy (Cambridge: Cambridge University Press, 2010), 182; Filippo Del Lucchese, *The Political Philosophy of Niccolò Machiavelli* (Edinburgh: Edinburgh University Press, 2015), 36–42. For an account of the degree to which Machiavelli's work more generally is structured by dialectical principles see McCanles, *The Discourse of Il Principe*; Banu Bargu, "Machiavelli after Althusser," in *The Radical Machiavelli: Politics, Philosophy, and Language*, ed. Filippo Del Lucchese, Fabio Frosini, and Vittorio Morfino (Leiden: Brill, 2015), 420–39; Catherine H. Zuckert, *Machiavelli's Politics* (Chicago: University of Chicago Press, 2017), 23. Also especially relevant in this respect is the work of Victoria Kahn. See, for example, Kahn, "Reduction and the Praise of Disunion in Machiavelli's *Discourses*"; Victoria Kahn, "Habermas, Machiavelli, and the Humanist Critique of Ideology," *PMLA* 105, no. 3 (1990): 464–76; Kahn, *Machiavellian Rhetoric*, 19.

political thinking. Machiavelli's conception of *fortuna*, to begin with, must be differentiated from the most well-known understandings of the meaning of fortune circulating during his time.[64] Machiavellian *fortuna*, considered in its necessary relation with that of *virtù*, refers us to the specifically human capacity to critically intervene in the world, altering its form of being through human action aiming at the introduction of completely new historical trajectories.[65] If we were to try to initially consider the concept of *fortuna* independently, we might characterize it as Machiavelli's representation of the being of the temporal world as flux. The degree to which *fortuna* speaks to worldly indetermination is clearly revealed, for example, in the poem "Of Fortune." Here Machiavelli writes: "Not a thing in the world is eternal; Fortune wants it so, and beautifies herself by it, so that her power be more discerned."[66] Fortune is Machiavelli's representation of the contingent and chaotic structure of the being of the world, the metaphysical representation of all that is beyond rational human control.[67] Fortune is thus neither a person, nor an object, nor a system, but an aesthetic representation of the indetermination of being.[68] And the objective manifestation of this contingency, of course, is itself always changing with the times, never taking on a determinate form, but throwing up

---

64 Especially relevant here are the formulations of Boethius and Dante. Although both theorize Fortune in terms of historical mutability, such mutability is immanent to Fortune itself, which is impervious to human intervention. See especially Boethius, *The Consolation of Philosophy*, trans. V.E. Watts (London: Folio Society, 1998), bk. 1.1, 1.3. Dante Alighieri, *Inferno*, ed. Giuseppe Mazzotta, trans. Michael Palma (New York: W.W. Norton, 2008), canto VII. 80–90.

65 Machiavelli's innovative articulation of the concept of fortune can lead to confusion when not recognized. Anthony Parel, for example, interprets Machiavellian *fortuna* in terms of Ptolemaic cosmology, reading it as identical with the heavens, and hence unsusceptible to any form of human intervention, and thus without political relevance. Anthony Parel, "Farewell to Fortune," *Review of Politics* 75, no. 4 (2013): 587–604.

66 Machiavelli, "Di Fortuna," in *Tutte le opere*, 978.

67 See, for example, von Vacano, *The Art of Power: Machiavelli, Nietzsche, and the Making of Aesthetic Political Theory*, 26.

68 Such has been pointed out by several readers. See, for example, Robert M. Adams, "Machiavelli Now and Here: An Essay for the First World," *American Scholar* 44, no. 3 (1975): 380. Mazzeo, "The Poetry of Power: Machiavelli's Literary Vision," 45–6; J.G.A. Pocock, "Machiavelli in the Liberal Cosmos," *Political Theory* 13, no. 4 (1985): 562; Lefort, *Machiavelli in the Making*, 195; von Vacano, *The Art of Power*, 26; Dillon, "Lethal Freedom."

new circumstances that confront the actor in perpetually new ways. Hence we also find in "Of Fortune" Machiavelli's emphasis on the ultimately unpredictable nature of worldly transformation: "She often keeps the good under her foot, the dishonest she raises up; and if she ever promises you anything, she never keeps it. / And she puts kingdoms and states upside down, according to how she feels, and deprives the just of the good that she offers the unjust freely. / This inconstant goddess and unstable deity often places the unworthy on a seat which to the worthy never comes."[69] There is thus no ultimate ground or foundation that would be capable of, if properly reflected upon and grasped in its complexity, allowing us to rationalize worldly movement.

Despite positing the indetermination of the world in such terms, Machiavelli will in the poem immediately go on to affirm, through a repetition of the famous river metaphor in *The Prince*, the ability of certain actors to jostle and push fortune. Through their resistance to its constraints they may succeed in impressing their will upon the world, a possibility precisely to the degree that this world lacks a stable form.[70] Contrary to those writers who interpret fortune as an omnipotent force, Machiavelli explicitly suggests that the perception of omnipotence is merely a reflection of the incapacity of certain individuals to assert themselves in such a way as to effect this worldly change. It is simply a manifestation of those who experience a disjunction between their modes and the times, and who in the face of this disjunction are incapable of adjusting through innovation. Hence Machiavelli writes: "This by many is called omnipotent, because whoever comes into this life, either late or early, feels her power."[71] One's arrival is capable of being transcended as an absolutely limiting boundary to the extent that individuals are endowed by their nature with the capacity for self-alteration. You as an actor will only be abandoned by fortune if you "cannot change your persona, nor leave behind the order that heaven endows you with."[72] The significance of this creative capacity to respond to the fluctuations of fortune through self-innovation, an innovation which is so strong that Machiavelli characterizes it in terms of an alteration of a God-given nature, will be returned to and explored in much greater

---

69 Machiavelli, "Di Fortuna," 976.
70 Ibid., 979.
71 Ibid., 976.
72 Ibid., 978.

detail in *The Prince*, where Machiavelli explicitly affirms the intertwinement of worldly contingency and creative action through these two categories of *fortuna* and *virtù*.

The most systematic articulation of this intertwinement appears in
chapter 25, entitled "How much fortune can be found in human affairs,
and in what mode it can be opposed." Machiavelli begins the chapter
by asserting that he is well aware of the various metaphysical doctrines
that interpret physical reality as a determined product of God or fortune, a product impervious to all human effort or mediation. If such
were indeed the case, Machiavelli concludes, human beings need not
expend too much energy worrying about human affairs and politics,
for they would be impermeable to merely mortal intervention. The
extent to which Machiavelli's concept of fortune is irreducible to such
formulations is immediately revealed, however, as he goes on to reject
all principles of structural determination by affirming the simultaneous
existence of fortune and human freedom. He writes, "so that our free
will is not eliminated, I judge it to be true that fortune is the arbiter of
half of our actions, but that she still leaves for us to govern the other
half, or near it."[73] Once again, fortune is theorized as a river, producing
shifts and displacements in the structure of the world, and once more it
is just this movement that generates spaces allowing for human intervention, here represented through the process of damming and diking:
"And I liken [fortune] to one of these ruinous rivers, which, when
angered, floods the plains, ruins the trees and the buildings, raises earth
from this part, puts it in the other; everyone flees before them, each
yields to their impetus without being able to oppose any part. And
although they are like this, it does not remain a fact that men, when
times are quiet, cannot provide precautions through dikes and embank-
ments, so that when they rise later, either they go to a canal or their
impetus is neither so wanton nor so injurious."[74] And indeed, if Italy
finds itself in such a wretched contemporary situation, seemingly overwhelmed at every instance by the worldly forces that it confronts, it is
because of a failure in this respect, for "if it had been diked by an appropriate virtue, like Germany, Spain and France, either this flood would
not have made the great variations that it has, or it would not have

---

73 Machiavelli, "Il Principe," chap. 25.
74 Ibid.

come to us."[75] In the river metaphor the seemingly either/or dichotomy of virtue-fortune is overcome, Machiavelli calling attention to the intermingling of the concepts through his appreciation of the ability to alter fortune through the exercise of virtue.

In theorizing a world open to human intervention so as to allow for the directed, if not determining, alteration of being, Machiavelli avoids two extremes that characterize much thinking on the nature of human freedom. The actor is not an autonomous subject whose relation to that exterior to him or herself takes the form of necessarily passive perception of a world impervious to human effort, but nor are the objects the actor confronts and works in and from the mere stuff of the actor's project, mere matter upon which a form can be unproblematically imposed. The capacity for action is constrained not by the limits of human imagination, but by those boundaries that characterize life in a historical world. Indeed, in the *Discourses* Machiavelli suggests that intellectual and material production is always conditioned by the form of its embeddedness, by its encounter with objective externalities: "as some more philosophers have written, the hands and tongues of men, the two noblest instruments for ennobling him, would not have worked perfectly nor directed human works to the height they have been directed to had they not been pushed by necessity."[76] Political creation, in particular, does not take place in a historical vacuum, but must work from and with existing matter. This is articulated in *Discourses* 1:25. Here Machiavelli concedes that if one wants to create a tyranny then one should endeavour to eliminate all vestiges of the prior way of life and "renew everything."[77] If one desires the establishment of "a political way of life," however, it is necessary to recognize the positive function of preserving existing orders for the sake of maintaining a minimal continuity of time.[78] The failure to ensure such preservation is the basis of Machiavelli's critique of Italian life prior to the rule of Theodoric, where "not only did the government and the prince vary, but the laws, the customs, the mode of living, the religion, the language, the dress, the names."[79] Machiavelli's critique of such arbitrary and destabilizing

---

75 Ibid.
76 Machiavelli, "Discorsi sopra la Prima Deca di Tito Livio," bk. 3.12.
77 Ibid., bk. 1.25.
78 Ibid.
79 Machiavelli, "Istorie fiorentine," bk. 1.5.

social movement reveals that innovation is irreducible to any model of political creation that affirms change merely for the sake of change, or better, that does not differentiate between modes of change, between change that is sensitive to social-historical context and change that is not.

One cannot build a free city on nothing, for people always have past experiences and modalities that form an essential part of their self-identity, the affirmation of which is a necessary condition of freedom. The new and free way of life is thus always historically situated and bound by the past in some way. The non-determining character of human embeddedness, as manifested in the dialectic of *fortuna* and *virtù*, is revealed in Machiavelli's concept of *occasione*.[80] If *fortuna* refers to the unstable and perpetually moving structure of the world, *occasione* refers to the spaces of action that such movement opens up, these spaces providing a ground from which the actor may launch a creative political project, provided he or she possesses the appropriate virtue to do so. What *occasione* speaks to is the fact that the political actor's creation always leans on external considerations, on an objectivity that eludes the subjectivity of the actor. This objective structuring is manifest even in those instances when Machiavelli recalls the political creation of the great and mythic legislator-founders. Moses, for example, could only have acted as he did if he had found the Hebrews enslaved in Egypt, while Cyrus needed to encounter a Median people beaten down and disenchanted by their rulers, and Theseus required a dispersed Athenian population for his creation.[81]

For Machiavelli the virtuous actor is he or she who is able to, through the deployment of a critical and reflective judgment, recognize these spaces of action that are opened up in the world, insert him or herself into them, and from them launch activity. The prince acts out of the opportunity that *fortuna* opens; hence the characterization of *occasione* as an encounter between a subjectivity and an objectivity that can never

---

80 In inserting the concept of *occasione* into the *virtù-fortuna* relation, we must again recall the co-determining form of the categories. As Thomas Berns notes, *virtù*, *fortuna*, and *occasione* "draw their respective meanings exclusively by relating to each other, thereby implying that none of them can have substantial value without the other two." Thomas Berns, "Prophetic Efficacy: The Relationship between Force and Belief," in *The Radical Machiavelli: Politics, Philosophy, and Language*, ed. Filippo Del Lucchese, Fabio Frosini, and Vittorio Morfino (Leiden: Brill, 2015), 207–8.

81 Machiavelli, "Il Principe," chap. 6.

be disentangled.[82] Neither is the prince capable of dominating fortune, nor is fortune capable of dominating the prince. The prince is not one who unitarily imposes his own will on an object and manipulates it to fit his design, but one who must reflectively alter his action in light of objectivity in order to seize the opportunity presented to him.[83] In the concluding chapter of *The Prince* Machiavelli maintains the state of contemporary Italy provides such a space, such an occasion, one from which a national project of unification and liberation can be initiated. The ruin of Italy has provided a ground for virtuous refoundation. Returning to the earlier discussion in chapter 6, Machiavelli reaffirms the delimitation of action by external conditions: "And if, as I said, it was necessary if wanting to see the virtue of Moses that the people of Israel be enslaved in Egypt, and to experience the greatness of spirit of Cyrus that the Persians be oppressed by the Medes, and to recognize the excellence of Theseus that the Athenians be dispersed, so at present, to want to realize the virtue of an Italian spirit it was necessary that Italy be reduced to the state she is in at present, that more enslaved than the Hebrews, more servile than the Persians, more dispersed than the Athenians, without a head, without order, beaten, despoiled, torn, overrun, and having suffered every sort of ruin."[84] Italy is thus just waiting for an actor to seize the historical moment, the opening or *occasione* that *fortuna* has provided: it is "ready and willing to follow a flag, provided that there is someone to raise it."[85]

---

82 The commingling of subjectivity and objectivity in the *virtù-fortuna* relationship is recognized by Agnès Cugno in Agnès Cugno, *Apprendre à philosopher avec Machiavel* (Paris: Ellipses, 2009), 51.

83 Hence Jérémie Duhamel writes that "*virtù* designates less the superior capacity of the act by which it would be able to dominate fortune, than the value of individual and/or collective effort that seeks to optimize the limited flexibility assigned to humankind." Jérémie Duhamel, "Machiavel et la vertu intellectuelle de prudence: étude du chapitre XXV du *Prince*," *Canadian Journal of Political Science* 46, no. 4 (2013): 835.

84 Machiavelli, "Il Principe," chap. 26.

85 Ibid. On *fortuna* providing the *occasione* for the actualization of freedom through the exercise of will see also Machiavelli's "Words to be Spoken on the Provision of Money": "Fortune does not change purpose where order is not changed, and the heavens do not want or are not able to support a thing that wants to collapse in any case. This I cannot believe in, seeing that you are free Florentines, and that your freedom is in your hands. For this I think you will have as much concern as those always have had who are born free and desire to live free." Niccolò Machiavelli, "Parole da dirle sopra la provisione del danaio, facto un poco di proemio et di scusa," in *Tutte le opere*, 13.

Freedom, then, does not lie in the unbounded capacity to master the world, in the ability to overcome being's contingent temporality through dictating form, but rather in the ability to spontaneously generate new realities out of the objective opportunities that the subject encounters. The world is not a formless mass that the virtuous actor is able to impose his or her will upon without resistance, but rather an irregular field of tensions and pressures that limits and circumscribes the possibilities for action.[86] In this sense Machiavelli's philosophical anthropology, as noted by Diego von Vacano, is tragic, "for it shows man's lot to be of necessity bounded by nature."[87] The being of the encounter between subject and object is perhaps expressed most clearly by Machiavelli when he writes: "here one may see extraordinary things without example, brought about by God: the sea has opened; the cloud has shown you the path; the stone has shed water; here has rained manna; everything has gathered for your greatness. The remainder you have to do yourself. God does not want to do everything, so as to not take from us free will and that part of glory that moves us."[88] The freedom of the historical actor is thus only actualized in the material encounter with a lived reality.[89] Free will is not reducible to the transcendental mastery of the inner life or soul, but is rather revealed in the human effort to partially impress one's will on social-historical being through the material specificity of the encounter.[90]

---

86 Needless to say, this resistant field is largely composed of the virtue of other actors. On fortune as the intersection of a multiplicity of human wills see Francesco Ercole, *La politica di Machiavelli* (Roma: Anonima Romana Editoriale, 1926), 17; McCanles, *The Discourse of Il Principe*, 113.

87 Von Vacano, *The Art of Power*, 25. Such a conclusion is also drawn in Mark Wenman, *Agonistic Democracy: Constituent Power in the Era of Globalisation* (Cambridge: Cambridge University Press, 2013), 38. And Machiavelli famously characterizes himself at one point as a tragedian. Machiavelli, "Lettere, 291, Niccolò Machiavelli a Francesco Guicciardini," in *Tutte le opere*, 1224.

88 Machiavelli, "Il Principe," chap. 26. See also Machiavelli, "L'Asino," 967.

89 As noted by Marcia Colish, Machiavelli certainly does not think that freedom is realized in the spontaneous activity of the mind, but rather in concrete material practice. Marcia L. Colish, "The Idea of Liberty in Machiavelli," *Journal of the History of Ideas* 32, no. 3 (1971): 327. On the various materialities that may potentially affect the encounter see Vittorio Morfino, *Il tempo e l'occasione: L'incontro Spinoza Machiavelli* (Milano: LED, 2002), 219.

90 That said, Machiavelli's emphasis on the human potential for creative self-activity may very well also have influenced certain representatives of the tradition of German idealism who posit the self's capacity for the spontaneous generation of

The content of the category of *virtù* will be explicated more in the following section, although we can already begin to see its specific meaning come into focus. *Virtù* speaks to the actor's ability to actively project his or her will externally, to the exteriorization of an originary psychic force. Recall that ambition is conceptualized by Machiavelli as a desire for transgressive value formation and is grounded in the instability and flux of the human psyche, as represented in the concept of *animo*. *Virtù* would here be the means by which this creative desire is actualized in the political sphere: the virtuous actor is he or she who is able to prudently recognize the *occasioni* opened by *fortuna*, and externalize his or her will through the active creation of new political realities. By tracing the expression of *virtù* to the activity of the psyche we are able to understand it as an element of Machiavelli's negative model of the human essence.[91] In a crucial passage in chapter 6 of *The Prince*, Machiavelli links together *fortuna, occasione, virtù*, and *animo* in a manner that will allow us to gather together and synthesize in a summary manner the various conceptual elements I have been calling attention to. Speaking of virtuous founders he writes: "examining their actions and lives, one does not see that they owed anything to fortune but the occasion, which gave them the matter to introduce the form they wanted; and without that occasion their virtue of spirit would have been eliminated, and without that virtue the occasion would have been in vain."[92] The new prince creates from the opportunity that is presented to him by fortune new political objects, these objects being the specific productive results of a process of value generation that is rooted in the desire of the spirit.

---

thought. Douglas Moggach, for example, claims that "Fichte finds in Machiavelli, in tension with the more authoritarian elements, a notion of free activity and self-transformation which accords with his own early philosophical principles." Douglas Moggach, "Fichte's Engagement with Machiavelli," *History of Political Thought* 14, no. 4 (1993): 577. In the words of Carl Schmitt, the recuperation of Machiavelli by figures such as Hegel and Fichte "belongs to the great work of historical justice and objectivity." Carl Schmitt, *The Leviathan in the State Theory of Thomas Hobbes: Meaning and Failure of a Political Symbol*, trans. George Schwab and Erna Hilfstein (Chicago: University of Chicago Press, 2008), 85.

91 Rarely is *virtù* seen as a manifestation of the human essence, but there are some readers who make this identification. John Bernard, for example, writes that "virtue is a fundamental component of human nature" that is manifest in "all social activities" that individuals undertake. John Bernard, *Why Machiavelli Matters: A Guide to Citizenship in a Democracy* (Westport: Praeger, 2009), 65.

92 Machiavelli, "Il Principe," chap. 6.

The concept of spirit (*animo*) refers us back to the originary structure of the psyche, its invariable and multiple organization seeking externalization via the energetic and ambitious expulsion of energy. The insatiability of desire is not frustrated after the initial generation of political order, however, for the instability of the world, represented in the concept of *fortuna*, necessitates that if the principality is to be preserved the prince must be perpetually active. The changing nature of the times requires the prince's dynamic and creative intervention, most commonly realized in the alteration in the image or form of appearance that the prince has constructed for himself.

Virtù and Performative Political Ethics

In the final instance historical creation, the *ex nihilo* production of new political forms, depends not entirely on virtue or entirely on fortune, but on what Machiavelli calls, in perhaps his most clear formulation regarding the dialectical codetermination of the two categories, "fortunate astuteness."[93] It is the centrality of the idea of political creation, and of that which is necessary to bring the new into existence, that has produced what is often taken to be the idiosyncratic nature of Machiavelli's ethics. The recognition of the double-indetermination of nature, of the openness of worldly and human being, serves as the foundation for the Machiavellian reorientation of ethics, for the displacement of traditional moralities structured around simple binaries of right and wrong. Such binaries must be overcome to the extent that they necessarily neutralize the potential for creative action, the construction of a fixed or universal system of morality schematizing – independently of any consideration of the historical demands of the empirical – the scope of human behaviour, thus erasing in advance the actor's capacity to critically respond to the opportunities generated by the shifting of *fortuna*. To possess *virtù* is not only to be able to recognize those spaces of action that open up in the world, but also to be able to judge what specific ethical qualities' adoption will permit one to from those spaces launch productive action that generates new realities. In short, the virtuous actor is the one who knows how to create, and who knows that in order to create one must be to some extent free from rigid moralities

---

93 Ibid., chap. 9.

that would restrict the scope of action. If *virtù* is considered in terms of its dialectical relationship with *fortuna* – its implication in a pre-existing world – then it must refer us to the power to critically adapt or be strategically fluid in the face of this concrete embededness.

Machiavelli's refusal to provide universal rules of behaviour is a manifestation of the need for methodological flexibility in the face of worldly contingency. It is in chapter 15 of *The Prince* that Machiavelli most explicitly rejects universalist moralizing that is grounded in the binary distribution of qualities along a predetermined axis. Machiavelli identifies what he takes as some of the traditional moral qualities and their corresponding vices: liberality and meanness; beneficence and rapacity; cruelty and mercy; faithfulness and treachery; cowardice and spiritedness; humaneness and arrogance; chastity and lasciviousness; straightforwardness and craftiness; agreeableness and hardness; levity and gravity; and religiosity and incredulousness.[94] According to Machiavelli if one wishes to succeed politically, that is, succeed in the effort to reinstitutionalize the social sphere through the creation of new political modes and orders, then one cannot possess all of the virtues exclusively: "And I know that everyone will confess that it would be a most praiseworthy thing in a prince to be all of the above qualities that are held to be good. But because he cannot have them, nor fully observe them, for human conditions do not permit it, it is necessary to be so prudent as to know how to avoid the infamy of those vices that will take away his state from him."[95] The prince who loses his state is the prince who ceases to be an actor, who no longer is effective in creating those new political realities that ensure the perpetuation of the regime. To possess *virtù* is to have the willingness and ability to alter one's mode of proceeding, an alteration that as we will see is characterized in terms of an alteration of nature, so as to be able to multiply activity. To be unvirtuous, on the contrary, is to adopt the position of the moralist. It is to be unwilling or unable to waver from an absolute set of universal standards of behaviour that close off the potential for activity through rendering the actor incapable of productively responding to the impermanency and flux of the temporal world, or what Machiavelli here calls "human conditions."[96] To be unvirtuous, in other words, is simply to be

---

94 Ibid., chap. 15.
95 Ibid.
96 Ibid.

unable to initiate activity, to be weak and passive, or to lack the ability to express the power of the will.[97]

A case study in the principle of virtuous adaptation, and of the danger of uncritically adhering to traditional moral categories regardless of circumstance or context, is undertaken by Machiavelli in chapter 16, through his interrogation of the qualities of liberality and meanness. Liberality is specifically identified as harmful to the actor when that actor becomes identified with it exclusively: "because if it is used righteously and as it ought to be used, it will not be recognized, and you will not avoid the infamy of its opposite."[98] If one is labelled liberal, and wants to maintain this identification, then one must be constantly exceeding one's prior liberality, necessitating an increasing expenditure of resources on lavish events and spectacles in the effort to confirm one's reputation. In order to do this, however, the prince requires funds, which must necessarily be extracted from his citizens: "It will be necessary in the end, if he wants to maintain a name for liberality, to burden and tax the people extraordinarily, and to do all those things that he can do to get money."[99] Excessive taxation of the people, though, will generate among them hatred of the prince. And should the prince attempt to reverse this hatred through eliminating public expenditures, he will immediately come to be identified as mean. In the process initiated by the desire to realize the value of liberality, then, this liberality consumes itself and turns into its opposite. The one-sided affirmation of the value is incapable of achieving the desired end. The prince should thus not concern himself with initially acquiring a reputation for meanness. Indeed, over time this identification, if the prince is able to prudently negotiate it, will also turn into its opposite as time moves forward: "Because over time he will be taken to be more and more liberal, it seen that with his parsimony his income is sufficient, he can defend himself from those who make war on him and he can undertake endeavours without burdening the people, so that he comes to use liberality with all those that he does not take from, who are countless, and meanness with all those to whom he does not give, who are few."[100] Meanness is thus

---

97 On virtue as a type of will to power see Negri, *Insurgencies*, 41; Honig, *Political Theory and the Displacement of Politics*, 67–75; Held, "Civic Prudence in Machiavelli," 121; Brown, *Manhood and Politics*, 82.
98 Machiavelli, "Il Principe," chap. 16.
99 Ibid.
100 Ibid.

the condition for providing a secure state for the citizens of the regime without having to exploit them. In Machiavelli's words, "a prince ought to care little of incurring a name for meanness, so as to not have to rob his subjects, to be able to defend himself, to not become poor and contemptible, to not be forced to become rapacious, because this is one of those vices that allows him to rule."[101] And significantly, through emphasizing the utilization of meanness as the condition for the perpetuation of an active rule, Machiavelli clarifies that what the prince is reproducing in this movement is not a static condition or organization of things, but rather the very capacity to act.

Although Machiavelli recognizes the necessity of the actor to be open to a diversity of strategic modes should political creation be successful, it is no doubt true that active as opposed to passive modes have a privileged position.[102] In *The Prince* this general ordering of types of modes is most clearly laid out in chapter 25. Again it is affirmed that the prince who has his security ruined is the one who is incapable of innovating his action so as to counter the shifting of fortune. Such innovation is realized in an interrogative process in which the actor may very well

---

101 Ibid.

102 The critique of absolute moral universalism and its generation of passivity is notably embodied in Machiavelli's well-known appraisal of Christianity. Whereas the ancient religions were fundamentally dynamic and active, the ferocity of the religious rites reproducing itself in the nature of people who were through their exposure to religion socialized to action, the Christian religion glorifies passivity, providing through such a glorification no space for the achievement of worldly virtue. Machiavelli, "Discorsi sopra la prima Deca di Tito Livio," bk. 2.2. Hence Nicole Hochner argues that Machiavelli's recuperation of the political potential of civil religion is to be found in the production of "new rites, new ceremonies and new symbolic gestures that can trigger a new civic virtuosity." Nicole Hochner, "A Ritualist Approach to Machiavelli," *History of Political Thought* 30, no. 4 (2009): 588. Even when commentators do try and make the case that Machiavelli's thought is strongly influenced by Christianity, this is an active Christianity that promotes the expression of vigour and vitality. On this point see, for example, de Grazia, *Machiavelli in Hell*; Ronald Beiner, "Machiavelli, Hobbes, and Rousseau on Civil Religion," *Review of Politics* 55, no. 4 (1993): 617–38; John H. Geerken, "Machiavelli's Moses and Renaissance Politics," *Journal of the History of Ideas* 60, no. 4 (1999): 579–95; Maurizio Viroli, *Machiavelli's God*, trans. Anthony Shugaar (Princeton: Princeton University Press, 2010). Indeed, even in his ostensibly Christian exhortation to charity Machiavelli praises the virtue of the active life, as opposed to the traditional emphasis on meekness and passivity. Machiavelli, "Exortatione alla penitenza," in *Tutte le opere*, 932–4.

need to "change his nature": "that prince who leans entirely on fortune is ruined as it varies. I believe, furthermore, that he is happy who adapts his mode of proceeding to the quality of the times, and similarly he is unhappy whose procedure is in discord with the times."[103] Two actors who proceed in the same mode may in fact achieve the same end, while two who proceed in identical modes might achieve opposite ends, and "this stems from nothing other than the quality of the times, which they conform to or not in their procedure."[104] As will be elaborated on shortly, there are thus no universal modes guaranteeing the actualization of specific results: "If one governs himself with caution and patience, and the times and things change in a way that his government is good, he is happy; but, if the times and things change, he is ruined, because he does not change his mode of proceeding."[105] It is therefore the case that in some instances the prudent actor might perceive the necessity of caution or patience, while in others he or she will foresee the need for boldness and impetuosity. The virtuous actor, because his or her character is not rigidly fixed, is capable of altering his or her nature in accord with the perpetually shifting realities of time, thus countering fortune's potentially adverse effects. Nevertheless, as summed up in the famous concluding lines of this chapter, precisely because of the active orientation of impetuosity, the latter is more friendly to subjective invention than caution, which when deployed must always be for the sake of innovation as opposed to mere passive preservation.[106]

The virtuous prince's self-affirmation is realized through the willingness to act, the will to make a decision.[107] In chapter 21 this will to action

---

103 Machiavelli, "Il Principe," chap. 25. Hence Skinner points out that in the final instance the ultimate failure of Maximilian, Cesare Borgia, and Julius II can be traced to the same error, this failure to accommodate personality to the times. Quentin Skinner, *Machiavelli* (Oxford: Oxford University Press, 1981), 17.

104 Machiavelli, "Il Principe," chap. 25.

105 Ibid.

106 Ibid.

107 Such a principle Machiavelli attempted to live according to himself. Hence writing to Francesco Guicciardini regarding the prospect of war in Italy and the potential forms of the relationship between Florence and France, he writes: "I declare a thing that will appear to you reckless or ridiculous; nevertheless, these times require bold, unusual, and strange decisions." Niccolò Machiavelli, "Lettere, 296, Niccolò Machiavelli a Francesco Guicciardini," in *Tutte le opere*, 1229.

or doing is juxtaposed with Machiavelli's critique of princely neutrality. Machiavelli writes that "a prince is further esteemed when he is a true friend and a true enemy; that is, when without any hesitation he declares himself in favour of one against another. This resolution will always be more useful than staying neutral."[108] For example, should the prince declare support for the winning party in a conflict, that party will have an obligation to him, and yet if he declares support for the losing party, the latter might nevertheless give him refuge. The danger lies in indecisive neutrality, in the passive mode. If the prince fails to make a decision the winner will become immediately suspicious of him, and should this party move against him the loser will not provide sanctuary as a result of his failure to provide aid. Indeed, the uselessness of neutrality is what the Romans attempted to convince the Achaeans of in their conflict with the Aetolians. Antiochus, allied with the Aetolians, urged them to remain neutral, while the Roman legate noted the truth of the matter. In the words of Livy, quoted by Machiavelli: "As to what they say, moreover, that you not intervene in the war, nothing is more alien to your interests; without thanks, without dignity you will be the prize of the victor."[109] In the final instance Machiavelli concludes that "irresolute princes, to escape present dangers, most times follow the neutral path, and most times are ruined."[110]

The prince's non-action as a general strategic mode, as represented in the utilization of a principle of neutrality, is one element of what Machiavelli takes to be a larger error: believing in the possibility of occupying a static place of safety secure from the vicissitudes of historical life.[111] Machiavelli writes: "Nor should any state ever believe that it can always make safe resolutions; rather, it should think that they all have to be doubted, because it is found in the order of things that one never tries to avoid one inconvenience without running into another one; but prudence consists in knowing how to distinguish the qualities of inconveniences and in taking up the less bad as good."[112] We have already

---

108 Machiavelli, "Il Principe," chap. 21.
109 Quoted in Machiavelli, *The Prince*, chap. 21.
110 Machiavelli, "Il Principe," chap. 21.
111 On Machiavelli's recognition of the impossibility of mastering reality, and how this sets him apart from modern governmental reason, see Robyn Marasco, "Machiavelli Contra Governmentality," *Contemporary Political Theory* 11, no. 4 (2012): 339–61.
112 Machiavelli, "Il Principe," chap. 21.

encountered in the previous chapter this language of inconvenience, and the extent to which it is one manifestation of Machiavelli's recognition of the contingency or instability of the being of worldly objects. It is this contingency or instability that princes who have lost their states have failed to grasp, they assuming on the contrary that the world is static, that the order of reality will not change, and hence that their passive orientation to the existent might be perpetually reproduced. And when they realize that this is in fact not the case, furthermore, they again, being incapable of action themselves, simply displace responsibility for reacting onto others: "having never thought that quiet times can change (which is a common defect in men, not to account, during the calm, for the storm), when then adverse times come they thought of fleeing and not of defending themselves."[113] What they fail to do, in other words, is affirm themselves and their will through the active making of a decision. Hence Machiavelli's final advice, that "one should never want to fall, believing that you can find someone to pick you up; because whether this happens or does not happen, it is not for you secure, for this defence is cowardly and does not depend on yourself. And only those defences are good, are safe, and are durable, that depend on yourself and on your virtue."[114]

As classically noted by Hannah Arendt, when Machiavelli says that a prince needs to learn how to not be good, this does not mean that he needs to learn how to be evil, but rather, that he needs to learn how to avoid all fixed or universal schemas of behaviour, or in other words, that he needs to learn how to decide.[115] Ethics is no longer identified with consistent adherence to rigid standards of conduct determined in advance of reflection on the concrete demands of the political situation, but with the active oscillation between multiple modes of doing, grounded in prudent consideration of the unstable structure of the world, and for the sake of the generation of new political modes and orders. This emphasis on multiplicity is here key, referring us once again to the ontological plurality that Machiavelli sees as characterizing the being of internal and external nature. As will be examined further

---

113 Ibid., chap. 24.
114 Ibid., chap. 25.
115 Hannah Arendt, "Some Questions of Moral Philosophy," in *Responsibility and Judgment*, ed. Jerome Kohn (New York: Schocken Books, 2003), 80; Hannah Arendt, *The Human Condition* (Chicago: University of Chicago Press, 1998), 77.

in the final chapter, the fact that the being of the people is multiple and hence unstable makes it the actor most suitable for engaging with or productively responding to the flux of history. Indeed, as pointed out by Filippo Del Lucchese, the prince is successful precisely to the degree that he is able to be like the people, that is, to the extent that he is capable of living as multiple and adaptable: "Only by continually adapting to changes is he able to achieve the kinds of results that the multitude, thanks to its multiple constitution, is naturally capable of accomplishing. The qualities that a single individual needs are various and even opposing."[116] It is in the context of this fact of multiplicity – which again, is a repetition of the multiplicity of nature – that we need to evaluate the image of Chiron the centaur that Machiavelli takes as a model of the teacher of the political actor. The centaur represents the necessity to affirm a principle of adaptation in the face of natural contingency through the capacity to become multiple or many.[117]

Chapter 18 of *The Prince* is extremely important from the standpoint of the Machiavellian account of subjectivity as active adaptation in the face of worldly contingency. Machiavelli begins by noting that there are two general forms of combat, the one that utilizes law and the one that utilizes force. Whereas combat through law is the mode proper to the human and combat through force is the mode proper to beasts, Machiavelli ultimately concludes that the first alone is insufficient to generate success, and hence "to a prince it is necessary to know well how to use the beast and the man."[118] Thus the good of Achilles and those other ancient princes who were raised by Chiron, the latter teaching the former how to oscillate between the sets of modes corresponding to each nature: "This does not mean anything other than, to have for a teacher a half-beast and half-man, that it is necessary for a prince to know how to use the one or the other nature; and the one without the other is not durable."[119] With respect to beastliness the actor must know how to be specifically both fox and lion, and when it is appropriate to imitate each one's nature. Specifically, both the fox and the lion overcome the deficiencies of the other, the fox being able to avoid snares through the recognition of the prudent necessity of not always keeping faith, and the

---

116 Del Lucchese, *Conflict, Power, and Multitude in Machiavelli and Spinoza*, 144.
117 Ibid., 142.
118 Machiavelli, "Il Principe," chap. 18.
119 Ibid.

lion being able to deter wolves through the external projection of princely power.[120] Although the modes of the fox and lion are initially framed in terms of a departure from humanity, what Machiavelli's subsequent discussion reveals is that human nature is actually located not in the one-sided affirmation of perpetual strategies, but rather in the ability to oscillate between different strategies. The original distinction between human and animal is thereby displaced, the former being redefined in terms of the capacity for virtuous adaptation.[121] This innovation can be especially well gleaned through contrasting Machiavelli's images of the fox and the lion with those of Cicero, whom he is ostensibly building from.[122]

Cicero will affirm a weak human difference in body and spirit through his account of the human being's capacity for playing roles, for adopting personas as on the stage. Regardless of individual personas

---

120 Ibid.

121 Emmanuel Roux notes that this is thus one element of Machiavelli's dialectical orientation: "This thinking is dialectical because it rejects *the conceptual separations that lead to alternatives whose terms are mutually exclusive.* Machiavelli thus refuses that it would be a contradiction for a prince to be both 'man' and 'animal.' The passage from man to the brutality of the lion and the simulation of the fox signifies that there is no political identity without dialectics." Emmanuel Roux, *Machiavel, la vie libre* (Paris: Raisons d'agir, 2013), 34. Original emphasis.

122 For a comparative analysis of use of the images of the fox and lion in Machiavelli and Cicero, specifically with respect to the question of the affirmation of the *vita activa* and its relation to classical philosophy, see J.J. Barlow, "The Fox and the Lion: Machiavelli Replies to Cicero," *History of Political Thought* 20, no. 4 (1999): 627–45. For an account of the way in which Machiavelli in *The Prince,* although seemingly imitating *On the Ideal Orator,* subverts Cicero, see Daniel J. Kapust, "Acting the Princely Style: Ethos and Pathos in Cicero's *On the Ideal Orator* and Machiavelli's *Prince," Political Studies* 58, no. 3 (2010): 590–608. Christina Christoforatau also calls attention to the ways in which Machiavelli subverts the traditional image of Chiron, and the latter's political significance. Christina Christoforatou, "Ontologies of Power in the Sovereign Politics of Pindar and Machiavelli," *Italian Culture* 33, no. 2 (2015): 97. For a reading that attempts to demonstrate how the lion–fox metaphor can be seen as situated within a specifically Lucretian as opposed to Ciceronian paradigm, see Tania Rispoli, "Imitation and Animality: On the Relationship between Nature and History in Chapter XVIII of *The Prince,*" in *The Radical Machiavelli: Politics, Philosophy, and Language,* ed. Filippo Del Lucchese, Fabio Frosini, and Vittorio Morfino (Leiden: Brill, 2015), 190–203. On the appropriateness of speaking of Machiavelli's political profiles in terms of personas see Michelle Zerba, *Doubt and Skepticism in Antiquity and the Renaissance* (Cambridge: Cambridge University Press, 2012), 184.

and the fact of this difference, however, there remains a fundamental substratum of universal nature. Our universal persona "is common, arising from the fact that we all have a share in reason and in the superiority by which we surpass brute creatures."[123] The legitimate scope of individual behaviour – the degree to which we can manifest our personas specific to us as individuals – is bounded by universal nature: "Each person should hold on to what is his as far as it is not vicious, but is peculiar to him, so that the seemliness that we are seeking might more easily be maintained. For we must act in such a way that we attempt nothing contrary to universal nature; but while conserving that, let us follow our own nature, so that even if other pursuits may be weightier and better, we should measure our own by the rule of our own nature."[124] For Cicero the modes of the lion and the fox, of force and deceit, are precisely those types of action that violate our fundamental nature, those which "seem most alien to a human being."[125] For Machiavelli, on the other hand, the form of activity characterized by the images of the fox and the lion does not represent a violation of human nature; rather, the very alternation between the two modes, undertaken as a result of critical reflection on the nature of political necessity, represents the highest form of human nature.[126] The shifting of appearances, possible to the extent that individuals possess a capacity for self-display and representation, is that which is necessary if one is to actualize the potential for action and assert one's status as a virtuous actor.[127]

_____

123 Cicero, *On Duties*, ed. M.T. Griffin and E.M. Atkins (Cambridge: Cambridge University Press, 1991), bk. 1.107.

124 Ibid., bk. 1.110.

125 Ibid., bk. 1.41.

126 For different perspectives on the specifically human features of these beastly figures see James A. Arieti, "The Machiavellian Chiron: Appearance and Reality in *The Prince*," *CLIO* 24, no. 4 (1995): 387; Eugene Garver, *Machiavelli and the History of Prudence* (Madison: University of Wisconsin Press, 1987), 88; Bernard Flynn, *The Philosophy of Claude Lefort: Interpreting the Political* (Evanston: Northwestern University Press, 2005), 24; Timothy J. Lukes, "Lionizing Machiavelli," *American Political Science Review* 95, no. 3 (2001): 561–75.

127 Machiavelli, "Il Principe," chap. 18. Hence Agnès Cugno writes: "The variability of the virtuous prince … is his only permanent virtue." Agnès Cugno, *Machiavel – Le Prince* (Paris: Ellipses, 2012), 58. On the extent to which Machiavelli himself performatively presents and negotiates his identity, and how such performance constitutes a theatrical act, see Guido Ruggiero, *Machiavelli in Love: Sex, Self, and Society in the Italian Renaissance* (Baltimore: Johns Hopkins University Press, 2007), 108–62.

The virtuous prince must know how "to be a great simulator and dissimulator."[128] This prince is conceptualized by Machiavelli as an actor in the aesthetic sense, as a performer upon the stage, playing many roles and wearing many masks.[129] The fact that Machiavelli constructs an aesthetics of politics, or thinks about politics in largely aesthetic categories, has often been pointed out by commentators.[130] What is of the utmost significance to recognize, however, is how this image of the prince as performing artist is specified through Machiavelli's reconceptualization of the political relation between means and ends. Such a reconceptualization has profound implications for Machiavelli's concept of action. Neal Wood could stand in for the large number of readers who correctly identify Machiavelli as a theorist of action: "Action in his sense suggests self-conscious and purposeful motion, self-directed doing for the accomplishment of the goals upon which the actor has deliberated."[131] In almost all instances, however, even when readers such as this recognize Machiavelli as a theorist of creative activity, they do not recognize this action for what I take it to be, a type of good-in-itself, instead subordinating it to the external goals that are pursued.[132]

---

128 Machiavelli, "Il Principe," chap. 18.

129 On the theatrical dimensions of Machiavelli's political thought see Jacobson, *Pride and Solace*, 27–8; Bernard, *Why Machiavelli Matters*, 41; Minogue, "Theatricality and Politics," 156; Zerba, *Doubt and Skepticism in Antiquity and the Renaissance*, 184; David Owen, "Machiavelli's *Il Principe* and the Politics of Glory," *European Journal of Political Theory* 16, no. 1 (2017): 49–50; Kahn, "Machiavelli's Afterlife and Reputation to the Eighteenth Century," 246; Charles D. Tarlton, "'Azioni in modo l'una dall'altra: Action for Action's Sake in Machiavelli's *The Prince*," *History of European Ideas* 29, no. 2 (2003): 139; Wayne A. Rebhorn, *Foxes and Lions: Machiavelli's Confidence Men* (Ithaca: Cornell University Press, 1988), 25.

130 In addition to the above, see also Edgar Quinet, *Les révolutions d'Italie, tome second* (Paris: Germer-Baillière, 1874), 37; Charles S. Singleton, "The Perspective of Art," *Kenyon Review* 15, no. 2 (1953): 169–89; Gérald Sfez, *Machiavel, Le Prince sans qualités* (Paris: Editions Kimé, 1998), 30; Smith, *Politics and Remembrance*, 69.

131 Neal Wood, "Machiavelli's Humanism of Action," in *The Political Calculus: Essays on Machiavelli's Political Philosophy*, ed. Anthony Parel (Toronto: University of Toronto Press, 1972), 34.

132 Although emphasizing the extent to which Machiavelli is concerned with the success of action, John Tinkler notes that nevertheless "Machiavelli is concerned with *virtù* for its own sake." John F. Tinkler, "Praise and Advice: Rhetorical Approaches in More's *Utopia* and Machiavelli's *The Prince*," *Sixteenth Century Journal* 19, no. 2 (1988): 197.

The prince is not an artist whose self-activity is considered in terms of the instrumental fabrication of an exterior aesthetic object, but rather in terms of a theatrical performance whose actualization is entirely internal to itself. It is Hannah Arendt who has clarified this most incisively. In her essay "What Is Authority?" Arendt interprets Machiavelli in the conventional manner, as a theorist of politics who emphasizes the instrumentality of foundation in such a way as to retroactively justify recourse to violence, should this violence as means successfully generate the end desired. According to this view of politics as making, "You cannot make a table without killing trees, you cannot make an omelet without breaking eggs, you cannot make a republic without killing people."[133] In "What Is Freedom?," however, Arendt gives a far more nuanced reading of Machiavelli's politics, interpreting them rather as a precursor of her own, a politics emphasizing not instrumental fabrication, but action as virtuous performance.[134] Here the aesthetic political content is not located in the art of production, but the art of performing, and hence contains its own end within itself. *Virtù* refers us to "an excellence we attribute to the performing arts (as distinguished from the creative arts of making), where the accomplishment lies in the performance itself and not in an end product which outlasts the activity that brought it into existence and becomes independent of it."[135] Politics cannot be seen as a plastic art, for as I will elaborate on in chapter 6, institutions are never complete, but are rather in need of constant

---

133 Hannah Arendt, "What Is Authority?," in *Between Past and Future: Eight Exercises in Political Thought* (New York: Penguin, 1993), 139. For a critical discussion of such an account of political constitution as an act of fabrication with respect to Machiavelli, see Thomas Berns, "Le retour à l'origine de l'état," *Archives de philosophie*, no. 59 (1996): 244–8. For a critique of Arendt's instrumental reading of Machiavellian political creation see Victoria Kahn, *The Future of Illusion: Political Theology and Early Modern Texts* (Chicago: University of Chicago Press, 2014), 91.

134 For an account of the performative dimension of Arendt's politics see Christopher Holman, *Politics as Radical Creation: Herbert Marcuse and Hannah Arendt on Political Performativity* (Toronto: University of Toronto Press, 2013).

135 Hannah Arendt, "What Is Freedom?," in *Between Past and Future: Eight Exercises in Political Thought* (New York: Penguin, 2006), 153. Contrary to Arendt, Wayne Rebhorn identifies the prince as practising the art of making, Machiavelli having a "vision of the Prince as an architect and mason." Wayne A. Rebhorn, "Machiavelli's *Prince* in the Epic Tradition," in *The Cambridge Companion to Machiavelli*, ed. John M. Najemy (Cambridge: Cambridge University Press, 2010), 81. See also Joseph D. Falvo, "Nature and Art in Machiavelli's *Prince*," *Italica* 66, no. 3 (1989): 323–32.

refinement in the face of the unstable temporality of the world. As opposed to the plastic arts, "the performing arts ... have indeed a strong affinity with politics. Performing artists – dancers, play-actors, musicians, and the like – need an audience to show their virtuosity, just as acting men need the presence of others before whom they can appear; both need a publicly organized space for their 'work,' and both depend upon others for the performance itself."[136]

As noted by a minority of commentators, Machiavelli's political thought actually constitutes a radical rejection of the logic of means and ends.[137] On the one hand, Machiavelli emphasizes the extent to which instrumental political logic is easily abstracted from any ethical content that could regulate the end for the sake of which it is deployed. In *Discourses* 1:34, in one manifestation of his critique of extraordinary modes, he thus writes: "for if one makes a habit of breaking orders for the sake of the good, then later, under that example, they are broken for the evil."[138] On the other hand, Machiavelli explicitly dissociates *virtù* from the successful actualization of the desired goal, locating glory not in the achievement of a result, but in the virtuous exercise of a capacity.[139] Machiavelli's most explicit rejection of instrumental political logic, however, takes place through the perpetually reoccurring critique of the hubristic attempt to discover means that would ensure or guarantee the actualization of specific ends.[140] Such a discovery is an impossibility

---

136 Arendt, "What Is Freedom?," 154. On the influence of Machiavelli on Arendt's idea of political performativity see Lawrence Hamilton, "Real Modern Freedom," *Theoria* 60, no. 4 (2013): 8–9; Faisal Baluch, "Arendt's Machiavellian Moment," *European Journal of Political Theory* 13, no. 2 (2014): 154–77. On the issue of Machiavelli's performativity, Yves Winter has gone so far as to interpret Machiavelli's theorization of war in terms of performance: "The battlefield resembles a stage on which a precise choreography must be enacted. War is a performance, or perhaps a dance." Yves Winter, "The Prince and His Art of War: Machiavelli's Military Populism," *Social Research* 81, no. 1 (2014): 183.

137 See, for example, Tarlton, "Azioni in modo l'una dall'altra: Action for Action's Sake in Machiavelli's *The Prince*," 139; Garver, *Machiavelli and the History of Prudence*, 84; Germino, "Second Thoughts on Leo Strauss's Machiavelli," 805; Shumer, "Machiavelli: Republican Politics and Its Corruption," 11; Kahn, *Machiavellian Rhetoric*, 38.

138 Machiavelli, "Discorsi sopra la prima Deca di Tito Livio," bk. 1.34.

139 See, for example, ibid., bk. 3.10; ibid., bk. 3.42.

140 This, notably, is the foundation of Machiavelli's critique of conspiracy as a form of political action. Conspiratorial activity is inadequate as a political mode to the extent

given both the unpredictability of worldly movement, and the incapacity of any human subject to escape that field of appearance which delimits their capacity to acquire knowledge of the object of investigation. I have already cited several passages that call attention to this impossibility, but it is perhaps summed up most concisely in the *Ghiribizzi*. Here Machiavelli writes that although the virtuous actor is one who is open to self-interrogation and changing one's modes in light of necessity, nevertheless there is no actor capable of perfectly mastering reality, even if we consider this reality to be objectively schematizable: "And truly, whoever were so wise as to understand the times and the order of things, and to accommodate himself to them, would always have good fortune, or he would avoid the bad, and it would come to be true that the wise could command the stars and the fates. But, because one does not find these wise, men being firstly short-sighted and then not able to command their nature, it follows that Fortune varies and commands men, keeping them under her yoke."[141] Machiavelli most certainly encourages the actor to act, to make a decision in light of prudent consideration of the opportunity presented; however there is no ultimate guarantee that such action will generate the desired result. This constitutes, as noted above, the tragic dimension of political action. To the extent that it is concretely grounded in the contingent materiality of existence, such action is always subject to chance and risk. What is essential to note is that in his various discussions of *virtù* Machiavelli highlights not necessarily the actor's terminal achievement of a concrete end, but rather the actor's ability to perpetually reproduce his or her capacity to act, to continually strive after political creation. Creative intervention in the world is potentially perpetual precisely because of the fact of political unpredictability. The prince's manipulation of appearance and his strategic adoption of multiple personas is ultimately for the sake of the continuation of action, for the sake of the maintenance of the prince's status as an actor.

---

that it necessarily presumes the human potential to master all elements of reality and marshal them toward the desired end. Such mastery, though, given the chaotic and variable form of being of the world, is clearly impossible. In the case of conspiracies an infinite number of contingencies can emerge, thus thwarting the design of the activity. Machiavelli, "Discorsi sopra la prima Deca di Tito Livio," bk. 3.6.

141 Machiavelli, "Lettere, 116, Niccolò Machiavelli a Giovan Battista Soderini," in *Tutte le opere*, 1083.

The Example of Cesare Borgia

It is in light of the above considerations that we might now attempt to make sense of what many commentators take to be the vexing problem of the contrast between two of Machiavelli's most notable examples in *The Prince*, those of Cesare Borgia and Agathocles the Sicilian. Is Cesare really the virtuous actor that Machiavelli seems to make him out to be, and what differentiates the quality of Cesare's virtue from that of Agathocles, who Machiavelli says at various times both does and does not possess *virtù*? I would like to briefly consider such questions through the recent contributions made by John McCormick on the subject. McCormick reads Machiavelli as the first significant theorist in the history of political thought to wholly support the interests of the people over those of the nobility, a support that is partially reflected in his celebration of Borgia: "Machiavelli suggests that Cesare, through his own accomplishments, earns the title 'duke' in the eyes of the people and, apparently, in the eyes of Machiavelli, as well. The people's judgment, *not* that of popes and kings, is what matters ultimately."[142] McCormick will go on to suggest that Machiavelli's use of the Borgia case study also provides an example of the extent to which the deployment of cruelty is subject to an essential limit. Specifically, the execution of henchman Remirro de Orco is taken as a concrete sign to the people that Cesare recognizes that extra-legal terror is incompatible with good government. The violence Cesare utilizes against Remirro and the nobility is thus codeterminate with a populist mode of political institutionalization: "Duke Valentino beat down the nobility who misruled the people for so long; he ended the arbitrary violence that continually plagued them; and he established judicial and representative institutions for them."[143]

---

142 John P. McCormick, "Prophetic Statebuilding," *Representations* 115, no. 1 (2011): 2. Compare McCormick here to a reader like Leo Paul S. de Alvarez, who agrees that Cesare is of the people, but argues that this being of the people is not accompanied by an adequate knowledge of the great. Leo Paul S. de Alvarez, *The Machiavellian Enterprise: A Commentary on The Prince* (DeKalb: Northern Illinois University Press, 1999), 33. According to de Alvarez it is this which ultimately causes Borgia's downfall, and which suggests the impossibility of his being a positive exemplar of a virtuous prince. Below I will attempt to show how this standard of success is no criterion for such an evaluation.

143 McCormick, "Prophetic Statebuilding," 9.

Such a reading seems indeed to be supported by the text. Borgia is initially presented as an example of one who acquires and loses power through fortune, yet one who nevertheless possesses the ability to secure oneself through virtue: he "acquired the state through the fortune of his father, and through that lost it, notwithstanding that he made use of every means and did all those things that a prudent and virtuous man must do to put roots in those states that the arms and fortune of others had granted him."[144] Crucially, however, Cesare's success is not identified by Machiavelli only with his ability to secure princely authority for himself, but with, as suggested by McCormick, providing a foundation of good government grounded in popular support, actualized first through the production of an internal social unity: "After having taken Romagna the duke found it had been commanded by powerless lords, who had sooner plundered their subjects than corrected them, and given them matter for disunion, not for union, so that the country was entirely full of thefts, intrigues, and every other form of insolence; he judged it was necessary, if he wanted to reduce it to peace and obedience to the regal arm, to give it good government."[145] This project of popular institutionalization is what is especially "worthy of notice and of being imitated by others."[146] Indeed, in his "Legations" Machiavelli recalls Borgia's declaration of his concern for the

---

144 Machiavelli, "Il Principe," chap. 7. Although here Machiavelli blames the fall of Cesare on the fortune of his father, he will later concede that Cesare did in fact err in allowing the creation of Pope Julius II. He forgot that "one who believes that new benefits to great personages will make them forget old injuries deceives himself. Therefore, the duke erred in this choice, and it was the cause of his ultimate ruin." Ibid. Although some readers of Machiavelli will take this as the latter's ultimate concession that Cesare cannot be seen as a virtuous actor, I prefer to read it in terms of Machiavelli's recognition that no political actor is capable of possessing an absolute knowledge that would perfectly guide their action with a precise certainty. As pointed out many times in this study, virtuous action is never enough to overcome or master the historical world within which the actor is embedded, a fact that is not revealed with any more clarity than in the example of Borgia. In an article, for example, emphasizing aging and death as particular limits on the capacity for adaptation, Timothy Lukes notes that even though Cesare possessed the seemingly requisite skills to succeed, he nevertheless was incapable of overcoming his own finitude. Timothy J. Lukes, "Fortune Comes of Age," *Sixteenth Century Journal* 11, no. 4 (1980): 45.
145 Machiavelli, "Il Principe," chap. 7.
146 Ibid.

popular interest: "he told me many things, which reduced to one, shows that he wants to make his stake here, and that he will not think about the past, but only about the common good."[147] Such is reasserted in the *Discourses on Livy*, where Borgia is brought up in the context of Machiavelli's discussion of how the seemingly sinful nature of peoples is rooted in the misrule of princes. The Romagna prior to the displacement of the local princes by Cesare "was an example of every most wicked life, because there one could see great slaughters and robberies following every slight cause. This was born from the wickedness of those princes, not from the wickedness of men, as [these princes] said."[148] Specifically, the laws in the Romagna were neither observed by princes nor applied and executed uniformly, while punishments were only inflicted in those instances in which princes thought there was a financial benefit to be extracted. From this situation "arose many inconveniences, and above all this, that the people were impoverished and not corrected; and those who were impoverished strove to prevail against those less powerful than themselves."[149]

Borgia's project, and the extent to which Machiavelli sees it as deserving of praise, must be partially understood in light of the recognition of both this particular social-historical context, and Cesare's desire to overcome it through the popular reinstitutionalization of the social order. Whereas initially the establishment of a non-arbitrary and legitimate order necessitated the utilization of force and violence, as manifested, for example, in the cruel means of Remirro de Orco, at a certain point Borgia realized that this "excessive authority" was no longer needed, and began to institute quasi-democratic civic reforms, such as the creation of a provincial court in which each town had a representative.[150] Cesare also recognized, however, that the institution of such a populist project needed to be accompanied by an explicit political distancing from earlier modes, in order to "purge the spirits of those people,"[151] Such was achieved through the execution of Remirro, the physical representative of these prior modes. The execution of Remirro will be a symbolic representation to the people of Cesare's recognition

---

147 Machiavelli, "Prima legazione alla corte di Roma," in *Tutte le opere*, sec. 30.
148 Machiavelli, "Discorsi sopra la prima Deca di Tito Livio," bk. 3.29.
149 Ibid.
150 Machiavelli, "Il Principe," chap. 7.
151 Ibid.

of the incompatibility of arbitrarily used extra-legal violence and civic life, and a declaration of his ultimate commitment to a political ethic of popular legitimacy.[152] Machiavelli famously writes of Cesare that after having "seized upon the occasion, in Cesena one morning he had him put in two pieces in the piazza, with a chunk of wood and a bloody knife beside him. The ferocity of this spectacle rendered those people at the same time satisfied and stupefied."[153] The execution of Remirro is from Machiavelli's perspective a performative political act meant to communicate to the people of the Romagna Cesare's commitment to them and to civil life in common.[154]

The example of Cesare in chapter 7 is immediately followed by that of Agathocles in chapter 8, where acquiring a principality through crime is identified as a mode distinct from acquiring it through fortune and virtue. And yet Machiavelli goes on to attribute the rise of Agathocles, achieved through clearly criminal acts, largely to his "virtue of spirit and of body."[155] After having distinguished himself in his military career to an extent that allowed him to rise to the position of praetor, he "decided to become a prince," a position that he was able to achieve after having ambushed the senators of the city and other social and economic elites, and killing them all at an assembly he had convened for the citizens of Syracuse.[156] After his appropriation of power

---

152 There is thus not necessarily a contradiction here between the utilization of brutal means and the affirmation of the common good. Hence Gennaro Sasso writes, "If then one looks more fully into the movement of *The Prince*, one sees that in the merciless and barbaric action of Cesare Borgia shines, in spite of everything, that awareness of the popular good that is the first element on the basis of which it is possible to distinguish the 'civil principality' from the 'absolute principality.'" Gennaro Sasso, *Machiavelli e Cesare Borgia: storia di un guidizio* (Rome: Edizioni dell'Ateneo, 1966), 82.

153 Machiavelli, "Il Principe," chap. 7. In the words of McCormick, in such a way Borgia "dismembers himself from the very body that signifies excessively cruel violence. He dramatically cuts himself off from the very em-bodiment of arbitrary violence." McCormick, "Prophetic Statebuilding," 8.

154 Diego von Vacano also calls attention to the fact that the killing of Remirro is an illustration of the performative nature of political action. Von Vacano, *The Art of Power*, 43. Michael McCanles, furthermore, reads Cesare's presentation of the murder of Remirro as a communicative act, as a discursive message transmitted to the people indicating, for example, his willingness to consider and respond to popular will. McCanles, *The Discourse of Il Principe*, 78.

155 Machiavelli, "Il Principe," chap. 8.

156 Ibid.

Agathocles reproduced his authority not through obligation, but the threat and application of non-consensual force. Through his criminality he was able to successfully consolidate his rule while defending his city from external Carthaginian encroachments, Agathocles surviving through his deployment of well- (as opposed to badly) used cruelties: "Well-used one can call (if of evil it is licit to speak well) those made in one stroke, out of the necessity to secure oneself, and then are not sustained but converted into the most benefit for the subjects as possible. Badly used are those which, although few in the beginning, grow more with time rather than be eliminated."[157] The seeming ambiguity in Machiavelli's treatment of Agathocles is that at the same time that he refers to the "well-used" cruelty and "virtue of spirit and of body," he also writes that "one cannot yet call it virtue to kill one's citizens, betray friends, be without faith, without mercy, without religion; these modes enable one to acquire rule, but not glory."[158] It seems as though in the final instance Agathocles's "brutal cruelty and inhumanity, with his infinite wickedness, do not permit him to be celebrated among the most excellent men. One cannot, therefore, attribute to fortune or to virtue that which he achieved without the one or the other."[159]

Readers of Machiavelli have attempted to explain this ambivalence in the deployment of the notion of *virtù* in chapter 8, and its relation to the articulation of the concept in the context of the example of Cesare Borgia in chapter 7, in a variety of ways.[160] As mentioned above,

---

157 Ibid.

158 Ibid.

159 Ibid.

160 Here we can list just a few notable examples. A typical interpretive strategy for reconciling the seeming Agathocles problem is to differentiate between two different forms of *virtù* operative in the chapter. Thus Michael McCanles, for example, argues that although it is true that Agathocles lacks Christian virtue, the evidence suggests that he possesses political virtue. McCanles, *The Discourse of Il Principe*, 62. Indeed, for McCanles this conceptual deployment is just one example of Machiavelli's discursive strategy, the meaning of the discourse being reversed through the shifting of textuality. Thus, "Agathocles' cruelty (and by the end of *Il Principe* any action) has no meaning at all, neither good nor evil, nor is it indeed *'crudeltà'* until men textualize the action and by the names they give the action set up semantic-logical entailments regarding the kind of discourse that can by thought, spoken, and written about." Ibid., 64. Contrasting the rhetorical strategy of Machiavelli with that of Cicero, Gary Remer claims that Machiavelli ultimately fails to uphold the division between the virtue of Borgia and the non-virtue of Agathocles, or even the differing types of virtue possessed by each, emptying the

however, here I would like to focus only on the democratic reading of John McCormick. In one of the most significant attempts to recuperate the legacy of Agathocles, McCormick argues that not only is the former considered virtuous by Machiavelli, but in fact Machiavelli sees his virtue as potentially exceeding even Cesare Borgia's.[161] Interrogating the facts of Agathocles's rise to power and rule is seen to reveal this worth. In short, Agathocles is interpreted as a revolutionary populist who succeeds in breaking the power of an oligarchic class that had earlier ended democratic rule, in the process never harming the people nor losing their support. Indeed, Agathocles's establishment of his principality is achieved through the wholesale elimination of Syracuse's *grandi*, who are killed "in full sight of the *popolo*."[162] It is this foundation of his rule in the people that allowed Agathocles to maintain his authority for so long, his citizens not having any inclination to conspire against him as a result of his defence of them. For McCormick Agathocles thus achieves his ultimately democratic end: he "initiates and guides the transformation of an oligarchic republic into a more democratic one."[163]

Although McCormick provides a compelling argument regarding the status of Agathocles in Machiavelli's text, particularly for those inclined to read Machiavelli through a democratic prism, I believe that it ultimately suffers to the extent that it reduces Machiavelli's politics to

---

concept of all substantive ethical content and losing any sense of the *honestum*. Gary Remer, "Rhetoric as a Balancing of Ends," *Philosophy and Rhetoric* 42, no. 1 (2009): 5–6. For Victoria Kahn, Agathocles's crimes cannot be called virtuous precisely to the extent that no one thing can be called *virtù*, there being no positive content that substantively fixes its meaning: "*virtù* is not a general rule of behavior that can be applied to a specific situation, but is rather, like prudence, a faculty of deliberation about particulars." Kahn, "*Virtù* and the Example of Agathocles in Machiavelli's *Prince*," 206. Kahn will later alter her interpretation of Agathocles, maintaining – contrary to my reading – that "Agathocles himself changed in response to the dictates of his reign," *virtù* being associated with the willingness to alter ones modes in light of changing circumstances. Victoria Kahn, "Revisiting Agathocles," *Review of Politics* 75, no. 4 (2013): 561. Nevertheless, Kahn now ultimately accepts Machiavelli's claim that Agathocles cannot be said to have achieved glory, as he failed to rise "to a Roman standard of greatness." Ibid., 569.

161 John P. McCormick, "The Enduring Ambiguity of Machiavellian Virtue: Cruelty, Crime, and Christianity in *The Prince*," *Social Research* 81, no. 1 (2014): 136.

162 John P. McCormick, "Machiavelli's Inglorious Tyrants: On Agathocles, Scipio and Unmerited Glory," *History of Political Thought* 36, no. 1 (2015): 32.

163 McCormick, "The Enduring Ambiguity of Machiavellian Virtue," 147.

the instrumental language of means and ends, evaluating the legacy of Agathocles solely in terms of his contribution to the establishment of an external state of being. As McCormick writes, "Agathocles initiates and guides the transformation of an oligarchic republic into a more democratic one. Both [Agathocles and Nabis] left their republics, by certain standards, in better civic and military condition than when they first usurped them."[164] Such a reading is perfectly adequate when considered from the standpoint of what I earlier identified as the transitional reading of the function of the new prince in relation to Machiavelli's normative defence of republican life. As I have suggested, however, *The Prince* operates on more than one register: the civil principality can be read as not only the prerequisite for the establishment of those social conditions necessary for the institution of the republic, but also as a model of human subjectivity. It is this double form that can be seen to account for the ambivalence in Machiavelli's treatment of Agathocles. Agathocles may very well be seen as a model prince to the extent that he purged his city of the nobles and grounded his authority in the people. He is not a model, however, for Machiavelli's ethics of self-activity as revealed in the articulation of the nature of performative *virtù*. McCormick writes: "There is virtually no difference between the crimes of Borgia and those of Agathocles."[165] This may very well be substantively true, however Machiavelli's condemnation of Agathocles is not grounded in the latter's willingness to utilize techniques of violence in order to secure political ends, but rather in his deployment of violence as a matter of principle, as a universally applicable political strategy. Agathocles errs in the same way as do the political moralists who demand that actors adhere to conventional ethical standards in every circumstance, although in an inverted way. What characterizes both is an inability to alter their mode of proceeding in order to respond to the shifting demands and necessities of fortune. Agathocles may have used cruelty well, but this good use is only a constituent element of a more fundamental ethic of virtue when reflectively combined with the prudent deployment of other political modes. Such a stratagem begins to

---

164 McCormick, "Machiavelli's Inglorious Tyrants," 40.
165 John P. McCormick, "Machiavelli's Agathocles: From Criminal Example to Princely Exemplum," in *Exemplarity and Singularity: Thinking through Particulars in Philosophy, Literature, and Law*, ed. Michèle Lowrie and Susanne Lüdemann (London: Routledge, 2015), 127.

be realized in the chapter's final paragraph, where Machiavelli discusses the necessity of doing injuries all at once so as to offend less, and of doing benefits little by little over time so as to be appreciated more consistently.[166] Already in this very crude account of the mixing of political modes do we find a radical departure from the singularity of Agathocles's technique.

Agathocles may very well have succeeded where Borgia failed, to the extent that he maintained his state. Virtue, however, is not defined exclusively in terms of such instrumental considerations. Cesare distinguishes himself from Agathocles through an openness to political flexibility grounded in prudent reflection on the always contingent nature of the field in which the prince acts.[167] Borgia is a pre-eminent example of an actor capable of comprehending the requirements of action, not relying on previously fixed schemas that structure behaviour in advance, but reflectively interpreting the historical situation and his place in it, and formulating a critical plan of action in light of this interrogation. And crucially, what this action aims at is not simply the reproduction of a state of being, in for example the perpetuation of one's rule, but the *ex nihilo* creation of new political realities.[168] Cesare Borgia is above all an innovator, a creator of new political forms. His political creation, though, was again possible only to the extent that he possessed a capacity for critical innovation with respect to political technique, neither refusing violence as a matter of principle nor affirming it as a singular mode. Violence, rather, was critically deployed in a creative project ultimately looking to benefit his citizens. The difference

---

166 Machiavelli, "Il Principe," chap. 8.

167 Indeed, that action must be grounded in such prudent reflection, and not merely the will to make a decision irrespective of rational consideration of historical possibility, must not be forgotten. Hence Machiavelli will locate the greatness of the Pope and the Duke in their interrogation of *occasioni* and their orientation of their action in light of it: "they are experts of the occasion and know how to use it very well; this opinion is confirmed by experience of the things carried out by them with the opportunity." Machiavelli, "Del modo di trattare i popoli della Valdichiana ribellati," in *Tutte le opere*, 15.

168 Indeed, for Althusser the figure of Borgia speaks to the emphasis on the *ex nihilo* form of creation in Machiavelli. Specifically, Borgia proves that a new prince can seemingly emerge from nothing, and hence that the radically new principality "is materially *possible*, and hence that it is not a dream or utopia." Althusser, *Machiavelli and Us*, 79.

between this project and that of Agathocles could not be more striking.[169]

In this chapter I have argued that through his emphasis on the performativity of political action, as represented in the characterization of the prince as an actor upon a stage theatrically embodying a multiplicity of diverse roles, Machiavelli reorients political activity as a good-in-itself.[170] The diversity of political actors and goals that Machiavelli chooses to highlight in *The Prince* is a manifestation of the central concern with the articulation of the form of political subjectivity, as opposed to that form of regime that is capable of generalizing this political subjectivity. In *The Prince* the process of creation itself is generally of far more significance than the precise object of creation. The prince deserving of praise is he who is able to, through the creative exercise of *virtù*, bring something new into the world, altering the structure of the world in some productive way. The actualization of human creativity is a normative good to be affirmed to the extent that it is grounded in a fundamental psychic orientation toward transgressive self-expression via the externalization of ambitious energy. *Virtù* is the human capacity that allows the actor to seize upon the *occasioni* presented by *fortuna* in order to generate new human realities. Political creation is a mode for the actualization of the negative human essence considered in terms of internal and external overcoming. This notion of *virtù* as performative self-expression allows us to more adequately contextualize Machiavelli's frequent deployment of the language of happiness in relation to the political self-activity of the prince. In chapter 6, for example, we first see the use of the term *felice*, the appearance of a concept of a specifically political happiness, a gratification realized in political creation: "These occasions, therefore, made these men happy, and their excellent virtue rendered the occasions known; hence their countries were ennobled and became very

---

169 In Lefort's words, "One unfolds entirely beneath the sign of violence; the other proves capable of being modified according to the imperatives created by the coexistence of the prince with his subjects." Lefort, *Machiavelli in the Making*, 135.

170 For a relatively early identification of the goodness that Machiavelli sees as internal to the creation of *ordini* see J.H. Whitfield, "On Machiavelli's Use of *Ordini*," *Italian Studies*, no. 10 (1955): 24.

happy."[171] Machiavelli's explicit identification of creative action and happiness, the latter term or a variation of it being most prominently displayed in chapter 25, where the Machiavellian theory of freedom is most clearly articulated in that text, is often obscured by his readers, who again tend to instrumentally focus on the prince's effort to actualize extrinsic conditions of being. A few commentators, however, have noted it, such as Wayne Reborn: "happiness essentially defines what he feels. For if princes do what they are supposed to do, if that is, they succeed – then they will be not only 'powerful, secure, honored,' but also, as Machiavelli adds, 'happy [*felici*].'"[172] Indeed, the penultimate chapter of *The Prince* abounds with terms such as *felice* and *felicitare*. Rebhorn argues that although often translated into the language of success and prosperity, such vocabulary would be more accurately rendered in terms of happiness, one of the overall lessons of *The Prince* being that their exists joy in action.[173] In the final instance, political creation, institutional expression as a mode for the externalization of human ambition, is thus seen to generate a type of gratification, and to this degree can be interpreted in performative terms as a sort of good-in-itself.

---

171 Machiavelli, "Il Principe," chap. 6.

172 Rebhorn, "Machiavelli's *Prince* in the Epic Tradition," 93.

173 Ibid. Such is recognized by a few other interpreters. Looking specifically at the *Art of War*, Elizabeth Frazer and Kimberly Hutchings note that virtuous action is "focused on glory and joy." Elizabeth Frazer and Kimberly Hutchings, "Virtuous Violence and the Politics of Statecraft in Machiavelli, Clausewitz and Weber," *Political Studies* 59, no. 1 (2011): 63. More generally, Roger Masters notes that a key element informing Machiavelli's normative thought is the affirmation of a principle of enjoyment. Roger D. Masters, *Fortune Is a River: Leonardo Da Vinci and Niccolò Machiavelli's Magnificent Dream to Change the Course of Florentine History* (New York: Free Press, 1998), 199. Crucially, furthermore, this joy in action is irreducible to a happiness acquired through command, an identification Machiavell never makes. Gennaro Sasso, "Problemi di critica machiavelliana," in *Studi su Machiavelli* (Napoli: Morano, 1967), 66.

PART THREE

Political Ontology

Chapter Four

Ambition and the People: The Popular Form of the Desire for Creation

In the previous chapter I argued that it is possible to read *The Prince* not only as a treatise on the being of a particular form of regime – the civil principality instituted by a new prince – but also as a treatise on the being of human subjectivity. In *The Prince* Machiavelli details what it would mean for the negative human desire for value formation – expressed through the concept of ambition – to be realized via the creative institution of new political modes and orders. According to my argument, reading the text in this way allows us to rearticulate the relationship between it and the *Discourses on Livy*. Specifically, in the *Discourses* Machiavelli attempts to theorize a form of regime that is democratic to the extent that all individuals, not merely princes, are capable of actualizing their potential for political creation. If *virtù* is the name given to the human capacity for such actualization, the *Discourses* provides an image of a political form of society in which all citizens are virtuous, a political form of society in which *virtù* is generalized. The suggestion that the popular virtue that Machiavelli defines in the *Discourses* is of the same quality as the princely virtue detailed in *The Prince* is one that would be rejected by most readers of Machiavelli, who prefer instead to qualitatively differentiate between the two expressions of *virtù*. A wide variety of scholars follow Friedrich Meinecke, who famously distinguished between heroic *virtù* and civic *virtù* – the latter, manifested in a concern for the common, being only a secondary derivation of the former, manifested in the creative form-giving activity of political elites. Ultimately civic *virtù* depends upon heroic *virtù* to the extent that only the truly great founder is capable of creating the conditions for the generation of republican life. In Meinecke's view, Machiavelli's privileging of heroic *virtù* "shows that he was a long way from

believing uncritically in the natural and imperishable virtue of a republican citizen, and that he viewed even the republic more from above,
from the standpoint of the rulers, than from underneath, from the
standpoint of broad-based democracy."[1] What all such differentiations
between types of virtue implicitly or explicitly affirm is a natural human
inequality, and in particular an inequality grounded in what is seen to
be a popular deficiency. Generally speaking, such deficiency is theorized in either one of two ways, although they are frequently combined
with each other. First, the people are often identified by readers of
Machiavelli as lacking the creative and ambitious desire to express
themselves in the world. Such a lack is the ground upon which the people are then justly excluded from certain political offices or roles, for
they do not possess any positive civic desire for political participation.
Political participation, in other words, is not a mode of activity the people crave to the extent that they lack an impulse to creative self-expression,
seeking as they do merely their own private security and well-being.
Second, even if and when the mass of citizens constituting the people is
seen to be in possession of an ambitious desire to participate in the
affairs of state, many commentators interpret Machiavelli as advocating withholding such participation on the grounds that they lack the
requisite intellectual or cognitive skills needed for prudent political
deliberation.

Contrary to such interpretations grounded in a perception of human
inequality, in this chapter I will attempt to locate in Machiavelli's
thought a double affirmation. On the one hand, Machiavelli provides
an affirmation of a radical human freedom, all individuals being seen

---

1 Meinecke, *Machiavellism*, 32. For further assumptions of a bifurcation of types of *virtù*
  see, for example, Hulliung, *Citizen Machiavelli*, 43; Skinner, *The Foundations of Modern
  Political Thought*, vol. 1: *The Renaissance*, 125; Michael Walzer, *The Revolution of the
  Saints* (Cambridge: Harvard University Press, 1965), 9; John Plamenatz, "In Search of
  Machiavellian *Virtù*," in *The Political Calculus: Essays on Machiavelli's Political Philosophy*, ed. Anthony Parel (Toronto: University of Toronto Press, 1972), 159; Markus
  Fischer, "Machiavelli's Political Psychology," *Review of Politics* 59, no. 4 (1997): 807,
  821; John H. Geerken, "Homer's Image of the Hero in Machiavelli," *Italian Quarterly*
  14, no. 3 (1970): 45; Ball, "The Picaresque Prince," 529; Neal Wood, "Some Reflections
  on Sorel and Machiavelli," *Political Science Quarterly* 83, no. 1 (1968): 81; R. Claire Snyder, "Machiavelli and the Citizenship of Civic Practices," in *Feminist Interpretations of
  Niccolò Machiavelli*, ed. Maria J. Falco (University Park: Pennsylvania State University
  Press, 2004), 217.

as inclined toward expressing a will to positively participate in public affairs, and this to the extent that they all desire an outlet for the expression of their essential ambition. And on the other hand, Machiavelli provides an affirmation of a radical human equality, all individuals being seen as potentially capable of possessing the intellectual capacities and skills required to make informed political decisions via the articulation of their desire in speech. After demonstrating in this chapter the extent to which Machiavelli theorizes the ambitious form of the popular desire for freedom and the equal capacity for popular political judgment, in chapter 5 I will demonstrate the extent to which the actualization of such freedom and equality has as its precondition the elimination of pronounced socio-economic stratification. Finally, in chapter 6 I will turn to look at the specific institutional form of Machiavelli's ideal republic, demonstrating how it is structured so as to give a positive expression to these two interrelated values of freedom and equality.

Social Difference and the Essentiality of Conflict

Machiavelli specifies the nature of the division between the humours of the great and the people in each of his three major political works. In *The Prince* he writes that "in every city is found these two diverse humours, and it stems from the fact that the people desire not to be commanded or oppressed by the great, and the great desire to command and oppress the people."[2] In the *Discourses* he grounds his early discussion of the productivity of social conflict in a recognition that there "are in every republic two diverse humours, that of the people, and that of the great,"[3] going on to specify the content of this bifurcation one chapter later, writing that "without doubt, if one considers the end of the nobles and of the ignobles, one will see in the former great desire to dominate, and in the latter only desire not to be dominated."[4] And in the *Florentine Histories* the division is articulated not in terms of a specification of its potential contribution to the establishment of freedom, but rather in terms of it as a source of corrupting factional conflict: "The grave and natural enmities between the people and the nobles,

---

2 Machiavelli, "Il Principe," in *Tutte le opere*, chap. 9.
3 Machiavelli, "Discorsi sopra la prima Deca di Tito Livio," in *Tutte le opere*, bk. 1.4.
4 Ibid., bk. 1.5.

caused by the wish of the latter to command and the former not to obey, are the cause of all the evils that emerge in cities; for from this diversity of humours all the other things that disturb cities take their nourishment."[5] This division, furthermore, is apparently considered to be grounded in a certain natural principle. Such is suggested by the seemingly inevitable emergence of conflict between the people and the *grandi* after the suppression of the factional conflict between the Guelfs and Ghibellines, Machiavelli writing that "there remained ignited only those humours that are naturally wont to exist in all cities between the powerful and the people; because, since the people want to live according to the laws, and the powerful to command them, it is not possible that they understand together."[6]

Machiavelli's emphasis on the division between these two humours, particularly the extent to which their interaction is implicated in the emergence of either productive or destructive social conflict, has been rightly taken to be a central issue by the majority of his readers. My contention, however, is that such readers err when they interpret this division in ontological terms, as speaking to a fundamental bifurcation of human nature or psychology, a bifurcation that closes off or limits the potential for democratic institutionalization through reading the being of the people in terms of an essential lack or incapacity. Typical in this respect is Anthony Parel, who writes that in the work of Machiavelli "political humors refer to desires and appetites natural to a social group."[7] Political potential, the possible range of institutionalization within the social body, is thus delimited by the biological realities of the primary humours, the body politic being thus reduced to a de facto organic entity: Machiavelli "makes a universal statement regarding the structure of political regimes, irrespective of whether they are principalities, republics, or oligarchies: in every city there are two opposed humors. The unity of a political regime, according to this statement, is organic."[8] The opposition between the humours cannot be overcome, for "these dispositions are natural, permanent, and necessary."[9] This

---

5 Machiavelli, "Istorie fiorentine," in *Tutte le opere*, bk. 3.1.

6 Ibid., bk. 2.12.

7 Parel, *The Machiavellian Cosmos*, 105.

8 Anthony Parel, "Machiavelli's Use of *Umori* in *The Prince*," *Quaderni d'Italianistica* 11, no. 1 (1990): 92.

9 Ibid., 93.

opposition, though, is mutually conditioning, the perception of this conditioning being rooted in the ancient medical science that understands the health of the organism in terms of the balanced opposition of the humoral elements.[10] The health of the body politic depends upon the mutual satisfaction of each humour in a relation of co-determination that is framed in terms of a law of organic necessity, such that we must conclude that "the real ends of politics are basically pre-moral and pre-rational."[11]

According to such a conception, the political task becomes one of balancing the parts of the city, identifying the political offices and roles that correspond to the biologically determined humours associated with each such part, and arranging them relative to one another so as to establish an internally proportionate unity that ensures to the greatest possible degree the stability of the body politic. Such a vision of the end of the state as being oriented toward the establishment of a peaceful internal coherence would be a common feature of civic humanist political thinking grounded in reflection on classical republicanism. Indeed, it was given perhaps an archetypal expression in Cicero's *De re publica*, which is worth quoting at length. Cicero writes: "In playing the lyre or the flute, and of course in choral singing, a degree of harmony must be maintained among the different sounds, and if it is altered or discordant a trained ear cannot endure it; and this harmony, through the regulation of very different voices, is made pleasing and concordant. So too the state, through the reasoned balance of the highest and the lowest and the intervening orders, is harmonious in the concord of very different people. What musicians call harmony with regard to song is concord in the state, the tightest and the best bond of safety in every republic; and that concord, can never exist without justice."[12] It is this tradition of theorizing republican life in terms of such a coordination of elements that many readers of Machiavelli take the latter to be participating in. According to such a model of republican life, the harmony of

---

10 Ibid. For a very different account of the extent to which Machiavelli was influenced by the medical science of his time, and in particular humoral theory, stressing the significance of social conflict as opposed to social harmony, see Marie Gaille-Nikodimov, *Conflit civil et liberté: la politique machiavélienne entre histoire et médecine* (Paris: Honoré Champion, 2004). See also Patapan, *Machiavelli in Love*, 112.

11 Parel, "Machiavelli's Use of *Umori* in *The Prince*," 99.

12 Cicero, "On the Commonwealth," in *On the Commonwealth and On the Laws*, ed. James E.G. Zetzel (Cambridge: Cambridge University Press, 1999), 56–7.

the political community is achieved to the extent that the direction of the humours within it are capable of being comprehensively mapped and channelled into modes that mutually satisfy them, in a relation of equivalent fulfilment. The determinate form of being of human appetite is thus the condition for the determinate form of being of the internally stable and harmonious republic.

There is very strong reason to doubt, however, that Machiavelli theorized either of these possibilities.[13] In chapter 2, for example, I attempted to show the extent to which human difference greatly exceeds the apparently natural division between the humours of the great and the people. In chapter 3 I attempted to show that Machiavelli theorizes human psychology in terms of an irregular and non-thematizable ambition that perpetually seeks an external expression through the transgression of existing realities. Indeed, it is the latter fact of inexhaustible human ambition that generates the former fact of inexhaustible human conflict. As was suggested in my presentation of Machiavelli's critique of contemplative historical understanding in chapter 1, the reduction of the image of the healthy city to one whose being is considered in terms of stability and self-identity was an ideological manoeuvre designed to cover up the fact of patrician domination. The humanist praise of civic harmony and unity functioned to mask a status quo where a minority derived political and economic privilege from the established set of social relations. Although the common good was praised, this good was interpreted as being realizable only through the benevolent application of wise policy by elites. The rejection of the potentially productive consequences of disunion was an ideological strategy for preserving patrician rule.

Machiavelli's affirmation of the productivity of conflict must not be read in terms of that conflict's potential resolution via the establishment

---

13 As is often the case, this fact was recognized with more clarity by certain of Machiavelli's contemporaries than by later readers, as suggested by Guicciardini's critique of Machiavelli, the former stating with reference to the latter that "praising discord is like praising a sick man's illness, because the remedy that has been used on him is the right one." Guicciardini, "Considerations on the *Discourses* of Niccolò Machiavelli," 393. For an additional example of Guicciardini's praise of internal social unity and his critique of discord and division see Francesco Guicciardini, *Dialogue on the Government of Florence*, ed. and trans. Alison Brown (Cambridge: Cambridge University Press, 1994), 81.

of an ordered relation of balance between the diverse elements seen to constitute the social field, but rather in terms of the irreducibility of conflict to a binary relation that is reconcilable in a static order of things.[14] Conflict in Machiavelli is a necessary condition of life given the multiplicity of forms of human being and doing. Filippo Del Lucchese is the contemporary reader who has done most to emphasize the significance of social conflict to Machiavelli's thought, and Machiavelli's rejection of universal models of the common human good. He notes, for example, that Machiavelli never speaks of the actualization of the common good as ensuring the realization of the good of every particular individual within the society.[15] The common good is thus not equivalent to the good of all, especially in social contexts marked by a division between the *grandi* and the people: "If what we mean by 'common good' means the good of all social groups, necessarily in conflict in the city (in Rome and in Florence), this good simply does not exist in the radically realistic thought of Machiavelli. If it is common, we might say, then it is not a true good."[16] Indeed, in *Discourses* 2:2 it is claimed that the common good can be realized where the few suffer, this few here being the grandees. The common good, in short, is irreducible to an organic conception of unity in which each part fulfils itself in its positive contribution to the well-being of the society. For Del Lucchese the impossibility of such a form of social closure is especially well revealed in the structure of the *Florentine Histories*, where the presentation of competing views on virtually all issues demonstrates both the conflictual nature of politics, and also the impossibility of reconciling competing visions in the realization of a good that is literally common to all.[17] Indeed, the very idea of justice is articulated through the conflict of interests that expresses the internal differentiation of society. Justice is not theorized in terms of the

---

14 This is sometimes recognized. See, for example, Wolin, *Politics and Vision*, 208; Mark Jurdjevic, *A Great and Wretched City: Promise and Failure in Machiavelli's Florentine Political Thought* (Cambridge: Harvard University Press, 2014), 103.

15 Del Lucchese, *Conflict, Power, and Multitude in Machiavelli and Spinoza*, 29.

16 Filippo Del Lucchese, "Machiavellian Democracy," *Historical Materialism* 20, no. 1 (2012): 242. On Catherine Zuckert's reading, when Machiavelli uses the phrase "common good" he means only "the good of the vast majority of the people who want the security government by law can provide without oppression. It does not include the good desired by the 'great.'" Zuckert, *Machiavelli's Politics*, 467.

17 Del Lucchese, *Conflict, Power, and Multitude in Machiavelli and Spinoza*, 32.

derivation of a specific order of things from a transcendent source, but is rather a conflictual claim articulated in a concrete historical context.

My argument is that multiplicity is itself the result of a basic fact of human existence: the negative human desire for creative self-expression. It is not that different groups of individuals have specifically fixed ends or purposes. On the contrary, all individuals are oriented toward the externalization of the same insatiable ambition. It is precisely because of the fact, though, that such ambition has no positive content that individuals attempt to realize it in such a diversity of conflicting modes, pursuing and valuing different objects.[18] The political question for Machiavelli then becomes: how can such necessarily conflictual diversity be given a social expression in a non-antagonistic way? In chapter 6 I will attempt to show how Machiavelli answers this question. First, however, it must be demonstrated that Machiavelli does in fact think the universality of the negative human desire for self-expression, that even the people, as opposed to simply the *grandi*, possess an active ambition that perpetually seeks exteriorization. My argument is that the distinction between the desire to oppress and the desire not to be oppressed is not grounded in a biological differentiation between differing human natures, but is simply a difference in the form of appearance of desire, a difference grounded in a divergence in the means by which individuals attempt to realize a universal negative human essence. Specifically, the great attempt to satisfy their ambition through the domination of others – that is to say, through denying others their capacity for ambitious expression. The people, on the other hand, do not participate in such a limitation, being content instead with a form of democratic institutionalization in which all citizens are able to express their creative desire. Whereas the people are satisfied to vent their desire through proper institutional outlets, the great attempt to vent their desire privately, and attempt to restrict such self-expression to themselves alone. The difference is thus not in the nature of desire, but rather in the mode of expression of desire.

---

18 On the necessary mutual intelligibility such a situation produces see Minogue, "Theatricality and Politics," 153; von Vacano, *The Art of Power*, 61–2.

The Ground of Freedom: The Active Form of Popular Desire

As suggested above, Machiavelli's identification of two humours always present in a city, one that seeks to oppress and one that seeks not to be oppressed, has often been interpreted by readers in terms of a fundamental bifurcation of human nature: whereas the great possess an active and spirited impulse to impress their will upon the world, the people are considered primarily as passive and static, seeking only the assurance of their own private security. Such a reading is common to a variety of intellectual traditions within Machiavelli studies, including neo-republican,[19] Straussian,[20] and even democratic.[21] In my view, however, such a polarization of desire (at least in the Straussian and the neo-republican cases, if not that of democratic readers) rests upon a conflation of the notions of domination and authority, as if the people's

---

19 Especially notable here is Skinner's stress on republican governments as those that provide the conditions for the realization of a negative liberty to undertake private pursuits, as "To be free, in short, is simpy to be unconstrained from pursuing whatever goals we may happen to set for ourselves." Quentin Skinner, "The Republican Ideal of Political Liberty," in *Machiavelli and Republicanism*, ed. Gisela Bock, Quentin Skinner, and Maurizio Viroli (Cambridge: Cambridge University Press, 1990), 302. See also Skinner, *The Foundations of Modern Political Thought*, vol. 1: *The Renaissance*, 125; Skinner, "Machiavelli on *Virtù* and the Maintenance of Liberty"; Philip Pettit, *Republicanism: A Theory of Freedom and Government* (Oxford: Oxford University Press, 1997), 28. For brief overviews of Skinner's attempt to reground republican liberty in negative freedom see Carl K.Y. Shaw, "Quentin Skinner on the Proper Meaning of Republican Liberty," *Politics* 23, no. 1 (2003): 46–56; Marco Geuna, "Skinner, Pre-Humanist Rhetorical Culture and Machiavelli," in *Rethinking the Foundations of Modern Political Thought*, ed. Annabel Brett, James Tully, and Holly Hamilton-Bleakley (Cambridge: Cambridge University Press, 2006), 50–72.

20 See, for example, Vickie B. Sullivan, *Machiavelli, Hobbes, and the Formation of Liberal Republicanism in England* (Cambridge: Cambridge University Press, 2004), 33; Vickie B. Sullivan, "Machiavelli's Momentary 'Machiavellian Moment': A Reconsideration of Pocock's Treatment of the *Discourses*," *Political Theory* 20, no. 2 (1992): 312.

21 Although stressing the active participation of the people in the republican regime, McCormick ultimately suggests that this participation is not driven by a desire for plebeian self-expression, but is rather a strategic response to the noble desire for domination: "The people and their plebeian magistrates must act in a more than a merely passive and reactive manner *if they are to contain and control* wily and well-resources social actors identified first and foremost by an insolent humor to oppress others." John P. McCormick, *Machiavellian Democracy* (Cambridge: Cambridge University Press, 2011), 94. Emphasis added.

apparent desire not to be dominated logically excludes the people's immanent desire to have a share in government. Such a position is a manifestation of an anti-democratic impulse that necessarily reads governance in terms of command or oppression. For Machiavelli, though, this identification is illegitimate. There is a popular desire to actively participate in legislative activities, and this desire is grounded in the universal vitality of the human psyche. The two primary humours are simply two different forms of appearance of the single desire for creative self-expression, two different modes for the realization of ambition. I will attempt to demonstrate the extent to which the people can be seen to possess such a desire through constellating several key episodes drawn from Machiavelli's writings.

There is certainly some precedent for thinking the presence of such a natural desire for participatory freedom in the people.[22] Most notable is a recent contribution by Mark Jurdjevic on Machiavelli's Florentine writings, specifically the *Florentine Histories* and the "Discourse on Florentine Affairs." According to Jurdjevic, we see in these writings a shift away from Machiavelli's earlier emphasis on the transformative power of single actors, toward an emphasis on the stimulating powers of collective action and mutual consent. In Jurdjevic's words, "we see a broad transformation in his way of thinking about power from an early focus on individuals to a later sociological analysis of power rooted in frank skepticism about the limit and utility of individual action."[23] Jurdjevic asks, for example, why in the Florentine writings there is not a single reference to the positive example of Rome, if not because Machiavelli abandoned the Roman model as a normative goal: "By 1520 Machiavelli has no intention of attempting or ever desiring to imitate the Roman model."[24] Significantly, this transition is thought in terms of a fundamental reconceptualization of the people and its desire. It is

---

22 Ugo Dotti, for example, links Machiavelli's affirmation of freedom to a specific form of naturalism, seeing freedom as grounded in the recognition of the specificity of human instinct. Ugo Dotti, *Niccolò Machiavelli: la fenomenologia del potere* (Milano: Feltrinelli Editore, 1979), 122–3. More recently, Erica Benner has identified the desire for freedom as a universal modality grounded in the natural human capacity for self-legislation, this universality explaining why certain peoples strive for freedom even without having any direct prior experience of it. Benner, *Machiavelli's Ethics*, 230.

23 Jurdjevic, *A Great and Wretched City*, 54.

24 Ibid., 73.

suggested that by this time Machiavelli no longer considers the people as capable of achieving satisfaction only through the guarantee of a secure space of negative liberty, but also as needing the attainment of an active participatory role in society. Hence "he repeatedly and explicitly warned that the people can only be satisfied by giving them an outlet in the government for the expression of their political ambitions and identity."[25] Popular desire is here oriented toward "action and participation for its own sake."[26] As a consequence of this identification of the nature of popular desire, Machiavelli is compelled to abandon his earlier differentiation of plebeian and noble humours, now reading both in terms of the same positive desire for political self-expression: "their desires are equally political, the problems they pose are identical, and the solutions are identical – realizing a form of government that gives both of them their voice and roles in the common enterprise of governing."[27] Hence, "In his later republicanism, the people have become irreducibly political."[28]

Although I think that Jurdjevic is absolutely correct that we can identify in Machiavelli's Florentine writings a popular political being considered in terms of a desire for self-legislation, I disagree with him that this being only emerges in these later works. I argue, instead, that there are several passages in the *Discourses* that suggest Machiavelli always identified plebeian desire with the will to participatory self-expression. The initial suggestion of the people's possession of an active ambition seeking exterior projection occurs early in the *Discourses*, in the defence of the socially productive consequences of Roman tumults in 1:4. After specifying the orientation of the two primary humours constituting the civic population, Machiavelli goes on to locate the institution of laws in favour of freedom in the conflictual confrontation of these humours, writing that "those who condemn the tumults between the nobles and the plebs seem to me to blame those things that were the first cause of keeping Rome free, and consider more the noises and the cries that these tumults created than the good effects that they brought."[29] What is immediately worthy of recognition is that Machiavelli does not claim

---

25 Ibid., 75.
26 Ibid., 76.
27 Ibid., 78.
28 Jurdjevic, "Machiavelli's Hybrid Republicanism," 1254.
29 Machiavelli, "Discorsi sopra la prima Deca di Tito Livio," bk. 1.4.

that these tumults constitute a good in themselves, but rather a good to the extent that they are articulated in a specific form, one that channels the humoral passions into modes that are not antagonistically violent, and for the sake of a specifically productive institutional creation. Regarding the former, on the non-violent character of the tumults, he writes: "from the Tarquins to the Gracchi, which was more than three hundred years, the Roman tumults rarely brought exile and very rarely blood. Therefore, these tumults can be neither judged harmful, nor a republic divided, which in such a long time sent into exile no more than eight or ten citizens due to its differences, and killed very few, and condemned not many more in fines."[30] If Machiavelli in defending the tumults was concerned exclusively with demonstrating that their continued existence did not preclude the establishment of a social field in which individuals could live without fear of interference, his narration might have ended here. He goes on, however, to note that the tumults generated in Rome a productive benefit associated with not only the creation of a negative security, but also the creation of positive institutional spaces allowing for the expression of a popular will to action.[31]

It is precisely the existence of popular ambition and the necessity of modes and orders capable of channelling this ambition that those who criticize the conflict of humours fail to recognize: "If anyone should say the modes were extraordinary, and almost savage, to see the people

---

30 Ibid.

31 Marco Geuna notes that the plebeian tumults that Machiavelli calls attention to were socially productive not only to the extent that they led to the generation of popular institutions in the first instance, but also all throughout the period that Rome lived in freedom. Marco Geuna, "Machiavelli ed il ruolo dei conflitti nella vita politica," in *Conflitti*, ed. Alessandro Arienzo and Dario Caruso (Napoli: Libreria Dante & Descartes, 2005), para. 1.2. Machiavelli says that Rome remained free from the expulsion of the Tarquins to the murder of Gaius Gracchus, a period of around 400 years, from 510 to 121 BCE. The tribunes were instituted first in 494 and then in 449, Machiavelli maintaining however that the tumults were the origins of laws in favour of freedom for long after this. What this suggests is that there is thus a permanent place for such activity in a democratic polity which is already directed toward plebeian good, to the extent that there is no constitutional form able to permanently reconcile social division, the latter being constitutive of the social order: "Looking at the thesis in this light shows that Machiavelli suggests indirectly that the tumults cannot be resolved once and for all, not even through the pure form of the mixed constitution. The tumults reemerging again and again and again must be managed by those who actively work in the politics of the republic. Even the perfect constitutional form cannot put them to an end." Ibid.

together shouting against the Senate, the Senate against the people, running tumultuously through the streets, the shops closed, all of the plebs leaving Rome, all things which frighten those who only read of them, I say that every city ought to have its modes with which *the people can vent its ambition*, and especially those cities that want to affirm the people in important things."[32] The people here are not merely reacting against the insolence of others who would seek to dominate them, but are actively looking to vent their own desire. Hence the tumults deserve to be commended to the extent that they were the stimulus to the creation of an institution that was capable of functioning as a stable medium for this active expression. The conflict between the great and the people is not praised in itself, but to the degree that it resulted in the creation of the tribunes as an order for the expulsion of plebeian ambition: "And if the tumults were the cause of the creation of the tribunes, they merit the highest praise; because, in addition to giving popular government its part, they were constituted as the guard of Roman freedom."[33]

The necessity of a specifically institutional form for the venting of ambition is articulated through Machiavelli's juxtaposition of the modes of "running tumultuously through the streets" and "leaving Rome," with participation in "important things." That which might constitute such participation in important things is suggested by the initial reference to the activity of the tribunes, but is immediately clarified in the following chapter, in relation to the newly introduced theme of the guard of freedom. The political question interrogated in 1:5 is perhaps the most significant in Machiavelli's thought. It is: what social institution of desire should be affirmed in the city? How should the political modes and orders be arranged so as to facilitate the expression of ambitious energy? Machiavelli approaches the question through his observation that any well-ordered republic requires a "guard of freedom."[34] The ostensible subject of the chapter is the question of who this guard should be placed in the hands of, the great or the many, the nobles or the people. The issue is initially approached through contrasting Lacedomonian and Venetian modes of institutionalization with the Roman one, the former two examples functioning as case studies in

---

32 Machiavelli, "Discorsi sopra la prima Deca di Tito Livio," bk. 1.4. Emphasis added.
33 Ibid.
34 Ibid., bk. 1.5.

constructing an aristocratic social economy of desire, the latter as a case study in constructing a democratic one. Machiavelli maintains that if one examines the matter from the standpoint of ends, then one should take the aristocratic position, for Sparta and Venice lasted longer than Rome. We know, however, that Machiavelli's criterion of political judgment is irreducible to merely instrumental considerations, such as the secure and stable reproduction of the political community in its self-identity, and hence the need for a more rigorous interrogation.

The aristocratic argument associated with the Spartan and Venetian models has two elements. The claim is that by giving the guard of freedom to the great you, first, allow them an outlet through which they are able to satisfy their ambition, and second, keep authority out of the restless and unstable hands of the plebs. The special significance of the latter claim has not been fully appreciated. What is recognized here by defenders of aristocratic order is that which most contemporary advocates of aristocratic rule (or more specifically, readers who reject the notion that Machiavelli was a democratic thinker affirming a popular will to political participation) deny: that popular desire is identical to noble desire, that is, that it is just as insatiable and perpetually directed toward additional acquisition.[35] Thus in Rome, where although "the tribunes of the plebs had this authority in their hands, it was *not enough* for them to have one plebeian consul, but they wanted to have both. From this they wanted the censorship, the praetor, and all the other offices of rule in the city; *nor was this enough for them*, for, carried away by the same *passion*, they with time began to adore those men who they saw as able to beat down the nobility."[36] In short, it is precisely the elite recognition of the plebs' possession of the same desire to acquire that they have which produces their belief in the necessity of closing off the former's access to major offices. The difference in desire lay not in the possession or non-possession of an ambitious appetite, but in the mode

---

35 On the identity of plebeian and noble nature see, for example, Alfredo Bonadeo, *Corruption, Conflict, and Power in the Works and Times of Niccolò Machiavelli* (Berkeley: University of California Press, 1973), 46; Giorgio Cadoni, *Crisi della mediazione politica e conflitti sociali: Niccolò Machiavelli, Francesco Guicciardini e Donato Giannotti di fronte al tramonto della Fiorentina libertas* (Roma: Jouvence, 1994), 37; Catherine Zuckert, "Machiavelli and the End of Nobility in Politics," *Social Research* 81, no. 1 (2014): 90; Coby, "Machiavelli's Philanthropy," 608–9; Del Lucchese, "Machiavellian Democracy," 239.

36 Machiavelli, "Discorsi sopra la prima Deca di Tito Livio," bk. 1.5. Emphases added.

by which this appetite is realized, as is made evident by the examination of the democratic argument. Defenders of the Roman model, including Machiavelli, thus maintain that the guard should be placed in the hands of those who are less likely to appropriate power for themselves alone: "And without doubt, if one considers the end of the nobles and of the commoners, one will see in the former great desire to dominate, and in the latter only desire not to be dominated; and, consequently, a greater will to live free."[37] It is not the case that the people have less of a desire to exercise political power, but rather that they have less of a desire to exercise it *exclusively*, appropriating authority for themselves alone and denying their fellow citizens the opportunity for political self-expression.

As I suggested in chapter 2 and as I will mention again in the following section in my discussion of popular political judgment, it is no doubt true that the popular desire for self-activity is one that can be largely repressed, and hence Machiavelli's identification of the corrupt multitude, the unshackled people who have not been self-educated to freedom, the people who lack forms of socialization that look toward the refinement of their critical-rational capacities.[38] Such a people were those that Machiavelli seemed to be primarily speaking of, for example, in *The Prince*.[39] Nevertheless, even under such conditions, even when the social economy of desire is organized in such a way that the majority of citizens appear to rest content with the existing order, and where only a few are capable of acting on the thirst for acquisition, the universal ambition which Machiavelli associates with value formation continues to exist as a subterranean current. That is, even in those instances where the people *seem* to be passive, conservative, interested only in the preservation of that which they already control, ambition is still present. Hence in 1:5, in the context of his articulation of the active form of being of plebeian desire, Machiavelli writes: "much disputed is which is the more ambitious, one who wants to maintain or one who wants to acquire; because easily one or the other appetite can be the cause of

---

37 Ibid.
38 Marie Gaille-Nikodimov argues that the particular form of expression of popular desire changes depending upon the context. Unlike in *The Prince*, where it is primarily a desire to be protected from the great, in the *Discourses* it takes the form of a desire for active participation in affairs of the city via self-government. Gaille-Nikodimov, *Conflit civil et liberté*, 44.
39 For an argument to this effect see Chabod, "*The Prince*: Myth and Reality," 63–5.

very great tumults. Yet nevertheless, more often than not they are caused by those who possess, because the fear of losing generates in them *the same desires* that are in those who desire to acquire; for it does not appear to men that they securely possess what they have, if they do not acquire something else new."[40] As Machiavelli puts it in *The Prince*, "It is truly a very natural and ordinary thing to desire to acquire."[41]

Machiavelli's belief in the universality of that human ambition which he attributes to the people in 1:5 is confirmed in various places throughout the *Discourses*. In 1:7, during his discussion of the function of accusation as a necessary mode to guard freedom, one of the two benefits associated with accusing is its creation of a field that allows for the expulsion of the always surplus energy of the people.[42] Such an expulsion, furthermore, is not identified as merely a reactive response to elite encroachments on the freedom of the republic. Indeed, in 1:50 Machiavelli maintains that the tribunate is a useful institution not only to the extent that it is able to guard against the ambition of the great being deployed against the plebs, but also to the extent that it is able to guard against the ambition of the people being deployed against itself: "Here one has to note, first, the utility of the tribunate, which was not only useful to moderate the ambition that the powerful used to control the plebs, but also that which they used among themselves."[43] In other words, Machiavelli is here positing the existence of a universal ambition that can be potentially directed toward others in an agonistic way, and which need not be associated exclusively with the *grandi*, who ostensibly alone possess the desire to oppress.

The orientation of desire toward the perpetual overcoming of the existent – that is, the insatiability of a general human ambition – is meanwhile affirmed in 1:29. Here Machiavelli, speaking of the universality of citizens, writes that "the nature of men is ambitious and suspicious, and does not know how to place a limit on its fortune."[44] This fact about human nature is what accounts for why a prince often feels the need to secure himself ungratefully against those subordinates who have distinguished themselves. Because of the ambitious nature of

---

40 Machiavelli, "Discorsi sopra la prima Deca di Tito Livio," bk. 1.5. Emphasis added.
41 Machiavelli, "Il Principe," chap. 3.
42 Machiavelli, "Discorsi sopra la prima Deca di Tito Livio," bk. 1.7.
43 Ibid., bk. 1.50.
44 Ibid., bk. 1.29.

individuals there is no ultimate achievement of a status, position, or state of being that would be capable of permanently satisfying their desire, thus terminating the quest for additional acquisition. Nevertheless, a republic, unlike a principality, may be structured so as to harness this vitality and deploy it toward ends beneficial to the city. One of the ends of a free city is the reproduction of the conditions of its freedom, a freedom which, as will be elaborated on in chapter 6, is considered in terms of this productive sublimation of ambition. One of the most common errors that republics make in the effort to maintain their freedom is offending those citizens that it ought to reward, and to suspect those that it ought to have confidence in.[45] Several chapters earlier Machiavelli identifies the necessity of rewarding those citizens who through the strength of their spirit are able to generate good works that benefit the city. Indeed, "although a republic be poor, and can give little, it ought not to abstain from that little; for always will every small gift, given to anyone in recompense for a good however great, be esteemed by whoever receives it as honorable and very great."[46] In sum, the republic errs when it treats these citizens as the prince does, for unlike the principality the healthy republic must provide opportunities for citizens to vent their desire without punishment, so long as this venting is generalized and directed toward socially productive objects. In this chapter, then, Machiavelli both identifies the universality of human ambition, and grounds the reproduction of freedom in the public recognition of those who have exercised such ambition for the sake of civic good, as opposed to private benefit. In the final instance, "although these modes in a republic that has come to corruption are the cause of great evils, and many times bring it more quickly to tyranny … nevertheless in a not corrupt republic they are the cause of great goods, and permit it to live free."[47]

The general insatiability of human desire is affirmed in three more significant places in the *Discourses*. In the Preface to Book Two it is identified again as the source of human dissatisfaction with the existent, a dissatisfaction that stimulates a perpetual drive toward innovation. Desire is here theorized as a surplus always in excess of the human capacity to acquire the objects of its cravings, largely as a consequence

---

45 Ibid.
46 Ibid., bk. 1.24.
47 Ibid., bk. 1.29.

of the contingent being of a world that does not present itself as open to human mastery: "besides this, human appetites are insatiable, for having, by nature, the power and the will to desire everything, and, by fortune, the power to attain little, the result is a continuous discontent in human minds, and a boredom with the things that they possess: this makes them condemn the present times, praise the past, and desire the future, even doing this if they are not motivated by any reasonable cause."[48] The foundation of what Machiavelli takes to be the human orientation toward innovation and creativity in this insatiability, furthermore, is confirmed in 3:21. The topic of the psychic fixation with the new is brought up in the context of a discussion of how it is possible that Hannibal could have acquired the reputation that he did in spite of the fact that, contrary to a figure such as Scipio, he deployed cruel and violent methods with regularity. Machiavelli writes that "thinking from whence this thing could emerge, there is seen several reasons for it. The first is that *men are desirous of new things*, so much so that most of the time those who are well off desire novelty as much as those who are poorly off; for, as was said another time, and it is true, men become bored in the good and grieve in the bad. Therefore, this desire opens the door to everyone who in a province makes themselves head of an innovation."[49]

The self-reference that Machiavelli makes above, in which he earlier speaks of the proclivity of individuals toward the new and their desire for innovation, is to be found in chapter 1:37, during the discussion of the conflict over the Agrarian law. And indeed, there is no passage within the *Discourses on Livy* that so clearly articulates the insatiable form of the plebeian desire for creative self-expression.[50] We begin again by noting both the natural orientation of human desire toward

---

48 Ibid., bk. 2, preface.

49 Ibid., bk. 3.21. Emphasis added.

50 Indeed, Luca Sartorello writes that in 1:37 "Machiavelli presents in a few passages of rare efficiency his theory of desire." Luca Sartorello, "L'urna sanza fondo machiavelliana e l'origine' della politica," in *Machiavelli: immaginazione e contingenza*, ed. Filippo Del Lucchese, Luca Sartorello, and Stefano Visentin (Pisa: Edizioni Ets, 2006), 208. Here we see the reappearance of the concept of ambition in a specifically popular form, and characterized by an infinite movement that perpetually exceeds the desired object. See also Giorgio Cadoni, *Crisi della mediazione politica e conflitti sociali: Niccolò Machiavelli, Francesco Guicciardini e Donato Giannotti di fronte al tramonto della Fiorentina libertas* (Roma: Jouvence, 1994), 35.

acquisition, and the incapacity of this desire coming to rest through being satisfied in objective possession: "nature has created men in a way that they can desire everything, and cannot attain everything; thus, since the desire is always greater than the power of acquisition, the result is discontent with that which they possess, and a lack of satisfaction with it. From this emerges the variability of their fortune; because some men desire to have more, and some fear to lose what has been acquired, they come to hostilities and war, from which arises the ruin of one province and the exaltation of the other."[51] What is essential to note, however, is that here Machiavelli will go on to explicitly identify this ambitious desire with the insatiable plebeian demand for opportunities for a specifically political self-expression relative to the *grandi*. Desire is not, as might be suggested by the above quotation, oriented only toward the acquisition of objects, but rather toward the actualization of a modality of political being. Machiavelli thus writes that "to the Roman plebs it was *not enough* to secure themselves against the nobles through the creation of the tribunes, to which *desire compelled it by necessity*; for having obtained that, it *immediately* began to struggle through ambition, and to wish to divide with the nobility honours and possessions, as the thing most esteemed by men."[52] It is within the context of this struggle over the social institution of desire, of the plebs' ambition to perpetually institute spaces allowing for creative legislation against the *grandi*'s ambition to limit the scope of freedom through restricting participation to it alone, that the Agrarian conflict must be understood.

The law ostensibly had two mechanisms oriented toward the maintenance of social equality, an equality that was considered essential as a ground for generalizing participation. The first was that no citizen could possess more than two *jugera* of land; the second was that the land appropriated from state enemies would be divided among the Roman people. The nobles were of course offended by both of these, "because those who possessed more assets than the law permitted (which was the greater part of the nobles), had to be deprived of them, and dividing among the plebs the assets of enemies removed from them the way to be enriched."[53] Over time the nobles

---

51 Machiavelli, "Discorsi sopra la prima Deca di Tito Livio," bk. 1.37.
52 Ibid. Emphases added.
53 Ibid.

temporized what they saw as offences through various means, with the original disputes ultimately subsiding as Roman territory expanded into isolated regions whose geographic location prevented plebeian intervention, the plebs being less desirous of distant and difficult-to-cultivate lands. As the debate over the law quieted down, the latter began to be no longer uniformly enforced, and it is here, not in popular insolence as defenders of aristocracy would suggest, that we can locate the root cause of the Agrarian scandal. Due to a general lack of enforcement over time, the sudden re-establishment of the law by the Gracchi had explosive consequences, and "ruined entirely Roman freedom."[54] Indeed, "it ignited so much hatred between the plebs and the Senate that they came to arms and blood, outside of every civil mode and custom."[55] The normal, legal, and regular enforcement of the law, by diverting passion through a publicly recognized legal order, would have minimized if not closed off the potential for extra-legal expulsion via the utilization of private modes of remedy. What the Agrarian episode ultimately demonstrates is not only that plebeian desire is insatiably oriented toward self-expression, but also that this ambitious self-expression, if it is not to be destructively released through antagonistic and private modes, must be productively channelled through the law. Law, in other words, does not exist in order to restrict or constrain desire, as was Machiavelli's position in "Of Ambition," but rather to provide a medium for the release of an always excess of desire, specifically the desire for freedom. This is a desire not just for any particular object, but for a mode of creative self-activity, and in this sense it is, to paraphrase Lefort, a desire not to have but rather to be.[56]

Such a desire is articulated particularly well in the *Florentine Histories* by a member of the Signori after Walter, Duke of Athens, had managed to install himself as de facto prince in Florence. After warning the duke of the dangers his extraordinary command would entail

---

54 Ibid.

55 Ibid.

56 Lefort, "Machiavelli and the *Verità Effetuale*," 112. Notably, however, whereas the desire "to be" is associated with the people and corresponds to the desire not to oppressed, the *grandi* possess instead a desire "to have" corresponding to their desire to oppress. See, for example, Claude Lefort, "Machiavel: la dimension économique du politique," in *Les formes de l'histoire: essais d'anthropologie politique* (Paris: Gallimard, 1978), 131.

to himself as a consequence of the hatred engendered by his private appropriation of power, the speaker goes on to posit the existence of that desire for freedom which, once again, is seen as manifest even in social contexts in which populations have no direct experience of free life itself: "That the time to consume the desires for freedom is not enough is most certain: for [freedom] is often taken up in a city by those who have never tasted it, but loved it only through the memory that their fathers had left them; and therefore, when recovered, they preserve it with every obstinacy and danger. And if ever their fathers had not remembered it, the public palaces, the places of the magistrates, the insignia of the free orders recall it: these things must be recognized with the utmost desire by the citizens."[57] And what is more, the positive form to this desire, the fact that it cannot be reduced merely to a negative desire to live secure in one's possessions, is suggested by the speaker's following claim that no amount of external goods, nor humane treatment or non-interference, is sufficient to counter it: "Which works of yours do you want to be a counterbalance to the sweetness of living freely, or to make men lose the desire for these conditions? Not if you were to add all of Tuscany to this dominion, and if every day you were to come back into this city triumphant over our enemies: for all of the glory would not be its, but yours, and the citizens would not acquire subjects, but fellow slaves, in which they would see their servitude reaggravated. And while your customs would be saintly, your modes benign, your judgments upright, they would not be enough to make you loved; and if you believe that they would be enough, you would deceive yourself, because to one accustomed to living untied, every chain weighs and every bond constrains him."[58] Popular desire thus exceeds the production of a space of negative liberty, this being here represented in the speaker's claim that bringing instrumental benefit to the city through benign modes and upright judgment, at least inasmuch as these are uninitiated by citizens or by those publicly authorized by citizens, is no substitute for self-determination. What the people desire is to be free, and this condition of being free can only be actualized in participatory political activity.

---

57 Machiavelli, "Istorie fiorentine," bk. 2.34.
58 Ibid.

The "Discourse on Florentine Affairs"
and the Democratic Imperative

Machiavelli's most concise articulation of this movement, from the recognition of the being of popular ambition to the demand for this ambition's actualization in concrete political participation, occurs in the "Discourse on Florentine Affairs." This text was written for Pope Leo X and is often dismissed as a compromised document from which no democratic lessons can be learned as a consequence of the multiple instances of overt Medici flattery, and the seeming guarantee of the perpetuation of a princely space within the proposed republican constitution. The "Discourse" can nevertheless be read, once these criticisms are properly situated within the social-historical context leaning upon Machiavelli, as an essential moment contributing important normative content to the Machiavellian theory of radical democracy. Such content, furthermore, to the extent that it articulates the form of relation between popular desire and popular rule, exceeds the common reading of the text as a representation of a potential transitional movement from the principality to the republic.[59] In the "Discourse" we can isolate two related democratic moments: the first in Machiavelli's recognition of the need for a popular institutional space for the venting of citizen desire, and the second in the call for a gradual deepening of this space through the enlargement of the sphere of popular participation over time.

Machiavelli begins by writing, "The reason why Florence has always varied frequently in its government, has been because it has been neither a republic nor a principality that has had its necessary quality; for one cannot call that principality stable where things are done according to the will of one, and decided with the consent of many; nor can one believe that republic to be enduring where those humours that need to be satisfied for the republic not to be ruined are not satisfied."[60]

---

59 See, for example, Gatti, *Ideas of Liberty in Early Modern Europe*, 28; Joseph Francese, "La meritocrazia di Machiavelli. Dagli scritti politici alla *Mandragola*," *Italica* 71, no. 2 (1994): 153–75; Luca Baccelli, "Political Imagination, Conflict, and Democracy," in *Machiavelli on Liberty and Conflict*, ed. David Johnston, Nadia Urbinati, and Camila Vergara (Chicago: University of Chicago Press, 2017), 359.

60 Niccolò Machiavelli, "Discursus florentinarum rerum post mortem iunioris Laurentii Medices," in *Tutte le opere*, 24.

Florence's oscillation between these two forms of regime as a consequence of each one's internal structural contradictions point to a fundamental polarity of government. Indeed, in the "Discourse" Machiavelli
maintains that when it comes to forms of state there are in fact only two
options, the principality or the republic: "no state can be ordered that is
stable if it is not either a true principality or a true republic, because all
of the governments between these two are defective."[61] This polarity,
however, is not an absolute one, there being a sort of dialectic between
the principality and the republic, the dissolution of each being achieved
through the tendency toward the other: "the principality has only one
way toward its dissolution, which is to descend to the republic; and so
the republic has only one way to being dissolved, which is to ascend up
to the principality."[62] The fact, however, that there is no principle or law
of motion that would direct the movement from one to the other demonstrates both Machiavelli's rejection of any type of cycle of government, as well as any form of government that could successfully
mediate between the two forms, such as in the classical image of the
mixed regime. Indeed, "All the other ones are useless and of very short
life."[63] According to this typology, then, there is simply popular government in which the people have an active role in rule, and all other
governments in which they do not, the vast plurality of non-democratic
regimes being collapsed into one category defined negatively in terms
of their shared lack. The republican criterion is here not simply found
in the existence of government oriented toward the institution of policies benefiting the common good, but toward concrete popular participation. This is why, for example, the government of Maso degli Albizzi
was bound to fail, for he attempted to order a "republic governed by
aristocrats," a fundamental contradiction in terms.[64] It would then be
correlatively the case that it is impossible to ground a long-lasting principality in the patronage of the people. As Giorgio Cadoni notes, "One
of the theses of the 'Discourse on Florentine Affairs' is that the only
possible principality is that which is founded on the support of the
grandi, and on the oppression of the masses."[65] If such is the case, then

---

61 Ibid., 26.
62 Ibid.
63 Ibid.
64 Ibid., 24.
65 Giorgio Cadoni, "Machiavelli teorico dei conflitti sociali," in *Machiavelli attuale /
    Machiavel actuel*, ed. Georges Barthouil (Ravenna: Longo Editore, 1982), 21.

Machiavelli's programmatic advice in *The Prince* regarding the need for a popular ground for foundation and preservation can only suggest the necessarily temporary form of the new principality.

Although Machiavelli initially claims that there is a foundation upon which one can judge the form of government that is most appropriate given existing social conditions, specifically the presence or non-presence of equality, there is a suggestion that there is a more primary ethical ground for his preference. The content of this ground is anticipated by Machiavelli's once more calling attention to the natural predilection that individuals have toward experiencing and enjoying the new: "Nor should one believe it to be true that men easily return to the old and customary mode of living, because this occurs when the old life is more pleasing than the new; but when it pleases less, they will not return if not forced, and then live for only as long as that force endures."[66] People are thus not only shackled to the past, to their already existent modes of doing and being, but are in fact open to and desirous of the new. This desire is given an outlet in the construction of a space within the proposed body politic for popular political creation. Although attempting to convince the Medici that establishing a principality in a city such as Florence would be not only difficult, but "inhuman and unworthy of anyone who desires to be held merciful and good," he nevertheless attempts to temper his proposal in their eyes, both through the suggestion that the movement toward republicanism would further esteem them, and through preserving a form of political inequality by ensuring that the highest offices would be occupied by elites.[67] We should not be misled, though, by the fact that Machiavelli's proposal grants the highest authority within the city to such seeming eminents – at least insomuch as the city contains citizens who "are arrogant and believe that they deserve to come before the others; to satisfy them is necessary in ordering a republic."[68] The historical reality of the contemporary Florentine situation thus structures the political possibility

---

66 Machiavelli, "Discursus florentinarum rerum post mortem iunioris Laurentii Medices," 26.

67 Ibid., 27.

68 Ibid. And although Machiavelli suggests that the three classes identified in Florence exist in all cities, earlier he concedes that it is possible to imagine a situation in which "all the nobility would have to be eliminated, and reduced to an equality with the others." Ibid. The potential for such an elimination will be further explored in the next chapter.

germinating within the city. For the grandees Machiavelli thus proposes a new Signoria composed of "sixty-five citizens of at least forty-five years, fifty-three for the major [guilds] and twelve for the minor; and they should remain in the government for life."[69] One member drawn from the Signoria should furthermore serve as Gonfalonier of justice for a fixed term of two or three years. This body minus the Gonfalonier would be divided into two groups of thirty-two, which would alternate governing on a yearly basis, and which would be further subdivided into groups of eight, rotating into and out of authority every three months. The second class of middling citizens, furthermore, would be satisfied through the institution of a permanently held Council of two hundred made up of individuals of at least forty years of age, one-hundred and sixty of whom would be selected from the major guilds and forty of whom would be selected from the minor guilds.[70]

After outlining the institutions meant to satisfy these elites and the middle group of citizens, Machiavelli turns to the largest group within the city, the people. Once again he emphasizes the insatiability of the desire of the people, and explicitly identifies its satisfaction with the establishment of a participatory space guaranteeing a popular role in government, a space furthermore that allows for the continual expression of ambition: "It now remains to satisfy the third and final class of men, which is the whole of the citizens: these are never satisfied (and whoever believes otherwise is not wise) if their authority is not restored or promised to be restored."[71] Each social class is seen as requiring its own institutional outlet to the extent that each possesses the same ambitious spirit seeking externalization. The people, contrary to various conservative or anti-democratic readings, is not an inert mass that is capable of being pacified through the guaranteed establishment of a private security, but rather an active force that seeks a concrete place in government in order to vent its ambition. Their participation would be achieved through the re-establishment of "the hall of the Council of one-thousand, or at least six-hundred citizens, who would distribute, in the same way that they had already distributed, all the offices and magistracies, except for the aforementioned Sixty-five, Two-hundred,

---

69 Machiavelli, "Discursus florentinarum rerum post mortem iunioris Laurentii Medices," 27.
70 Ibid., 28.
71 Ibid.

and Eight of the *balía*."[72] Because the people possess the same participatory desire for self-expression as do the other groups of citizens, they will never be contented through the preservation of their security alone, but rather require an active place in government. Hence, "Without satisfying the whole of the people, it is not possible to render a stable republic. The whole of the Florentine citizens will never be satisfied unless the hall is reopened."[73]

In addition, Machiavelli also calls – "in order that the whole of the people … is satisfied" – for the establishment of sixteen citizen provosts, four of which would be chosen by lot to hold office for one month at a time.[74] The provosts would scrutinize the elite institutions in order to ensure no decision contrary to the common good would be enacted, Machiavelli writing that "the thirty-two would not be able to decide anything without the presence of said provosts," and that "nor could the Council of two-hundred do anything, if there were not at least six of the sixteen provosts."[75] Through such institutions common citizens have the ability to not only accuse others who might transgress civil life in common, but also are given an additional field for the expulsion of their creative energy. Machiavelli thus writes: "It is also not good that citizens who have a hand in the state should not have someone who observes them, and makes them refrain from activities that are not good, removing from them that authority that they use badly. The other reason is that, through removing from the universality of the citizens, by raising up the Signoria as you do today, the power of being Signori, it is necessary to restore to them an office that resembles that which is taken away: and this [new office] is greater, more useful to the republic, and more honourable than that [old office]."[76]

After articulating the need for a popular venting of desire, in the final pages of the "Discourse" Machiavelli suggests a will to intensify his seemingly modest democratic reforms after the death of Giovanni de' Medici. He speaks, for example, of the existing proposals as meant to be instituted within "the life of Your Holiness," even writing that as "Your Holiness and the most reverend monsignor are living, [the state] is a

---

72 Ibid., 28–9.
73 Ibid., 29.
74 Ibid.
75 Ibid.
76 Ibid., 29–30.

monarchy, because you command all the arms, you command the criminal judges, you have the laws in your breast."[77] Machiavelli is both flattering the Medici in the hopes that they will overlook the fully democratic potential germinating in the reforms, while at the same time expressing a wish for the further entrenchment of democracy, which would receive a popular demand after the death of Giovanni. Machiavelli thus writes: "We do not yet see how the universality of the citizens cannot be satisfied, seeing restored that part of the distributions, and seeing the others *little by little fall into their hands*."[78] Such would ultimately be of the highest benefit to the city, and generate additional reputation for the reformers, and this because "I believe that the greatest honour that men can have is that voluntarily given them by their homeland: I believe that the greatest good that one does, and the most pleasing to God, is that which one does to one's homeland. Besides this, there is no man so exalted in any of his actions, as are those who with laws and institutions reform republics and kingdoms: these are, after those who have been Gods, the first praised."[79] If Giovanni does not seek after his glory through the initial movement toward genuine republican life, the city will never be free of threats and ills. Machiavelli, though, is aware that it is not possible to order a perpetual republic, to construct a system of orders that is capable of fixing the being of the polity and eliminating all accidents and dangers. That said, the form of regime most able to successfully ward off such dangers is one structured according to a principle of self-government, that is, one ordered "in a way that it administers itself."[80] In such a state "it is enough that Your Holiness keeps half an eye facing it."[81] In the final instance the healthiest city is one that has orders and institutions structured such that "each person will have a hand in them,"[82] that is to say, such that each person will have an opportunity to actively participate in political life, thereby achieving satisfaction through the expulsion of creative energy.

---

77 Ibid., 30.
78 Ibid. Emphasis added. In framing his proposal in this way, Machiavelli, always aware of the historical conditions that structure potentiality, thus "adjusts to the reality of the present." Cadoni, *Crisi della mediazione politica e conflitti sociali*, 161.
79 Machiavelli, "Discursus florentinarum rerum post mortem iunioris Laurentii Medices," 30.
80 Ibid., 31.
81 Ibid.
82 Ibid., bk. 31.

The Ground of Equality:
The Competency of Popular Judgment

In the previous two sections I attempted to demonstrate that Machiavelli locates in popular desire an ambitious impulse to self-expression. Democratic participation can thus not be rejected as a Machiavellian ideal as a consequence of the people's lack of such an impulse. There is, however, another ground upon which readers attempt to deny Machiavelli's democratic ethics. This denial is based on the assumption that the people, regardless of whether or not they possess an ambitious desire that looks to realize itself through political participation, lack the requiste cognitive ability, either as individuals or as a collectivity, to initiate informed and reasoned policy decisions.[83] The fact that members of the people lack certain critical-rational faculties necessitates that they should be entrusted only with that minimal amount of authority that they are capable of exercising competently, matters of legislation, for example, being left to political elites.

Hence, for example, the influential reading of Strauss, who argues that to the extent that the people are moved by mere appearances they are incapable of penetrating to the truth of objects in themselves, and thus must be guided to act by wise and prudential leaders: "The true issue becomes visible once one reflects on the fact that the multitude or the plebs needs guidance. This guidance is supplied ordinarily by laws and orders which, if they are to be of any value, necessarily originate in superior minds, in the minds of founders or of princes."[84] Whereas princes are superior in creating new laws and orders, the people are superior only in maintaining them, and this because whereas princes are rational and innovative, the people are conservative and traditional: "The people is the repository of the established, of the old modes and orders, of authority."[85] Even if the republic is oriented toward the actualization of the common good or the good of a majority, the people should not have access to legitimate institutions of rule: "The majority

---

83 For examples of readers who affirm popular ambitious desire yet see essential differences in individuals' capacities for the realization of this desire, see Gilbert, *Machiavelli and Guicciardini*, 187; Fischer, "Machiavelli's Political Psychology," 790; Fischer, "Machiavelli's Rapacious Republicanism," xlviii.
84 Strauss, *Thoughts on Machiavelli*, 129–30.
85 Ibid., 130.

cannot rule. In all republics, however well ordered, only a tiny minority ever arrives at exercising functions of ruling. For the multitude is ignorant, lacks judgment, and is easily deceived; it is helpless without leaders who persuade or force it to act prudently."[86]

It is not simply readings influenced by Strauss, however, that reject popular political competency. Even those readers of Machiavelli who emphasize his normative concern with the good of the people and the desire for popular civic participation still tend to minimize the potential for concrete rule on the part of common citizens. Hence, for example, Alfredo Bonadeo writes that Machiavelli "was aware of the limitations inherent to the actual and potential political power and value of the people," the most notable such limitations being the people's lack of leadership and practical knowledge.[87] Similarly, and despite the fact that she stresses a universal human desire for self-legislation, Erica Benner nevertheless still locates in Machiavelli's work a recognition of the need for a differentiation of political tasks grounded in a disparity of political capacity: "In all his main works Machiavelli stresses the need for a clear division of political labor between the few who exercise authority and the many who obey."[88]

The passage most often pointed to as problematizing this affirmation of a strict inequality of intelligences in Machiavelli's thought is *Discourses* 1:58, entitled "The multitude is more wise and more constant than a prince." Machiavelli frames the chapter as a critique of Livy's assertion regarding the inconstancy and vanity of the multitude. In this

---

86 Ibid., 260. Following Strauss, Vickie Sullivan argues that even in those instances in which Machiavelli seems to be democratically oriented, such is a merely instrumental dissimulation meant to pacify the common citizens who are always a majority within the city. Sullivan, *Machiavelli, Hobbes, and the Formation of Liberal Republicanism in England*, 40.

87 Alfredo Bonadeo, "The Role of the People in the Works and Times of Machiavelli," *Bibliothèque d'Humanisme et Renaissance* 32, no. 2 (1970): 375.

88 Benner, *Machiavelli's Ethics*, 270. Many further manifestations of such a position could be presented. See, for example, Burnham, *The Machiavellians*, 51; Germino, "Second Thoughts on Leo Strauss's Machiavelli," 810; Orr, "The Time Motif in Machiavelli," 208; Eugene Garver, "After *Virtù*: Rhetoric, Prudence, and Moral Pluralism in Machiavelli," *History of Political Thought* 27, no. 2 (1996): 212; Janara, "Machiavelli, Elizabeth I and the Innovative Historical Self," 484; Nomi Claire Lazar, "Must Exceptionalism Prove the Rule? An Angle on Emergency Government in the History of Political Thought," *Politics and Society* 34, no. 2 (2006): 256; Balot and Trochimchuk, "The Many and the Few."

judgment, Machiavelli maintains, Livy is entirely within the main-stream of the Western tradition of thought, whose representatives have almost always posited a stark distinction between the intellectual capacities of the few and the many. In attempting to refute the legiti-macy of this distinction Machiavelli knows that he is staking out a scan-dalous position, writing that "I want to defend a thing that, as I said, has been accused by all the writers."[89] Such accusations are from his perspective ungrounded, though, to the extent that they are ahistorical, the writers not situating their analyses of popular capacity in reflection on the concrete social-historical conditions within which subjectivity is developed. Specifically, when comparing the qualities of peoples to those of princes, we must begin by attempting to equalize the condi-tions of evaluation to as great a degree as possible. If such an equaliza-tion is achieved, we can only conclude that there exists a general equality between peoples and princes, the critics of popular judgment simply arbitrarily selecting the objects of analysis without any consid-eration of the contingent background conditions that structure an always negative human nature. Such an abstraction is for Machiavelli theoretically illegitimate. He hence claims that "as to that defect of which the writers accuse the multitude, they can accuse all men par-ticularly, and above all princes; for everyone who is not regulated by the laws would make those same errors as the unshackled multitude."[90] Indeed, one could easily proceed in the investigation from an opposite route, selectively examining the being of princes who act contrary to apparent reason, Machiavelli noting that "there are and there have been many princes, and the good and wise ones have been few."[91]

---

89 Machiavelli, "Discorsi sopra la prima Deca di Tito Livio," bk. 1.58.
90 Ibid.
91 Ibid. Just as he will challenge Livy's assessment of the deliberative capacities of the people most generally, so too will Machiavelli challenge Livy's assessment of the deliberative capacities of the common soldier more particularly, maintaining that Livy is mistaken in thinking that Roman growth owed more to the virtue of the city's captains than its soldiers. Indeed, in many of Livy's own accounts are we able to find evidence of the spontaneous ability of the soldiers to self-generate modes and orders independent of elite guidance. Ibid., bk. 3.13. Hence, for example, the Roman army's recovery and self-organization in Spain after the death of its two leaders and subsequent securing of Roman rule. Indeed, when Machiavelli two chapters later maintains that when it comes to matters of war it is useless to divide com-mand among many, this imperative is not grounded in any observation regarding an inequality of capacity. The need to identify a source of final authority is grounded in

Already in chapter 2 I identified the error of those readers of Machia-velli who attempt to abstract the particular manifestation of human being from the historical context within which it is articulated, positing a mere appearance as a transcendental universal applicable in all times and places. Against such totalizing theoretical tendencies Machiavelli rejects the vision of both fundamental human goodness and fundamen-tal human badness, locating the appearance of both in concrete social facts of existence, in whether or not individuals have been institution-ally socialized to civility. The demand for the same contextualization of evaluation is made during Machiavelli's discussion of popular judg-ment in 1:58. One cannot compare, as Livy and the other classical authors do, a prince of a well-ordered city with an unshackled multi-tude lacking regulation: "for the comparison ought to be posed with a multitude regulated by the laws such as [those princes] are; and there will be found in it the same goodness that we see to be in them, and it will be seen to neither dominate arrogantly nor meekly serve: as was the Roman people, who, while the Republic was uncorrupted, *never served meekly nor dominated arrogantly*; indeed, with its orders and mag-istrates it held its position honourably."[92] The italicized portion of the above quotation is especially significant, for it simultaneously reveals that the people are neither naturally passive, nor is their energy when mediated through certain institutional channels naturally oriented toward the actualization of self-interest. On the contrary, the form of popular participatory action is structured by its institutional back-ground conditions, a good organization of civic life being one that is able to productively direct ambition, a direction that depends in the first instance on the fundamental human capacity for reflective self-activity.

The potential range of forms of this self-activity is wide in scope, Machiavelli mentioning in this chapter a few of the political tasks that the people are potentially capable of excelling at. They can, for exam-ple, demonstrate a legislative ability surpassing that of princes, being able to critically reflect on the demands of the situation and formulate prudent policy in light of their consideration and comprehension of the

---

the specificity of military technique alone, for although many individuals might be capable of performing the task competently, the number occupying the position at any one time must be limited for practical reasons. Ibid., bk. 3.15.

92 Machiavelli, "Discorsi sopra la prima Deca di Tito Livio," bk. 1.58.

conditions within which they act. When the situation demands creative intervention they initiate new modes, while respecting the legislative authority of others when appropriate. Hence "when it was necessary to move against a powerful person, it did so, as is seen in Manlius, in the Ten, and in others who sought to oppress it," and yet "when it was necessary to obey the dictators and the consuls for the public safety, it did so."[93] The popular capacity for critical interrogation also manifests itself in the people's superior ability to judge between competing claims: "As to judging things, one sees very rarely – when [the people] hears two speakers taking different sides, and when they are of equal virtue – that [the people] not take up the better opinion, and not understand the truth that it hears."[94] It is this ability to make prudent judgment after representing and mediating between conflicting positions that makes the people also better suited to choosing magistrates than the prince, the latter having a tendency to be persuaded by powerful and corrupt individuals. Machiavelli thus notes that "in so many hundreds of years, in so many elections of consuls and tribunes, it did not make four elections of which it had to repent."[95]

Machiavelli provides a more detailed account of this phenomenon in *Discourses* 3:34, where he poses the question as to how individuals go about judging potential magistrates, stating initially that "the people in its distributing goes according to what is said of one through public voice and fame – when his works are not otherwise known to it – or through the presumption or opinion that it has of him."[96] These opinions "are caused either by the fathers of these, for being great and valiant men in the city it is believed that their sons ought to be like them, until such time as through their works [the people] perceive the opposite; or it is caused by the modes taken by he of whom we are speaking of. The best modes that can be taken are: to keep company with serious men, of good customs, and reputed wise by everyone."[97] Although perhaps initially suggesting an aristocratic affirmation of a principle of heredity, Machiavelli here is actually implicitly recognizing the power of positive socialization, noting that if one keeps good company one

---

93 Ibid.
94 Ibid.
95 Ibid.
96 Ibid., bk. 3.34.
97 Ibid.

has the strong potential to be educated to that company's good modes. More notably, however, Machiavelli identifies as the greatest source of public recognition the explicit doing of virtuous works. The people are seen as capable of prudently judging the virtue of others according to all three of these above-mentioned modes (through consideration of the actor's legacy, the actor's current company, and the actor's good works): "the people, when it begins to give a position to one of its citizens, by relying on those three reasons written above, does not found itself badly."[98] And later, when virtue is further generalized through increased democratic institutionalization, the people "can almost never be deceived."[99]

For Machiavelli the key criterion for competent human judgment is not the possession of any intrinsic skill or capacity, but rather access to those facts of existence that constitute the historical present. If people have access to such facts they will generate decisions of equal or superior worth than princes. Machiavelli is thus concerned with thinking about the construction of institutional orders that allow the people to acquire the knowledge of the world needed to make informed judgments.[100] And indeed, once these orders are in place they will err less than princes, to the extent that the latter's counsellors, lacking the people's diversity of perspective, are inferior to popular orders and deliberative spaces as modes of knowledge acquisition. Machiavelli thus writes: "And because it can be that peoples might be deceived about the fame, the opinion, and the works of a man, esteeming them greater than they are in truth – which would not happen to a prince, because he would be told and he would be warned by those who council him – so that peoples also do not lack these councils, good orderers of republics

---

98 Ibid.

99 Ibid.

100 Cary Nederman contrasts this discursive republicanism with that of James Harrington, for whom "public decision-making must be conducted in accordance with a strict principle of right reason, accessible only to a wise few, who therefore take it upon themselves to serve as guardian of the people for the sake of common benefit." Nederman, "Rhetoric, Reason, and Republic," 266. Indeed, Harrington himself in *The Commonwealth of Oceana* perceives Machiavelli's hostility to the idea of a privileged noble class, going on to defend the central place that the nobility should have in popular government as a corrective to Machiavelli's view. James Harrington, "The Commonwealth of Oceana," in *The Commonwealth of Oceana and A System of Politics*, ed. J.G.A. Pocock (Cambridge: Cambridge University Press, 1992), 15.

have ordered that when they have to create the supreme offices of the city, where it would be dangerous to put inadequate men, and seeing the popular will directed at creating something that would be inadequate, it is lawful to every citizen, and is attributed to his glory, to publicize in speech the defect of that one, so that the people, not lacking knowledge of him, can judge better."[101] Machiavelli in this passage is certainly not denying that democratic life does not necessitate a division of political tasks, that there are not certain political roles that require a particular skill that not all possess as a consequence of divergent educations and upbringings. However, in these cases the people are seen as having ultimate responsibility for choosing who fills these offices, the form of this choosing extending well beyond the aristocratic mode of election to include more comprehensive interrogation and scrutiny. Such interrogation depends upon the people possessing a critical rationality that allows them to fully represent to themselves the spectrum of opportunity and comprehend the demands of the political situation.

The quality of the people's selection, the fact that it is grounded in a highly reflective scrutiny of the necessity of the objective circumstances, is revealed in the fact that they do not uncritically or reactively elevate members of their own class to positions simply as a result of their social affiliation. Hence in *Discourses* 1:47 Machiavelli notes a key event in the plebeian confrontation with the noble appetite, here expressed through the exercise of consular authority. The Roman people, reflecting on their role in the city, determined that they deserved consular representation, and in response the nobility agreed to create a limited number of tribunes with consular power, tribunes that would be open to both nobles and plebs. Revealingly, however, despite the fact that the plebs had potential access to this office, the Roman people elected all nobles: "It appeared generally to the Roman plebs that it deserved the consulate, because it had more part in the city, because it carried more danger in wars, because it was that which with its limbs kept Rome free, and made it powerful. As it appeared to it, as was said, this desire was reasonable, it turned to obtaining this authority in any mode. But as it had to make judgment on its men particularly, it recognized the weakness of them, and judged that none of them deserved that which all of them

---

101 Machiavelli, "Discorsi sopra la prima Deca di Tito Livio," bk. 3.34.

together appeared to merit."[102] Although here plebeian desire for political self-expression is clearly evident, the people demonstrate a willingness for self-limitation in light of their consideration of the specificities of the political occasion.

What all of these examples of the competency of popular political judgment reveal to Machiavelli are not any natural facts about the unique being of the people, but rather the general fact of human equality. The distinctions that Machiavelli calls attention to are not grounded in essential differences of intellect or understanding, but are entirely reducible to historical circumstances of socialization. Hence a shackled people will show a more refined judgment than either an unshackled people or an unshackled prince. The fundamental nature of all, however, is equivalent: "the variation in their proceeding *does not stem from a diverse nature*, because all are in one mode; and if there is advantage of good, it is in the people, but from having more or less regard for the laws, within which both the one and the other live."[103] In this passage Machiavelli simultaneously reveals the identical nature of the people and the great (here represented in the figure of the prince), but also provides us with the means to comprehend the meaning of the distinction between the desire to oppress and the desire not to oppress. As I have attempted to show, both the people and the great possess the same fundamental ambition, an ambition that is partially expressed in the demand for outlets for political self-expression. The two humours thus cannot be grounded in a biological differentiation of psychic desire. On the contrary, they are two different forms of appearance of the single desire for ambitious expression. The difference between the two forms lies in the fact that whereas the people seek to satisfy their desire within the boundaries of a legal order that has been self-instituted and which all are subject to, the great have no such respect, believing themselves entitled to an exclusive satisfaction that knows no institutional limitations. In chapter 6 I will further explore the nature of this type of elite insolence within the context of the distinction between the modes of republican life detailed by Machiavelli in the *Florentine Histories* and the *Discourses on Livy*. For now, however, we can simply note that Machiavelli's distinction between a wise and an unwise people lay in

---

102 Ibid., bk. 1.47.
103 Ibid., bk. 1.58. Emphasis added.

this respect for the legitimacy of a democratic order in which all individuals are provided spaces for the expulsion of their creative energy. A wise people, in other words, is one that understands that it cannot will what it desires irrespective of consideration of the being of other citizens. Genuine freedom is thus constituted in autonomous self-regulation, for "a people that can do whatever it wants is not wise."[104]

It is because forms of institutionalization are capable of filtering popular desire so as to transform it into an articulate and self-conscious deliberative force that Machiavelli claims that the people "have one mind in the *piazza*, and another in the *palazzo*."[105] It is within the context of the need for a city to construct a system of institutions that would provide a stable space from which popular ambition can be vented that we must understand Machiavelli's image of "a multitude without a head," which he identifies as politically useless.[106] More often than not this appraisal is taken to be a manifestation of Machiavelli's anti-democratic tendencies, his belief that plebeian political intervention is only capable of becoming a consciously reflective and articulate force when it is directed by an elite leader in possession of a unique skill or intelligence.[107] This, though, does not seem to be the case. In *Discourses* 1:44 the multitude's lack of a head is identified with the multitude's lack of those institutions necessary for the deliberative expression of political will, the installation of a head in this instance being associated with the recreation of the military tribunes during the final period of the rule of the Ten.[108] This is explicitly confirmed by Machiavelli in 1:57 when the Virginia incident and the tribunes are once again invoked. Here Machiavelli argues that the transformation of the people into an active political force necessitates a process of institutionalization that is able to provide safe spaces of action from which each participant is able to self-articulate their political desire with security: "For there is nothing, on the one hand, more formidable than an unshackled multitude without a head; and, on the other hand, there is nothing more weak; for even

---

104 Ibid.
105 Ibid., bk. 1.47.
106 Ibid., bk. 1.44.
107 For example, Nikola Regent has recently claimed that the image of the multitude without a head is a symbol of the fact that "great individuals are needed to organize a republic, and to lead it." Nikola Regent, "Machiavelli, Empire, *Virtù* and the Final Downfall," *History of Political Thought* 32, no. 5 (2011): 755.
108 Machiavelli, "Discorsi sopra la prima Deca di Tito Livio," bk. 1.44.

though it has arms in hand, it is easy to diminish it, as long as you have a refuge where you can avoid the first surge. For when spirits have cooled down a little, and everyone sees that they have to return to their home, they begin to doubt themselves, and to thinking about their safety through flight or through conciliation. Therefore a multitude so excited, wanting to avoid these dangers, has immediately to make from itself a head to correct it, to hold it united, and to think of its defence."[109] Machiavelli is here suggesting that the head is not an exalted individual in possession of a unique rationality or intelligence, but simply the institution, providing a concrete example of such a process of subject formation when stating that it occurred in Rome after the death of Virginia, when the plebs self-instituted the twenty tribunes.

Indeed, against the seemingly elitist model of single-person political transformation suggested by the transitional reading of the relation between *The Prince* and the *Discourses*, Machiavelli here gestures toward a dialogical model of self-transformation made possible as a consequence of the receptivity of the people to rational argumentation. Hence in 1:58 Machiavelli claims that even an unshackled people can be returned to a good mode if it is "spoken to by a good man," and that "to cure the illness of the people words are enough."[110] In 1:54, where Machiavelli begins to overturn his more critical view of the people as expressed in earlier chapters of the *Discourses*, the multitude's capacity for achieving self-understanding through an openness to argumentation is again affirmed, Machiavelli tracing the root of reverence to an actor's ability to rationally persuade a critical people of the good of a policy. The example given is that Francesco Soderini, who during a factional dispute between the Frateschi and Arrabbiati inserted himself into a group of participants in an attempt to prevent further violence: "immediately after he heard the noise and saw the crowd, he put on his most honourable clothes, and over them his episcopal rochet, met those who were armed, and with presence and with words stopped them; this thing was celebrated and noticed throughout the whole city for many days."[111] In short, the people are seen as making prudent decisions when given the requisite access to information via reasoned argumentation.

---

109 Ibid., bk. 1.57.
110 Machiavelli, "Discorsi sopra la prima Deca di Tito Livio," bk. 1.58.
111 Ibid., bk. 1.54.

Such a position is only one manifestation of Machiavelli's affirmation of the transformative potential of dialogical activity, an activity that could potentially be developed as a ground from which to construct an alternative model of political change than the one suggested by the transitional reading. Many examples on this point could be provided, and not only from the *Discourses*. I have already, for example, called attention to the example of Philopoeman in *The Prince*, his critical scrutiny of his contextual situation containing a dialogical component grounded in the interrogative demand to give an account. Speaking of his relationship with his advisers, Machiavelli writes: "and he proposed to them, moving along, all the contingencies that can occur to an army; he perceived their opinions, said his own, supported it with reasons; so that through these continual cogitations there could never, while he guided the army, emerge any accident for which he did not have the remedy."[112] In chapter 23 of *The Prince* Machiavelli further highlights the necessarily dialogical form of prudent, princely decision making. The prince's advisers should be encouraged to speak freely to the former, and in turn "he ought to ask them about everything, and hear their opinions, and then decide for himself, in his mode."[113] The prince's right to make a final determination regarding a policy decision certainly does not degrade the authenticity of the deliberation. Machiavelli stresses that dialogue between the prince and his advisers must be authentic and substantive, the prince neither accommodating mere flatterers nor feigning interest in his council.[114] On the contrary, he must actively engage with and demonstrate a legitimate will to learn from others. Such an active ability to receive counsel is even identified as a constitutive part of princely virtue, Machiavelli writing that "a prince who is not wise in himself cannot be counselled well, unless indeed by chance he defers to one alone, who is a very prudent man, who governs entirely."[115] Dialogue meanwhile is not unidirectional, the prudence of the prince acting as a check on the counsel he receives, preventing the

---

112 Machiavelli, "Il Principe," chap. 14.
113 Ibid., chap. 23.
114 It should be noted that in *The Art of War* Machiavelli will go so far as to maintain that the authority of the ruler in a principality should be highly limited, the prince having executive right only in military matters. Machiavelli, "Dell'Arte della guerra," in *Tutte le opere*, 19.
115 Machiavelli, "Il Principe," chap. 23.

latter from manifesting the merely private interest of the adviser. If the prince lacks a wisdom of his own, "of the advisers, each will think of his own interest; he will not know how to correct or understand them."[116] Good counsel does not generate prudence, but counsel can become good only where the prince is prudent: "Thus one concludes that good counsel, from wherever it comes, should stem from the prudence of the prince, and not the prudence of the prince from good counsel."[117] Dialogue is ultimately a synthetic confrontation between two wisdoms, the quality of each allowing for a form of reciprocal exchange that deepens the understanding of both parties.

Machiavelli's readers have for many years attempted to highlight the extent to which the former's writings, in both form (e.g., through a discursive and conversational mode of presentation) and content (e.g., through the emphasis on the refinement of the critical-rational capacities of princes and peoples that results from discourse and deliberation), establish dialogue as a normative value. Such a value is operative not only in Machiavelli's explicitly republican writings but in *The Prince* as well.[118] Excepting perhaps the sum of his personal correspondence[119], however, the text in which Machiavelli's formal commitment to dialogical processes of learning and knowledge acquisition is most clearly articulated is *The Art of War.*[120] Unlike the false dialectic that moves

---

116 Ibid., bk. 23.

117 Ibid., chap. 23.

118 On the dialogical form of *The Prince*, for example, see John Parkin, "Dialogue in *The Prince*," in *Niccolò Machiavelli's The Prince: New Interdisciplinary Essays*, ed. Martin Coyle (Manchester: Manchester University Press, 1995), 65–88; Jean-Louis Fournel, "Is *The Prince* Really a Political Treatise? A Discussion of Machiavelli's Motivations for Writing *The Prince*," *Italian Culture* 32, no. 2 (2014): 85–97; Erica Benner, *Machiavelli's Prince: A New Reading* (Oxford: Oxford University Press, 2013).

119 For example, citing Machiavelli's most famous letter to Vettori in particular, Linda Zerilli highlights the extent to which Machiavelli here articulates an image of political theory as dialogical converstation, as "a transhistorical dialogue that links the voices of the present with those of the past in a discourse concerning the meaning of public life." Linda Zerilli, "Machiavelli's Sisters: Women and 'The Conversation' of Political Theory," *Political Theory* 19, no. 2 (1991): 252. For a comprehensive evaluation of the significance of the Machiavelli-Vettori letters see John M. Najemy, *Between Friends: Discourses of Power and Desire in the Machiavelli-Vettori Letters of 1513–1515* (Princeton: Princeton University Press, 1993).

120 As is often pointed, it is essential to recognize the extent to which the text's setting in the Rucellai gardens refers us to Machiavelli's own practical education in the transformative power of dialogue in the Orti Oricellari. In the first phase of

Platonic dialogues, for example, in which the protagonist is always in possession of the terminal knowledge in advance of the conversation, in *The Art of War* Fabrizio demonstrates a genuine openness to reflective alteration of his position as a consequence of his exposure to new evidences.[121] The emphasis is not on the unidirectional communication of a fixed, positive knowledge, but rather on the perpetually open process of learning and refinement. In Benedetto Fontana's words, "the conversation is in the process of becoming as it is carried forward by the questioning and the answering."[122] And even in those many instances when Fabrizio is seen as possessing the truth of a matter, that truth becomes properly established as truth only when his interlocutors autonomously affirm it themselves after rational consideration. As Erica Benner writes, "Although Fabrizio is much more experienced in war and politics, he urges his interlocutors not to accept uncritically anything he says. They must question him from many angles, and judge for themselves whether Fabrizio would know how to return to the ancient modes he praises. It is essential that they trust their own judgment more than his or anyone else's because they, in the end, must take responsibility for military and civil orders in their city."[123] The goal

---

meetings in the gardens, hosted by Bernardo Rucellai and his sons, the political spirit was strongly aristocratic, the participants being contemptuous of the perceived popular persecution of elite citizens. In the second phase, however, hosted by Bernardo's grandson Cosimo, and including the presence of Machiavelli, the spirit turns republican, despite the fact that the participants were still young aristocrats. Miguel Vatter writes that "no one knows exactly what Machiavelli said in his informal lessons, but we do know that some of the aristocrats in his audience, perhaps seduced by the mixed messages regarding the virtues of the plebeians contained in Machiavelli's lectures, were later accused of conspiring to eliminate the Medici and set up a new republic in Florence." Vatter, *Machiavelli's The Prince*, 11. For a short history of the Rucellai meetings see Felix Gilbert, "Bernardo Rucellai and the Orti Oricellari: A Study on the Origin of Modern Political Thought," *Journal of the Warburg and Courtland Institutes* 12 (1949): 101–13.

121 For an account of an example of this openness see Christopher Lynch, "The *Ordine Nuovo* of Machiavelli's *Arte della guerra*: Reforming Ancient Matter," *History of Political Thought* 31, no. 3 (2010): 423–4.

122 Fontana, *Hegemony and Power*, 113. For a contrary reading, which interprets *The Art of War* in terms of the discourse of systematic utopia, allegedly looking toward the construction of an internally coherent and totalizing form, see Rinaldo Rinaldi, "Appunti su utopia (tra Moro e Machiavelli)," *Forum Italicum* 21, no. 2 (1987): 217–25.

123 Benner, *Machiavelli's Ethics*, 112.

of Fabrizio and Machiavelli is thus to stimulate their interlocutors to think and act for themselves, not to contribute to the elevation of any single or group of individuals to the position of ultimate arbiter of authority based on a superior knowledge or capacity.

Although it is important to recognize the extent to which Machiavelli highlights the popular capacity for political judgment grounded in reflection and dialogue on historical conditions of existence, we should not be thereby misled into thinking that the criterion of proper political determination is for Machiavelli one of rightness, considered in terms of a decision's correspondence with some transcendent standard of truth. The specific content of the judgment is not to be assessed by its conformity to an exterior measure of rationality.[124] Rather, the legitimacy of the judgment is rooted in the extent to which it was formulated within a political context that is able to provide spaces for the mediating of competing positions, and the subsequent acquisition of a certain degree of knowledge of the relevant facts of social-historical existence. A judgment is correct, in other words, if it was made by the people in as full a light as possible of all the relevant evidences. What Machiavelli, in emphasizing the institutional conditions of competent popular judgment, is calling attention to is the extent to which the expression of the desire of the people must exceed mere voluntarism, the immediate and unrefined expulsion of will. It is not the content of the decision that is essential, but rather that the decision was made under deliberative conditions allowing for the actualization of the participants' critical and rational human faculties, faculties that they share with all others. The standard of correct political determination is no longer one of rationality, but rather one of desire.[125]

We already know that for Machiavelli it is impossible for a human subject to perfectly thematize the objective contours of reality, because

---

124 For a similar line of thought see McCormick, *Machiavellian Democracy*, 136.

125 Hence Claude Lefort's judgment that in chapter 25 of *The Prince* we see "suggested the idea that the power of man does not reside only (nor perhaps principally) in the exercise of intelligence, but is due to the initiative of the desiring subject." Claude Lefort, "Machiavel et les jeunes," in *Les formes de l'histoire: essais d'anthropologie politique* (Paris: Gallimard, 1978), 154. As noted by Ruth Grant, Machiavelli is concerned with demonstrating the impossibility of instituting a rational political theory grounded in a dispassionate consideration of interest. Ruth W. Grant, *Hypocrisy and Integrity: Machiavelli, Rousseau, and the Ethics of Politics* (Chicago: University of Chicago Press, 1997), 52.

of both the limitations of human conceptual appropriation and the chaotic and irregular form of the being of the world. Machiavelli never suggests that the people can transcend such limitations, only that the extent to which these limitations lean on them is no greater than in the case of others. He hence writes: "I conclude, therefore, against the common opinion which says that the people, when they are princes, are varying, mutable, and ungrateful, affirming that they are *not otherwise* in these sins than are particular princes."[126] The competency of popular judgment (or indeed of any judgment) does not lie in the fact that the people have access to a privileged knowledge discerned through the exercise of a perfect rationality, but rather in the fact that they are capable of articulating their desire in light of their reflective consideration of worldly possibility, or the effectual truth of the thing. They are capable of communicating their political will through speech, and of understanding the political will of others, this double capacity being in fact the foundation of Machiavelli's affirmation of freedom and equality.

The Ciompi Affirmation of Freedom and Equality

The ethical foundation for democratic life is grounded in Machiavelli's recognition of human equality, of the fact that the people are in possession of the same ambitious desire for self-expression as the great, and that they possess the same capacity for reflective judgment as the great. In the words of Filippo Del Lucchese, "If nature is the same for everybody, if the prince cannot lay claim to a superior political rationality, then the multitude can demand its entrance onto the political scene on par with the other players."[127] And indeed, the fact that the people need to be considered as meaningful actors is revealed through Machiavelli's perpetual effort to give a voice to popular political demands, an effort most notably expressed in the *Florentine Histories*.[128] Perhaps in no other place is Machiavelli's double affirmation of freedom and

---

126 Machiavelli, "Discorsi sopra la prima Deca di Tito Livio," bk. 1.58. Emphasis added.

127 Del Lucchese, *Conflict, Power, and Multitude in Machiavelli and Spinoza*, 123.

128 Erica Benner calls attention to Machiavelli's effort to give a voice to the entire plurality of elements within the city, such an effort speaking to the mutual implication of its citizens in a shared life. Benner, *Machiavelli's Ethics*, 34.

equality articulated with such passion as in his account of the revolt of the Ciompi.[129] What is unique in Machiavelli's retelling of the narrative is that the perspective of the lower class[130] becomes one worthy of being taken into account, its conflicts with other groups providing impetus to the movement of the republic. Unlike, for example, Plato's giving time to the sophist, Machiavelli does not let the worker speak in order to simply dialectically refute his argument and replace it with a superior one, but evaluates its legitimacy and respects it on its own terms.[131] Although many commentators question the precise degree to which, or whether at all, Machiavelli sympathizes with the insurrectionaries, the very fact that he provides an opportunity for the former to speak for themselves suggests at the very least a recognition of their human ability to articulate their political demand for equality, demonstrating the fact of the latter in this very movement.[132] The significance

129 For Niccolò Rodolico, in narrating the events of the revolt Machiavelli keeps alive a sense of the specificity of the political passions of the era, a sense which in fact would soon be lost. Niccolò Rodolico, *I Ciompi: una pagina di storia del proletariato operaio* (Firenze: G.C. Sansoni, 1945), x.

130 It should be noted that in keeping with the articulation of social division in terms of a primary distinction between two humours, Machiavelli does not undertake a detailed class analysis of the various gradations to be located within the labouring groups that lack guild association. As Michel Mollat and Philippe Wolff point out, members of the *sottoposti* were highly diverse with respect to economic and social status. For example, although there was a large group of sub-subsistence labourers, many of whom were recently peasants, there were also some who were economically of the same status as many guild members. In the final instance, "sociologically, it is impossible to regard the *sottoposti* as a whole, including the Ciompi, as a homogeneous class in the modern sense of the term." Michel Mollat and Philippe Wolff, *The Popular Revolutions of the Late Middle Ages*, trans. A.L. Lytton-Sells (London: George Allen and Unwin, 1973), 158. The fact that Machiavelli largely glosses over such internal distinctions reveals the extent to which the Ciompi stand in for the people and their desire most generally.

131 Martine Leibovici, "From Fight to Debate: Machiavelli and the Revolt of the Ciompi," *Philosophy and Social Criticism* 28, no. 6 (2002): 648, 655.

132 In this sense Machiavelli anticipates the recent democratic contributions of Jacques Rancière, who theorizes democratic practice in terms of the demonstration of an equality of intelligences, in terms of an excluded group's struggle to reveal its human capacities through speaking and thinking. Especially revealing here is Rancière's rereading of the first plebeian secession in Rome, where in response to the patrician denial of their being as humans, the plebs set out to assert themselves and their intelligence through their self-activity. Jacques Rancière, *Dis-Agreement: Politics and Philosophy*, trans. Julie Rose (Minneapolis: University

of the fact that Machiavelli's account of this event, despite any seeming ambivalence within it, goes against the current of all Florentine scholarship of the time, cannot be overstated. Michel Mollat and Philippe Wolff note that commentators on the revolt "are nearly all hostile to the Ciompi."[133] Indeed, with respect to his own historical context Machiavelli's sympathy with the Ciompi cause is singular. Hence Jurdjevic writes that "the Florentine historical tradition leading up to Machiavelli spoke with one voice in condemning this revolt. Machiavelli's humanist predecessors in the Florentine chancery, including Coluccio Salutati and Leonardo Bruni, consistently portrayed the Ciompi as an irrational, anarchic, and destructive mob, susceptible to the worst manifestations of demagoguery in the city's history."[134] This diagnosis is seen by such commentators as being not necessarily specific to the Ciompi case, but rather the tendencies and features identified and criticized are interpreted as necessary symptoms of any democratic movement. Hence Francesco Guicciardini's claim that in the time of the Ciompi Florence was "in the arbitrary and licentious power of the populace."[135] Licentiousness and arbitrary rule are of the essence of democratic politics to the aristocratic mind.

It is such thinking that Machiavelli's account attempts to counter. The centrepiece of this account is certainly the revolutionary speech of the anonymous Ciompo in book 3:13, the worker seeming to stand in for Machiavelli himself to the degree that he articulates various Machiavellian lessons and insights. For Yves Winter, Machiavelli's imagination of this speech is a key element that indicates his larger democratic and egalitarian commitments, and if readers of Machiavelli tend to ignore it, this is a consequence of their failure to comprehend the latter.[136] Indeed, in "rejecting aristocratic doctrines of natural hierarchy

---

of Minnesota Press, 1999), 24–5. Significantly, this episode as recalled by Rancière is also identified by Emmanuel Roux as belonging to the tradition of democratic action that Machiavelli is situated in and advancing. Emmanuel Roux, *Machiavel, la vie libre* (Paris: Raisons d'agir, 2013), 183–4. On the proximity of Machiavelli and Rancière see also Gaille, *Machiavel et la tradition philosophique*, 143.

133 Mollat and Wolff, *The Popular Revolutions of the Late Middle Ages*, 142.

134 Jurdjevic, *A Great and Wretched City*, 110–11.

135 Guicciardini, *Dialogue on the Government of Florence*, 135.

136 Winter, "Plebeian Politics," 737. Other democratic readers, on the contrary, have certainly recognized the speech's centrality. See, for example, John P. McCormick, "Machiavelli and the Gracchi: Prudence, Violence, and Retribution," *Global Crime* 10,

and inequality, the Ciompo makes the most radical claim for human equality in Machiavelli's work."[137] The affirmation of equality in the passage, however, is not expressed exclusively through the substantive claims regarding the being of the people, but rather has a double register. At the same time that the demand for political equality is made through a recognition of the conventional form of social hierarchy and the universality of human being, the speaker simultaneously, through his mode of action, manifests his equality via a clear demonstration of the type of human virtue detailed in *The Prince*. Regarding the former we may quote the best-known part of the speech, in which the Ciompo locates the existing forms of economic and political stratification in merely contingent facts of existence. Speaking to his fellows he states, "And do not be overawed by that antiquity of blood with which they reproach us; for all men, having had one same beginning, are equally ancient, and *by nature they have been made in one mode*. Strip us all naked: you will see that we are alike; dress us in their robes, and they in ours; without doubt we will appear noble and they ignoble, because only poverty and riches make us unequal."[138] The Ciompo makes the case that the superior social status of the nobles is not grounded in any special capacity or merit, or indeed in any type of particular qualification whatsoever, but rather in a mere accident of birth or circumstance. Even if it might appear that one's privileged position has a legitimate foundation in some sort of demonstration of superior capacity, such as in the ideological image of the self-made person, the Ciompo makes it clear that such an elevation is achieved only through a willingness to subvert established modes of social behaviour: "But if you will notice the mode of proceeding of men, you will see that all those with great riches and great power have arrived at them either through fraud or through force;

---

no. 4 (2009): 301; Dotti, *Niccolò Machiavelli: la fenomenologia del potere*, 10; Filippo Del Lucchese, *The Political Philosophy of Niccolò Machiavelli* (Edinburgh: Edinburgh University Press, 2015), 99. Compare such readings with that of Timothy Lukes, who speculates that in the Ciompi episode it is the figure of Niccolò who stands in for Machiavelli himself, possessing as he does, as opposed to the various hasty and unreflective members of the plebs not yet ready for republican life, a capacity to descend to the particulars in deliberative activity. Timothy J. Lukes, "Descending to the Particulars: The Palazzo, The Piazza, and Machiavelli's Republican Modes and Orders," *Journal of Politics* 71, no. 2 (2009): 10.

137 Winter, "Plebeian Politics," 746.
138 Machiavelli, "Istorie fiorentine," bk. 3.13. Emphasis added.

and these things, later, that they have usurped with deception or with violence, to conceal the ugliness of acquisition are made legitimate under the false title of earning."[139] The Ciompo seems to here, speaking in the midst of the entrenchment of relations of merchant capitalism in Florence, provide a proto-theory of primitive accumulation, noting the extent to which the original acquisition of wealth necessitates acting in a "rapacious and fraudulent" manner, or as Marx would say, through the methods of "blood and fire."[140]

The anonymous Ciompo, however, not only makes in his speech a call for equality, but demonstrates it through his very action. He thus actualizes that capacity for reflective self-activity which Machiavelli had identified in *The Prince* as a condition of virtuosity. The speech opens with an appeal to the people that the most effective course of action is one that adopts the modes of robbery and arson. Such an adoption, however, would certainly be no reactionary or voluntaristic response to an external stimulant, but the result of a considered decision preceded by intensive deliberation on the available options and their likely effects. The need for such reflective deliberation, the need to represent and mediate between potential trajectories of action, is affirmed multiple times. The first sentence of the speech, for example, reads: "If we had to *deliberate* now whether to take up arms, to burn and to rob the homes of citizens, to despoil the churches, I would be one of those who would *judge* it a choice to *think over*."[141] And a few sentences

---

139 Machiavelli, "Istorie fiorentine," bk. 3.13.

140 Ibid.; Karl Marx, *Capital: A Critique of Political Economy*, vol. 1, trans. Ben Fowkes (London: Penguin, 1976), 875. Also interpreting the Ciompi revolt in the theoretical terms of Marx, Simone Weil defines it as the first proletarian insurrection. Simone Weil, "A Proletarian Uprising in Florence," in *Selected Essays: 1934–43*, trans. Richard Rees (Oxford: Oxford University Press, 1962). More generally, Althusser refers to Machiavelli as one of the "true precursors of Marx," historically articulating as he does the form of appearance of class struggle at a particular conjuncture. Louis Althusser, "The Facts," in *The Future Lasts Forever: A Memoir*, ed. Olivier Corpet and Yann Moulier Boutang, trans. Richard Veasey (New York: New Press, 1992), 361. Such was also suggested by Lev Kamenev, who labels Machiavelli a "dialectician of brilliance," writing that "in the works of Machiavelli emperors, popes, kings, lords, bankers and merchants walk without masks, and by their actions confirm the truth of the historical views of the founders of dialectical materialism." Lev Kamenev, "Preface to Machiavelli," *New Left Review*, no. 1/15 (1962): 40, 42.

141 Machiavelli, "Istorie fiorentine," bk. 3.13. Emphases added.

later he states: "We must therefore look for two things and have, in our *deliberations*, two ends: the one is not to be able to be castigated for the things done by us in recent days, and the other is to be able to live with more freedom and more satisfaction than we have in the past. We should, therefore, so *it appears to me*, if we want to be forgiven for our old errors, to make new ones, redoubling the damages, and multiplying the arson and the robbery … To multiply damages, then, will make ourselves find forgiveness more easily, and will give us the way to getting those things that, for our freedom, we desire to have."[142] Contrary to his humanist counterparts who read the violence of the Ciompi as arbitrary and irrational, Machiavelli goes to great lengths to demonstrate that the recourse to violent modes was the productive result of a deliberative activity in which the actors evaluated strategies in light of their understanding of prior facts of history, and in light of the specific goals that they hoped to achieve, specifically their desire "to live with more freedom and more satisfaction."[143]

Contrary to an actor like Agathocles, for whom violence is deployed singularly as a universal political technique, the Ciompo makes it clear that the people's utilization of these methods in this instance is informed by their understanding of the concrete facts of the social-historical situation, not because the deployment of force is seen as exhausting the range of political possibility. In other words, force is deployed to the extent that it is what necessity requires given the objective situation of the Ciompi and of Florence as a whole at that time: "One ought therefore to use force when the occasion is given to us. There can be no better offered to us by fortune, citizens being still disunited, the Signoria uncertain, the magistrates dismayed: so that they can, before they unite and harden their spirit, be easily suppressed."[144] Indeed, in the second half of the speech the Ciompo provides a concise summary of the significance of the concept of *occasione* in Machiavelli's thought, highlighting the extent to which the seizing of the opportunity necessitates the actor's adoption of those specific modalities of action – again articulated through the contrasting of the ways of force and fraud – required given the existing state of the being of the world.[145] And similarly to the

---

142 Ibid. Emphases added.
143 Ibid.
144 Ibid.
145 Ibid.

virtuous prince, furthermore, the Ciompo realizes that in an unstable world perpetually in flux, should the occasion opened up by *fortuna* be seized it is necessary to act in a bold and decisive way: "The opportunity that the occasion brings us is fleeting, and it is in vain, when it has fled, to try and recapture it."[146] Such a popular display of boldness is certainly no marker of rashness or irrationality, but is a component of that critical and reflective human orientation that Machiavelli associates with *virtù*. Hence the Ciompo's articulation of the bold willingness to make a decision in the face of danger in terms of the exercise of a faculty of judgment: "I confess this choice to be bold and dangerous; but when necessity compels, boldness is judged prudence."[147]

In addition to the anonymous Ciompo's call for and demonstration of equality, the second significant detail to be noted in Machiavelli's narrative is the primacy of the political as the field for Ciompi self-expression. It might be tempting to read the episode in primarily economic terms, as being stimulated by a grievance with respect to material distribution and looking only toward the satisfaction of this grievance in a mere rearrangement of an economic pattern of things. Machiavelli thus writes of "a hatred that the lesser people had for the rich citizens and princes of the guilds, it not appearing to them that they were being satisfied for their labour in accordance with what they believed they justly deserved."[148] It soon becomes clear, however, that the popular dissatisfaction is not merely a reactive response to the perception of material inequality, and hence potentially reconcilable through different forms of economic redistribution, but is actually a specifically political dissatisfaction with the lack of outlets for the expression of the people's will. Hence Machiavelli's stress on the existing composition of the guild system, the fact that certain groups, through being excluded from self-organization in a guild, lacked a mode through which they could direct their activity on their own terms: "in the ordering of the bodies of the guilds many of those practices in which the lesser people and the lower plebs laboured were without their own bodies of guilds, but were subject to various guilds suited to the quality of their practices. It arose that when they were either not satisfied for their labours, or in another way oppressed by their masters, they did not have

---

146 Ibid.
147 Ibid.
148 Ibid., bk. 3.12.

somewhere else to take refuge from the magistrate of that guild that governed them; from this it did not appear to them that they were granted that justice which they judged appropriate."[149]

Machiavelli thus theorizes in this chapter a sophisticated co-determination of economic and political inequality,[150] grounding the former partially in the latter, and perceiving protest over the former as a potential stimulant to the latter. This second movement is further explicated by Martine Leibovici. Leibovici notes that although the Ciompi's original concerns were economic in nature, this mutated into a specifically political demand (or better: the social extension of an already political demand articulated in an economic context) grounded in a desire for freedom: "Even if their motivation was economic in the first place, that struggle had begun to change them into politically autonomous actors. From now on, they would not content themselves with claiming better means of earning their living; they would also raise the question of their involvement in sharing political power itself."[151] As I have already noted, the action of the protesters was not indiscriminate or indeterminate revolt, but calculated action looking toward a concrete political end: "Parallel to the chain of violence, the people are acceding to the formulation of their desire for freedom; instead of undifferentiated robbery, we put forward new propositions of organization necessarily specific and definite."[152] Specifically, the call for the reorganization of the guilds – which again, is already partially political in nature – morphs into a call for explicit political power at the societal level, as initially represented, for example, in the demand for not only the creation of the new guild bodies, but for them to have their own Signori.[153] Hence, Mollat and Wolff write: "What was new and original in July and August was that the Ciompi adopted an organization of their own initiative with a view to seizing power."[154] Although the Signoria

---

149 Ibid.

150 On the extent to which the Ciompi revolt reveals the degree to which Machiavelli thinks the interrelationship of political and economic inequality and conflict see Filippo Del Lucchese, "Crisis and Power: Economics, Politics and Conflict in Machiavelli's Political Thought," *History of Political Thought* 30, no. 1 (2009): 75–96.

151 Leibovici, "From Fight to Debate: Machiavelli and the Revolt of the Ciompi," 649.

152 Ibid., 656.

153 Machiavelli, "Istorie fiorentine," bk. 3.15.

154 Mollat and Wolff, *The Popular Revolutions of the Late Middle Ages*, 143.

originally attempted to pacify the uprising through reprimanding certain government elites and rehabilitating some select Ghibellines, given the nature of the participatory desire such temporizing was insufficient to prevent the revolutionary explosion in July, which culminated in the seizing of the Palazzo Vecchio, the reassignment of Gonfalonier of justice, and the creation of new guilds and a new *balìa*. And: "Lastly, on 29 July, with a view to making permanent the movement of the commune toward democracy, the Ciompi burned the 'purses' containing the names of candidates for the magistature which were to be drawn by lot. New and enlarged lists had to be drawn up."[155]

Of all these events that speak to the existence of the popular positive desire for freedom and participatory self-expression, the most significant is the appointment of Michele di Lando to the position of Gonfalonier of justice. Machiavelli's account of di Lando reveals that ambiguity in his thought which I have referred to at several times in this study, and which is articulated most clearly in the transitional interpretation of the relationship between the principality and the republic. According to this view, which Machiavelli clearly promulgates in multiple places, the founding institution of good civic modes and orders is dependent upon the action of a sole individual who alone is able to create the institutional forms necessary for socializing individuals to a free way of life. Machiavelli repeats this position in his account of the revolt of the Ciompi. Di Lando's assent to the position of Gonfalonier of justice was wholly the result of a plebeian exercise of will, the people voluntarily, through a political act of delegation, consenting to have him function as an institutional representative for them. Speaking of di Lando's selection Machiavelli writes: "turning to the multitude, [Michele] said: 'You see: this palace is yours, and this city is in your hands. What do you think that you should do now?" To which all responded that they wanted him as Gonfalonier and lord, and to govern them and the city as it appeared best to him."[156] The election of di Lando is a signal of the people's recognition that the venting of its desire, if it is to be stably reproduced through time, requires a concrete outlet, a positive expression in the orders of the city. In this sense it is representative of the democratic necessity of sublimating popular

---

155 Ibid., 151.
156 Machiavelli, "Istorie fiorentine," bk. 3.16.

ambition through institutional channels that are able to give it a productive and socially beneficial expression.

The people soon learn, however, of the instability of all political
forms – that there is no terminal modality of political being capable of
indefinitely regulating human affairs – when di Lando violates his
mandate to express their will and desire in his new office. Specifically,
Michele in restructuring the orders of the city would give too many
titles and offices to the people's patrician enemies, enemies who still
harboured a humour to oppress and desired the expulsion of the people from public life. Thus "it appeared to the plebs that Michele, in
reforming the state, had been too partisan toward the greater people; it
neither appeared that they had as much a part in government as was
necessary to maintain and defend themselves; so, pushed by their usual
boldness, they again took up arms and tumultuously, under their
ensigns, came into the piazza."[157] What will occur next is a clear display
of plebeian self-institution. Disgusted by di Lando's subsequent cen-
sure of them in the face of their grievance, "the multitude, incensed
with the palace, settled at Santa Maria Novella, where they ordered
among themselves eight heads, with ministers and other orders that
gave them reputation and reverence; thus the city had two seats and
was governed by two different princes."[158] The delegates of the people
began to make further policy demands and decisions, undertaking a
bold attempt at redistributing the offices of the city in order to re-establish
a genuinely popular system of orders: "They took away from Messer
Salvestro de' Medici and from Michele di Lando all that in their other
decisions had been granted them; they assigned to many of themselves
offices and subsidies, to be able to maintain their position with dignity."[159] For a second time, then, the people demonstrate a capacity to
articulate their political desire, and outline a system of orders that they
deem capable of giving this desire a positive expression in the political
sphere.

Despite his sympathy for the plebeian cause, it seems clear that in
this dispute between the people and Michele di Lando Machiavelli
clearly comes down on the side of the latter, even going so far as to
write of him that "in spirit, in prudence, and in goodness he surpassed

---

157 Ibid., bk. 3.17.
158 Ibid.
159 Ibid.

any citizen of that time, and he deserves to be counted among the few who have benefited their homeland," and that "his goodness never let come into his mind a thought that would be contrary to the universal good."[160] Nevertheless, in providing his account Machaivelli demonstrates the existence of that popular capacity that renders the idea of singular institutionalization unnecessary as a mode of political foundation. The people themselves demonstrate during the revolt of the Ciompi their ability to autonomously institute political modes and orders that would be capable of actualizing their desire for freedom. And significantly, the development of such a will to participatory freedom is nurtured and expressed in a poorly ordered social context, thus demonstrating the extent to which the people are capable of transcending their one-sided private being in an autonomous way. What the revolt of the Ciompi seems to prove, in other words, is that political elites are not required in order to lead the people out of their corrupted state, but that the intrinsic popular desire for participatory self-expression, manifested in the concrete affirmation of the values of freedom and equality, is capable of being self-actualized.[161]

In this chapter I have argued that Machiavelli thinks about the being of the people and the being of the *grandi* in an identical way: although there exists no positive human nature that permanently outlines the structure of human life, it is nevertheless true that all individuals possess the same negative drive toward creative self-expression, this drive being that which accounts for the people's desire for participation in legislative political modes. At the same time, furthermore, Machiavelli also recognizes that all individuals are in possession of a certain political competency, an ability to articulate their will and formulate prudent

---

160 Ibid.

161 I thus disagree with readers such as Kiran Banerjee and Mauricio Suchowlansky, who argue that the Ciompi episode reveals Machiavelli's "pessimism concerning the plebs as agents of political innovation." Kiran Banerjee and Mauricio Suchowlansky, "Citizens, Subjects or Tyrants? Relocating the People in Pocock's *The Machiavellian Moment*," *History of European Ideas* 43, no. 2 (2017): 196. This is one manifestation of the now common reading which interprets the *Florentine Histories* as constituting a theoretical break in the Machiavellian oeuvre, initiating a more conservative and sceptical orientation toward the people most generally.

policy decisions in light of their internal deliberation on the opportunities for realizing this will. It is this double affirmation that is the ground for Machiavelli's ethical affirmation of democracy as the preferred political form of being.

The fact that Machiavelli has such a political preference, and that this preference is rooted in his belief in a fundamental human equality, is a fact that was certainly not lost on various of his contemporaries. Guicciardini, for example, clearly recognizes the democratic implications of Machiavelli's defence of popular rationality. Indeed, he criticizes Machiavelli for overestimating the political intelligence of the people and providing them with the most significant role to play in the reproduction of the life of the city. For Guicciardini the good of "a government of aristocrats" lay in the fact that it is ruled by "the most qualified men in the city," who "govern it with greater intelligence and wisdom than the masses."[162] There is simply a natural intellectual difference between the wise and the many that closes off in advance the possibility of effective popular government. However, unlike many other antidemocratic republicans who combine the rejection of popular political competency with an affirmation of the fundamentally passive and singular form of human desire, Guicciardini simultaneously recognizes the active and creative being of the people, as well as the people's fundamental plurality. Both of these latter facts, given the assumption of the inferiority of popular judgment, produce particularly pernicious civic effects. Regarding the first, Guicciardini writes that the people have a perpetual "desire for innovation."[163] This unstable desire seeking outward expression often leads to social persecution, a particular problem when directed against elites with the potential to improve the life of the city. Regarding the second, the "disharmony of minds," which concretely manifests itself in the production of "differing judgments, differing ideas, and differing ends," closes off the potential for the actualization of deliberative consensus produced via a mutually intelligible process of deliberation.[164]

---

162 Guicciardini, "Considerations on the *Discourses* of Niccolò Machiavelli," 389.

163 Ibid., 423.

164 Ibid., 422. Hence "to speak of the people is really to speak of a mad animal gorged with a thousand and one errors and confusions, devoid of taste, of pleasure, of stability." Francesco Guicciardini, *Maxims and Reflections of a Renaissance Statesman*, trans. Mario Domandi (New York: Harper, 1965), sec. C 140.

Like Guicciardini, Machiavelli also believes that the being of the people is multiple and fickle. This is a result of the fundamental form of human ambition, of the human desire to innovate, change, and overcome the existent. Unlike Guicciardini, however, this popular being is not differentiated from elite being in any originary way. There is no superior group of individuals in possession of a unique intelligence that would allow them to transcend their temporality. The type of perfectly rational deliberation that Guiccardini takes as a political ideal is for Machiavelli simply an ideological veil masking a form of contingent domination without any natural foundation. As I showed in this chapter, for Machiavelli princes are just as inconstant and variable as peoples. At the same time, peoples are potentially just as prudent and wise as princes. It is this double equality that Machiavelli's political thought is aimed at negotiating. The political question that Machiavelli's republican writings seek to answer is: what form of political regime is capable of harnessing the universal capacity for reflective judgment for the sake of the affirmation of the universal desire for creative self-overcoming?

Chapter Five

Social Equality and the Contingent Being of the Great

In the previous chapter I noted how Machiavelli's account of the revolt of the Ciompi suggested a co-determination of political and economic equality, the actualization of the former being seen as inconsistent with the preservation of the latter. In this chapter I will further explore this idea through situating Machiavelli's contention that the healthy republic must aim to equalize the distribution of economic resources – classically expressed in the formulation that maintains the necessity of keeping the public rich and the citizens poor – within the context of what remains a largely underdeveloped potentiality in his thought: that of the elimination of the *grandi* as an organized social class embodying a particular shared humour. Contrary to those readers, democratic and otherwise, who seemingly eternalize the existence of the *grandi*, defining popular participatory activity negatively in terms of its opposition to the activity of the great, I argue that Machiavelli unhinges the being of the great from any natural psychological considerations. If it is true that the people and the great share the same nature then there can be no essential ground distinguishing them, their opposition on the contrary being merely conventional. Machiavelli ultimately theorizes the *grandi* not in terms of a particular psychic orientation unique to them, but in terms of a contingent class composition. The great are those individuals who are able to consolidate themselves into a social group united in their end, which consists in leveraging their economic wealth to advance their own particular position within the city through excluding others from political modes and orders. The noble humour – the will to dominate expressed through conscious social action – only emerges with this consolidation. As I will stress below, the *grandi*'s desire to oppress considered as a humour only emerges in a class context, the concept of *umore* not referring to the direction of individual will.[1] The elimination of economic inequality thus presupposes the elimination of the *grandi* as a social class. After outlining the democratic deficits of those readings that eternalize the noble humour, and outlining some of the manifestations of Machiavelli's defence of economic equality, I will conclude this chapter by gesturing toward the potential for the abolition of the *grandi*, and hence the conflict between it and the people. As I will again stress, however, such is not to suggest that all conflict itself may be eradicated. The persistence of conflictual relations between particulars is ultimately a necessity given the fact of human difference and the plurality of modes of human doing and being. Indeed, as we shall see in chapter 6, Machiavelli's democratic politics derives its energy precisely from such conflictual relations.

The Originary Division of the Social in Democratic Readings of Machiavelli

For several decades the dominant democratic interpretation of Machiavelli was that initiated by Claude Lefort, which achieved its most comprehensive form of expression in his *Le travail de l'oeuvre Machiavel*.[2] Lefort's reading of Machiavelli must be understood in light of his critique of the impulse to totalitarian domination, the latter being an attempt to in a sense recolonize the space of sovereignty, although in a now limitless form, after the emergence of modern democracy and the disentaglement of the principles of power, law, and knowledge.[3] With the breaking apart of the medieval order the concept of sovereignty, which had previously been incarnated in the body of the monarch, was disincorporated of right and emptied of its positive content. Power

---

1 Such is implicitly suggested by Étienne Balibar when he writes that the term *umori* is "notoriously difficult to translate in modern languages since it refers at the same time to classes, interests, and regimes of passions." Étienne Balibar, "*Essere Principe, Essere Populare*: The Principle of Antagonism in Machiavelli's Epistemology," in *The Radical Machiavelli: Politics, Philosophy, and Language*, ed. Filippo Del Lucchese, Fabio Frosini, and Vittorio Morfino (Leiden: Brill, 2015), 354.

2 Throughout this study I have been citing the slightly abridged English translation. Lefort, *Machiavelli in the Making*.

3 For a brief attempt to situate Lefort's reading of Machiavelli within his overall political and philosophical trajectory see Knox Peden, "Anti-Revolutionary Republicanism: Claude Lefort's Machiavelli," *Radical Philosophy*, no. 182 (2013): 29–39.

took on the appearance of an empty place, a symbol of the non-identity of the social order. In Lefort's words, "Democracy inaugurates the experience of an ungraspable, uncontrollable society in which the people will be said to be sovereign, of course, but whose identity will constantly be open to question, whose identity will remain latent."[4] Totalitarianism is the attempt to refill this space, to embody sovereignty through the imposition of a new identity on the social order via the construction of an image of the People-as-One, a people escaping internal division or differentiation.[5] The significance of Machiavelli for Lefort lies in the former's effort to give an account of the perpetually divided being of the political community. On Lefort's reading, though, this division is articulated through the opposition of society's two primary classes – defined in terms of the orientation of their humour: toward oppression and toward the avoidance of oppression – which co-constitute each other through the mutual implication of their desire.

Lefort claims that the division between those whom Machiavelli labels the people and the *grandi* is an originary one present in every social order, and thus has "universal application."[6] The key question resulting from the perception of this universality is that regarding the negotiation of the conflictual bifurcation: "Either it engenders a power that rises above society and subordinates it entirely to its authority – as in the princedom – or it is regulated in such way that no one is subject to anyone – legally at least – as in liberty – or it is powerless to resolve itself into a stable order – as in license."[7] What the political observer is incapable of hoping to achieve, however, is a termination of the conflict between the humours through the reduction of the social order to a homogeneous unity grounded in a universality of desire. Society can never be reduced to such a unity precisely because each class's desire – the one to oppress and the other to not be oppressed – is insatiable and ineradicable. Indeed, it is the dynamic relation between these two

---

4 Claude Lefort, "The Image of the Body and Totalitarianism," in *The Political Forms of Modern Society: Bureaucracy, Democracy, Totalitarianism*, ed. John B. Thompson (Cambridge: MIT Press, 1986), 303–4.

5 Claude Lefort, "The Logic of Totalitarianism," in *The Political Forms of Modern Society: Bureaucracy, Democracy, Totalitarianism*, ed. John B. Thompson (Cambridge: Cambridge University Press, 1986), 287.

6 Lefort, *Machiavelli in the Making*.

7 Ibid., 139.

desires that structures the existence of each class. The grandees are the *"natural* adversary" of the people, "the Other who constitutes them as the immediate object of its desire."[8] If originary division is a universality inscribed into every political society, we nevertheless can analyse the precise form of its articulation in specific social-historical contexts: hence Machiavelli's typology of regimes in chapter 9 of the *The Prince*. If in the principality it is subordinated to the authority of the prince and in a state of licence it is desublimated independently of political order, in the *Discourses* originary division is the condition for the actualization of a concrete freedom, through the institution of a political life in which each person or faction is incapable of appropriating power for itself, and in which human desire is able to be expressed through law.

It is the conflictual interaction of desire between the co-constitutive classes that prevents the closure of society via one party's occupation of a site of power. Instituted in this movement, law is not that which restricts the expulsion of desire, but rather that which gives it an expression through the creation of a space that allows for the actualization of the will to freedom. In Lefort's words, "Law cannot be thought beneath the emblem of measure, nor traced to the action of a reasonable authority, which would come to put a limit to the appetites of man, nor conceived as the result of a natural regulation of those appetites imposed by the necessity of group survival. It is born of the excessiveness of the desire for freedom, which is doubtless linked to the appetite of the oppressed – who seek an outlet for their ambition – but does not reduce to it, since strictly speaking it has no object, is pure negativity, the refusal of oppression."[9] Precisely because the people's desire is to not be oppressed, there is no potential for the objective satisfaction of it: "it detaches the subject from any particular position and binds him to an infinite requirement."[10] The universality of originary division is located in this articulation: the conflict between the classes is incapable of being definitively reconciled to the extent that it is not a contestation over an exterior object whose possession is capable of terminating desire. To the

---

8 Ibid., 141.
9 Ibid., 229. On the negativity of desire see also Miguel Abensour, "'Savage Democracy' and the 'Principle of Anarchy,'" in *Democracy against the State: Marx and the Machiavellian Moment*, trans. Max Blechman and Martin Breaugh (London: Polity Press, 2011), 122.
10 Lefort, *Machiavelli in the Making*, 455.

degree that the conflict of desire cannot be eradicated, political struggle is a permanent condition of human reality. In the *Discourses on Livy* this conflict serves as the foundation for a specifically democratic practice: the existence of modes and orders that allow the plebs to respond to the actions of the grandees permits for the perpetuation of a power open to contestation, the dynamic relation of desire serving as the ground for the production of the new through its continual negotiation and renegotiation in law. Democratic activity, rooted in the non-identity of the social order, in an irreconcilable economy of desire, is presented as a form of perpetual interrogation, a refusal to yield to a static order of things that would freeze the political field, terminating that explicit conflict of humours which is the source of the liberty of the people. The city must thus be structured so as to give an expression to this double movement or division of desire. The ethical question is not whether desire is abolished, an impossibility, but whether desire is given a productive expression through ordinary modes: "What makes the virtue of the institution is not, then, that it eliminates error and injustice at the same time that it disarms instinct; it replaces private with public violence."[11]

What later radical democratic readers of Machiavelli influenced by Lefort would more clearly articulate than the latter is one of the consequences of such a theorization of originary division. The polarization of the multiplicity of desire that characterizes life in a shared world into what might appear as a quasi-metaphysical opposition between two transhistorical terms present in every society seemingly universalizes an oppressive humour, reactively defining the will to freedom in its opposition to this former tendency. The democratic non-occupation of the site of power does not exclude, in fact cannot exclude, the perpetuation of oppression, and hence Lefort's claim that the people can never become free of domination.[12] Because of the always-present opposition of the two primary desires, freedom and domination are inseparably linked, freedom in fact emerging in opposition to the desire for domination. In the words of Miguel Abensour, "In short, for Machiavelli politics and domination are at once different and closely interrelated; the one, in its negativity, born from the fact that it resists and opposes

---

11 Ibid., 236.
12 Lefort, "Machiavelli and the *Verità Effetuale*,"" 135.

the other and, in its affirmation, asserts that a human world is possible, provided that the many cease being oppressed by a minority of the great."[13] To the extent that the plebeian will is oriented toward resisting the encroachments of the grandees – that is, to breaking up the attempt at unifying the conflict of humours through fixing the form of society under one law – its orientation is essentially negative. It is realized not through institution, but rather through the struggle against all institutionalizing tendencies, which attempt to schematize the social field via the distribution of places and functions in the name of an artificial harmony that legitimates the domination of many by some.

The contemporary interpreter who has done the most to advance the non-institutional reading of Machiavelli's democratic theory is Miguel Vatter, who like Lefort grounds his analysis in a recognition of an originary social division between the desires of the great and the people. He thus speaks of the "two totally heterogeneous desires with totally opposite relations to the principle of rule."[14] The significance of the relation between the trajectory of desire and rule is here essential. The republic cannot be thought of in terms of the institutionalization of the rule of the people because the people do not desire rule, but only no-rule. Machiavelli's account of social discord, then, does not refer us to a positive institutionalization of a state form now able to provide a space for regulating competition: "the republic, as a political form, does not exist and will never exist because the *res publica* is not a political form (*res*) at all but denotes an iterable event in which forms of legitimate domination are changed in a revolutionary fashion."[15] The people's very real and active desire for freedom is the desire to replace rule by no-rule, and is thus a negative one eschewing a positive instauration in an order of things: "the desire for freedom as no-rule transcends every given social and political form that imposes a distinction between who commands and who obeys. In a literal sense, the people's desire not to be commanded or oppressed is an extra-constitutional desire that can never be integrally realized in any form of government or stabilized in any legal order of domination."[16]

---

13 Miguel Abensour, "Machiavel: le grand penseur du désordre," *Le Monde*, 11 April 2006, 8.

14 Vatter, *Between Form and Event*, 101.

15 Ibid., 6.

16 Ibid., 95.

Even though the multiplicity of negative desire cannot be positively organized into a political form capable of realizing it, it nevertheless can lead to the demand to reorder the political form, exposing the being of the latter as merely contingent and subject to history. What must not be forgotten is simply that there is no end to any chain of reorder, no ultimate discovery of a political form capable of actualizing political freedom as a permanent condition of existence: "every realization of freedom as no-rule is also its reification, that is, any given form is bound, in the course of time, to stop counting as an acceptable response to the question posed by the desire for freedom as no-rule."[17] Vatter thus concludes that Machiavelli's republic cannot be interpreted as a form of state, even if its constitution allows for the expression of popular desire through specific counter-institutions: "The people enter political life through special institutions, like that of the Tribunate, that contrast the proper activity of the state, i.e., the administration of rule. These institutions of political contrast, or counter-institutions, carve up the state so as to clear a space in which to voice and act out the demands of no-rule."[18] The particularity of such counter-institutions can be seen, for example, through examining the function of the Tribunate. The Tribunate is the society's guard of freedom because its function is to suspend the relation of rule.[19] For Vatter all counter-institutions operate in this way: all are opposed to the positive force of the established law of the state, the corruption of the free society occurring precisely where the people are used as a ground for the construction of a government: "To make the people serve as the foundation of the state is equivalent to the process of giving substance or reality to the desire for freedom as no-rule, thereby denying what is most proper to this desire: its capacity to transcend factual political and legal order and suspend its validity."[20] Again, the desire of the people is incapable of being embodied in a positive order of law, for its free expulsion is articulated in its confrontation with and interruption of the noble desire to rule. Hence, "the political body is alive only when it is discordant with itself, when it makes space for the people and their desire for freedom in opposition to the desire for domination expressed by the noble elements of the body."[21] Vatter

---

17 Ibid., 96.
18 Ibid., 99.
19 Ibid., 104.
20 Ibid., 122.
21 Ibid.

ultimately reads the corruption of the body politic in terms of the reification of plebeian desire, as expressed for example in the modern state's attempt to pacify desire through instituting it in a system of negative liberty looking toward the achievement of a universal security. Indeed, according to Vatter all modern political theory turns on this operation: "The state can be founded only on the basis of the security of the people, that is, only on condition that the negativity of freedom as no-rule is neutralized and co-opted by realizing it as a system of negative liberties or rights that is both secured by, and securing for, the political and legal order of domination."[22]

The recent democratic reading of Machiavelli produced by John McCormick can be largely framed in terms of an alternative to such radical democratic interpretations that emphasize the merely negative and disruptive form of plebeian activity. McCormick writes: "Through the tribunes and in their assemblies, Machiavelli demonstrates unequivocally that the plebeians participate in rule," but McCormick insists that such participation is not of a radical democratic quality.[23] On his reading Machiavelli advocates ruling and being ruled in turn, but not "no-rule"; that is, he advocates "a dispersal of rule but *not* a dissolution of rule as such."[24] Contrary to readers like Vatter, who see democracy and positive institutionalization as incompatible with each other, McCormick understands political institutions to be a necessary element of democratic life and expression, not the "inherent antithesis of democratic vitality."[25] Indeed, through their hostility to the concepts of rule and institutionalization, "the scholars who today champion democracy most boldly may, in fact, undermine it most seriously."[26] Curiously enough, however, McCormick nevertheless himself reduces plebeian political activity to that same reactive principle seemingly affirmed in the radical democratic positing of originary division, an originary division that structures the very rejection of the institution that McCormick criticizes. McCormick also eternalizes a will to domination when he writes that "Machiavellian Democracy then capitalizes on *ever-present* moments of aristocratic oppression by seeking and putting in place

---

22 Ibid., 129.
23 McCormick, *Machiavellian Democracy*, 204n11.
24 Ibid.
25 Ibid.
26 McCormick, "Defending the People from the Professors."

institutional arrangements through which the people vigorously and effectively respond to the grandi's repressive schemes and actions."[27] Indeed, on McCormick's reading the self-activity of the people is not grounded in an intrinsic participatory desire, but rather emerges in a reactive manner in the face of elite encroachments and transgressions.[28] To the extent that there is always an oligarchic element within the republic, Machiavelli always looks to elite compromise rather than the abolition of the oppressive desire. Hence the fact that he does not propose to replicate Swiss republicanism, which does not provide noble incentives: "The Swiss model provides the popolo with liberty and equality without in any way compensating the grandi for this fact."[29] The noble desire to oppress is curbed but not eliminated, the *grandi* continuing to have access to the most prominent civic offices.

My own democratic reading of Machiavelli is distinct from both those of Lefort and the radical democrats as well as McCormick, and is intended to overcome the aporias of each.[30] Although agreeing with Lefort that the popular desire for freedom is perpetually surplus, an insatiable orientation toward a mode of existence or being, I disagree that this desire is actualized in a merely negative confrontation with an external power that attempts to constrain it through incorporating it within a necessarily repressive institutional order of things. On the contrary, I agree with McCormick that the institution can be thought of as being capable of giving an expression to the popular desire for freedom. This desire, though, cannot be reduced simply to a wish to avoid domination at the hands of the great. It is rather immanent to human being itself, a manifestation of the orientation of the ambitious will for creative self-expression. This will for self-expression must be seen as present regardless of its relation or non-relation to a dominating force exterior to

---

27 McCormick, *Machiavellian Democracy*, 31. Emphasis added.

28 For similar criticisms of McCormick see Arlene W. Saxonhouse, "Do We Need the Vote? Reflections on John McCormick's *Machiavellian Democracy*," *The Good Society* 20, no. 2 (2011): 179; Lawrence Hamilton, *Freedom Is Power: Liberty through Political Representation* (Cambridge: Cambridge University Press, 2014), 62.

29 McCormick, *Machiavellian Democracy*, 59.

30 For a recent attempt to demonstrate that neither the institutional nor the no-rule approach to democratically reading Machiavelli is adequate on its own see Boris Litvin, "Mapping Rule and Subversion: Perspective and the Democratic Turn in Machiavelli Scholarship," *European Journal of Political Theory*, advanced online publication (2015): 1–23, doi:10.177/1474885115599894.

it. This is thus to suggest that readers are incorrect in naturalizing the division of humours that Machiavelli presents, eternalizing the will to domination through grounding it in a fundamental opposition of desire universal to all cities. Although Machiavelli himself never provided a definitive answer to this question, in this chapter I will attempt to briefly suggest that he gives us enough conceptual resources to at least think about the possibility of instituting a social situation in which the *grandi* are eliminated, thus dissolving the originary division of the social and making it easier to grasp the essential form of the human desire for ambitious expression, as well as the extent to which this ambitious expression can be realized not in terms of its opposition to a now non-existent social class, but through the very institutional life of the free city.

Social Equality as the Precondition for Political Self-Creation

Machiavelli primarily speaks about the great in terms of the orientation of their humour, which looks toward the oppression of the people. Such, however, is not sufficient to establish a definition of the *grandi*. After all, Machiavelli provides – particularly in the *Florentine Histories* – several examples of individual members of the people, as well as popular groups who emerge from the *popolo*, who act according to a seeming will to domination, looking to exclude others from public life and monopolize political authority for themselves alone. There is thus a second definitional feature of the category of great: not only are the *grandi* individuals whose will looks toward political command and exclusion, but they are also those who are able to, through combining into a class conscious of their desire and united in their end, leverage their privileged social position so as to actualize this shared desire through a definite mode of activity. Specifically, the great are those who are able to deploy their disproportionate economic wealth in order to advance their political position relative to those who lack such wealth, a position which is then in turn exploited so as to further augment the relations of material inequality which they benefit from.[31] A

---

31 Hence McCormick notes that in *Discourses* 1:5 Machiavelli uses the term "the great" in order identify the oligarchic element in every republic. McCormick, *Machiavellian Democracy*, 45. Indeed, McCormick reads Machiavelli's account of the conflict over the Agrarian Laws, for example, as indicating the latter's understanding of the significance of economic inequality and the conflict that it gives rise to as being central

consideration of the place of the *grandi* in the city is thus impossible independently of a consideration of the place of the distribution of wealth and resources.

In the previous chapter I demonstrated the relationship between political and economic inequality as revealed through the events of the revolt of the Ciompi. In the *Discourses on Livy* the political need to overcome the latter inequality can be approached initially through a consideration of Machiavelli's famous contention that "well-ordered republics have to keep the public rich, and their citizens poor."[32] Such a statement is not to suggest that the healthy republic has need of maintaining its people at a certain determinable level of material subsistence, the concept of poverty being deployed by Machiavelli to indicate not one pole of a social relationship marked by an inequality of wealth, but rather 1) the very levelling of such relationships, along with 2) a reorientation of citizens' attitudes toward wealth accumulation. Maurizio Viroli implicitly calls attention to the former through linking the concept of poverty less to a certain degree of economic or substantive well-being, and more to a principle of social equality: "When [Machiavelli] said he was born in poverty, he meant he had not been born to a prominent, well-to-do family and therefore could not have hoped to be elected to public office or to make a fortune in business."[33] To generalize poverty is not to generalize Machiavelli's own

---

to domestic political struggle. What the episode reveals is that the *grandi*, contrary to the common Straussian reading, are not motivated only by their love of glory and honour, but rather by their desire for wealth. McCormick, "Machiavelli and the Gracchi," 302. The plebs seem to recognize that a condition for the actualization of their demand for an increased share in honours and institutions in the city is a reduction of material inequality and a limitation of the noble pursuit of wealth. John P. McCormick, "'Keep the Public Rich, but the Citizens Poor': Economic and Political Inequality in Constitutions, Ancient and Modern," *Cardozo Law Review* 34, no. 3 (2013): 890. For a further reading of economic inequality and the Gracchi case see Benedetto Fontana, "Machiavelli and the Gracchi: Republican Liberty and Conflict," in *Machiavelli on Liberty and Conflict*, ed. David Johnston, Nadia Urbinati, and Camila Vergara (Chicago: University of Chicago Press, 2017), 235–56. On conflict between the great and the people as being primarily grounded in economic inequality see also Tejas Parasher, "Inequality and *Tumulti* in Machiavelli's Aristocratic Republics," *Polity* 49, no. 1 (2017): 54–5.

32 Machiavelli, "Discorsi sopra la prima Deca di Tito Livio," in *Tutte le opere*, bk. 1.37.

33 Maurizio Viroli, *Niccolò's Smile: A Biography of Machiavelli*, trans. Antony Shugaar (New York: Hill and Wang, 2000), 6.

experience of political exclusion, but is rather to eliminate such a potential through the equalization of wealth, through the abolition of the economic conditions that sustain elevated social positions that allow some to extract surplus private benefits that are denied others. Julie L. Rose, meanwhile, highlights the latter through her attempt to demonstrate that the republican need to keep its citizens poor refers not only to the maintenance of a fixed level of poverty (and hence equality), but more importantly to the maintenance of a particular psychic orientation toward poverty. Specifically, it is "a prescription for particular *attitudes* citizens must hold toward poverty and wealth."[34] According to Rose there are three main elements to Machiavelli's preferred attitude to poverty and wealth: citizens must not ground their judgment of other citizens on the basis of wealth; citizens must not value private wealth more than the public good; and citizens must not allow private objects to distract them from public matters.[35]

Both elements of Machiavelli's affirmation of poverty are revealed through his account, already mentioned in chapter 2, of the material life of the German free cities. In addition to the passages already cited from the *Discourses*, in his "Report[s] on the Affairs of Germany" Machiavelli explicitly associates living freely with living an austere mode of life, a mode of life in which citizens do not aggrandize themselves through ostentatious displays of wealth meant to mark their social superiority. Indeed, their mutual equality in poverty generates the richness of the society in an economic dialectic that seemingly dissolves the conventional opposition and co-relation of the categories of rich and poor. He writes: "And if I say that the people of Germany are rich, so it is the truth. And they are made rich in large part because they live as poor, for they do not build, nor dress, nor furnish their houses expensively, and it is enough that they abound with bread and meat, and have a stove wherein to take refuge from the cold. Those who do not have other things do without them, and do not seek for them … none take account of what they lack, but only of that of which they have need; and their needs are much less than ours. And because of these customs it results that money does not leave their country, they being content with that which their country produces, and in this they enjoy their rough and

---

34 Julie L. Rose, "'Keep the Citizens Poor': Machiavelli's Prescription for Republican Poverty," *Political Studies* 64, no. 3 (2016): 737.

35 Ibid., 10.

free life."[36] Machiavelli here gives an expression to his non-belief that civic life is capable of being enriched through a generalized drive toward the private accumulation of wealth on the part of individuals.[37] Machiavelli produces a critique of the debilitating effects of the asymmetrical distribution of wealth and its production of the ideal of luxury, which is stimulated by and stimulates the emergence and entrenchment of a psyche obsessed with the self-differentiation of one from others. In the *Florentine Histories*, for instance, Machiavelli grounds social corruption in a certain type of decadent and conspicuous consumption that accompanies the institution of pronounced economic inequality: "Of which emerged in the city those evils that are most of the time generated in peace; for the young, more unshackled than usual, were spending to excess on dress, on banquets, and on other similar wantonness, and being idle, they consumed time and substance in games and in women; they studied to appear splendid in dress and to be witty and clever in speech, and the one who was most deft at biting the others was more wise and more esteemed."[38] In response to such displays "the good citizens thought that it would be necessary to put a stop to it, and with a new law they set a limit on clothing, burials, and banquets."[39]

What Machiavelli admires in these German people's acceptance of austere living is the rejection of material acquisition as a mode for the actualization of social distinction. We have already seen that in the *Discourses* such is one of the two causes of the generation of civic goodness among the citizens. The second, meanwhile, is identified as a general

---

36 Machiavelli, "Rapporto delle cose della Magna fatto questo di 17 giugna 1508," in *Tutte le opere*, 65.

37 See Hans Baron, *In Search of Florentine Civic Humanism: Essays on the Transition from Medieval to Modern Thought*, vol. 1 (Princeton: Princeton University Press, 1988), 255–6; Bonadeo, *Corruption, Conflict, and Power*, 46; Eric Nelson, *The Greek Tradition in Republican Thought* (Cambridge: Cambridge University Press, 2004), 77; Amanda Maher, "What Skinner Misses about Machiavelli's Freedom: Inequality, Corruption, and the Institutional Origins of Civic Virtue," *Journal of Politics* 78, no. 4 (2016): 1003–15.

38 Machiavelli, "Istorie fiorentine," in *Tutte le opere*, bk. 7.28. For further insight into Machiavelli's perception of the nature of the idle classes see Machiavelli, "Capitoli per una compagnia di piacere," in *Tutte le opere*, 930–2.

39 Machiavelli, "Istorie fiorentine," bk. 7.28. Machiavelli repeats the critique of such forms of conspicuous consumption in various places. See, for example, his account of the meeting of Castruccio Castracani and Taddeo Bernardi in Machiavelli, "La vita di Castruccio Castracani da Lucca," in *Tutte le opere*, 627.

hostility on the part of the people toward those whom Machiavelli labels gentlemen: "The other cause is that those republics where a political and uncorrupt life is maintained do not allow that any of their citizens be or live in the way of a gentleman; indeed, they maintain among themselves a level equality, and to those lords and gentlemen in that province they are extremely hostile. And if by chance they receive some in their hands, they put them to death as the beginnings of corruption and the cause of every scandal."[40] In this chapter Machiavelli seems to define the category of gentleman in a straightforward way, identifying members of this group as seeming relics of a feudal order who, although they may or may not be able to command political allegiance from a vassal population as a result of their holdings, are nevertheless able to extract economic advantage from their landed property independently of any self-activity. He writes, "I say that those are called gentlemen who live idly from the rents of their abundant possessions, without having any care either for cultivation or for other labour necessary to live. Such as these are pernicious in every republic and in every province, but more pernicious are those that, in addition to the aforementioned fortunes, command from a castle and have subjects who obey them."[41] In regions with gentlemen "there has never emerged any republic or political life, for such types of men are entirely hostile to every civilization."[42] Hence "one who wants to make a republic where there are many gentlemen, cannot do it unless he first eliminates all of them."[43]

Machiavelli's account of gentlemen in 1:55 has aroused much scholarly attention, and indeed, such attention has mostly tended to emphasize the implicit critique of feudal or rentier modes of obligation and accumulation.[44] Many commentators will go even further, suggesting that Machiavelli's critique can also be understood as an implicit defence of advanced free market relations or a specifically capitalist mode of

40 Machiavelli, "Discorsi sopra la Prima Deca di Tito Livio," bk. 1.55.
41 Ibid.
42 Ibid.
43 Ibid.
44 For a reading of *Discourses* 1:55 as Machiavelli's critique of rentier capitalism see Jérémie Barthas, "Machiavelli, Public Debt, and the Origins of Political Economy," in *The Radical Machiavelli: Politics, Philosophy, and Language*, ed. Filippo Del Lucchese, Fabio Frosini, and Vittorio Morfino (Leiden: Brill, 2015), 288–9.

production and exchange.[45] The conceptual delimitation of the category would then seem to preclude its extension so as to be able to serve an explanatory function with respect to other relations of inequality, most specifically that between the nobles and the people. I would argue, however, that such an operation misses what is the essential core of Machiavelli's critique. What needs to be interrogated in the first instance is whether, as most commentators assume, there exists a clear analytical distinction between the very categories of noble and gentleman.[46] There are indeed several instances in which Machiavelli deploys the latter term in an ambiguous way, or at least one that is apparently distinct from its specific usage in *Discourses* 1:55.

During a discussion of the foundation of the Venetian state in *Discourses* 1:6, for example, he notes that in Venice the term gentlemen referred to "all those who can hold administration," that is to say, to a specific class of social elites who are marked off against the people and who, unlike the majority of the population, participate in government.[47] In the "Discourse on Florentine Affairs" Machiavelli repeats his belief that if one wants to order a republic in a city with inequality "it would be necessary to eliminate all the nobility, and reduce it to an equality with the others; for between them they act so extraordinarily that the laws are not enough to restrain them, but you need a living voice and a royal power to restrain them."[48] Conversely, if one wants to institute a princedom where there is a general equality, "it would be necessary to first order inequality, and make for yourself many nobles of castles and villas, who, together with the prince, would keep the city and the whole province in subjugation with their arms and adherents."[49] What is

---

45 See, for example, Kocis, *Machiavelli Redeemed*; Lionel A. McKenzie, "Rousseau's Debate with Machiavelli in the *Social Contract*," *Journal of the History of Ideas* 43, no. 2 (1982): 209–28; Jo Ann Cavallo, "On Political Power and Personal Liberty in *The Prince* and *The Discourses*," *Social Research* 81, no. 1 (2014): 107–32. On Machiavelli's anticipation of the "market liberal tradition" see also Brandon Turner, "Private Vices, Public Benefits: *Mandragola* in Machiavelli's Political Theory," *Polity* 48, no. 1 (2016): 109–32.

46 Erica Benner, for example, gives voice to a common ground for such distinction, identifying the nobles as those who possess privilege through birth, and the gentlemen as those who possess privilege through wealth. Benner, *Machiavelli's Ethics*, 273.

47 Machiavelli, "Discorsi sopra la prima Deca di Tito Livio," bk. 1.6.

48 Machiavelli, "Discursus florentinarum rerum post mortem iunioris Laurentii Medices," in *Tutte le opere*, 27.

49 Ibid.

interesting in this passage from the "Discourse" is not only that Machiavelli repeats the need to eliminate gentlemen as a pre-condition for the
establishment of a genuine republic, but also that he uses the terms
noble and gentleman interchangeably, the term gentlemen being associated with the nobility most generally, who support the prince as a
means to advance their own self-interest. This arrangement is "seen in
all the states of a prince, and especially in the kingdom of France, where
the gentlemen lord over the people, the princes the gentlemen, and the
king the princes."[50]

In an important contribution, Alfredo Bonadeo suggests that the conceptual distinction between noble and gentlemen is largely illusory.
Bonadeo notes that Machiavelli was writing in a historical context in
which the term grandee was used synonymously with terms such as
nobile, *potente*, and *gentiluomo*, and that "this reveals a connection
between the concepts of power, nobility, and 'grandigia.'"[51] Indeed, by
the end of the thirteenth century the term noble was not exclusively
deployed in reference to an individual's hereditary status, but was
applied also to those wealthy commoners who had become rich through
commerce, acquiring power and status that was previously reserved
for the feudal nobility. They thus also achieved the rank of grandee,
alongside that older class of gentlemen that readers of Machiavelli
associate with the explicitly idle group of expropriating lords. What
Bonadeo points out is that the terms noble, great, and gentleman all
refer to the same individuals, individuals not necessarily defined in
terms of membership in an economic or political class precisely specified, but rather simply in terms of their articulation in a relationship of
general inequality in which they extract surplus political benefit: "'gen-
tiluomini,' 'nobili,' 'signori,' 'ottimati,' 'potenti,' 'ricchi,' 'principali,'
'grandi,' and similar terms appear with the same meaning. All designate people who may be noble, either by extraction or by acquisition, or
may not be noble; but they are wealthy and either have political power
or are seeking it as socially prominent citizens."[52] As noted in the previous chapter, it is important to remember that Machiavelli does not see
himself as articulating a precise class analysis, whether in the ancient
Roman or the Florentine case, the category of the people subsuming

---

50 Ibid.
51 Bonadeo, "The Role of the 'Grandi' in the Political World of Machiavelli," 10.
52 Ibid., 11–12.

several other distinctions, just as the category of the great or noble does.[53]

What Machiavelli is calling attention to is social inequality as such, and the extent to which it militates against the establishment of a free way of life considered in terms of the generalization of public participation. The asymmetrical distribution of wealth and resources provides the few with the concrete conditions necessary for the actualization of their desire for domination. Hence his critique, not of any particular mode of social production and exchange, but disproportionate material accumulation in itself, and his subsequent contention that republican life is capable of being instituted only in a social context marked by distributive equality. Hence also his affirmation of equality as a conditional element or principle of justice: "[Justice] defends the poor and the powerless, restrains the rich and the powerful, humbles the arrogant and the impudent, curbs the rapacious and the avaricious, castigates the insolent, and scatters the violent; it generates in the state that equality which, in order to maintain them, is desirable in every state."[54] As Filippo Del Lucchese suggests, the "wonderful equality" that

---

53 This is noted by John Najemy, who suggests that Machiavelli is not concerned with providing his readers with a precise sociological account of the nature of class division in ancient Rome, but is rather locating in the categories of the great and the plebs a means to analyse the key contemporary social division of the Florence of his time, that between the *popolo* and the *grandi*. John M. Najemy, *A History of Florence: 1200–1575* (Oxford: Blackwell, 2008). Indeed, the term *popolo* had multiple meanings itself in Florence, at its most expansive referring to all Florentines, although it most often was intended to simply designate non-elites: "When Florentines spoke of the popolo in specifically political contexts, they usually understood it as synonymous with the large majority of guildsman who did not belong to elite families." Ibid., 35. Discussing the distinction between the concepts of the people in pre- and post-eighteenth-century political contexts, McCormick notes that whereas in modern republics the idea of the people refers to the homogenized sum of all individuals in society, possessing as they do identical abstract formal rights, prior to this the people referred to not simply the citizen body as a whole, but to the poor and non-elite elements of the city. John P. McCormick, "People and Elites in Republican Constitutions, Traditional and Modern," in *The Paradox of Constitutionalism: Constituent Power and Constitutional Form*, ed. Martin Loughlin and Neil Walker (Oxford: Oxford University Press, 2007), 107.
54 Machiavelli, "Allocuzione fatta ad magistrato," in *Tutte le opere*, 36. For a situation of Machiavelli's "Allocution Made to a Magistrate" within what is seen as his broader understanding of the conventional form of political justice, see A.J. Parel, "Machiavelli's Notions of Justice: Text and Analysis," *Political Theory* 18, no. 4 (1990): 528–44.

Machiavelli famously references in the *Florentine Histories* refers to "an economic situation more favorable to a popular government and to freedom, a position Machiavelli consistently holds throughout his intellectual production."[55] This economic equality would be achieved through "the destruction of the rich and the reappropriation of the richness by the many."[56]

Referring in particular to the "Discourse on Florentine Affairs," Bonadeo argues that it is evident that the establishment of a republic depends upon the realization of a certain type of equality, this realization including both the elimination of social and political class distinctions, as well as the generation of a space for plebeian participation in government through, not just the exclusion of the grandees from certain institutions, but the very elimination of the *grandi* itself. In his words, "to establish a republic it is necessary to wipe out all the nobility and bring it to a level with the other citizens."[57] Such a possibility is suggested, even though it was never realized in the Roman case, in the *Discourses on Livy*. It can be counterposed to what is often pointed out to be one of Machiavelli's preferred solutions to the problem of the internally destructive orientation of noble desire: its external redirection. In such redirection an outlet is given for the satisfaction of the *grandi*'s will to dominate via the city's imperial expansion.[58] This was indeed the preferred mode in the Roman case, although in *Discourses* 3:16 it is acknowledged that there is another option that republics may take. Machiavelli begins the chapter by noting that "it has been always,

---

55 Filippo Del Lucchese, "Freedom, Equality and Conflict: Rousseau on Machiavelli," *History of Political Thought* 35, no. 1 (2014): 42.

56 Ibid., 46. For a recent account of Machiavelli's critique of economic inequality in the *Florentine Histories* and its implication in the fact of political corruption see Amanda Maher, "The Power of 'Wealth, Nobility and Men': Inequality and Corruption in Machiavelli's *Florentine Histories*," *European Journal of Political Theory*, advanced online publication (2017): 1–20, doi:10.1177/147885117730673.

57 Bonadeo, *Corruption, Conflict, and Power*, 104.

58 Nikola Regent sums up the position of several readers on the question of republican expansion, writing that for Machiavelli "*the highest possible aim*" of political life is the establishment of a "long-lasting empire which expands." Regent, "Machiavelli, Empire, *Virtù* and the Final Downfall," 753. Original emphasis. For perhaps the most systematic and thorough attempt to demonstrate that one cannot separate Machiavelli's commitment to internal Florentine liberty from his commitment to Florence's external imperial expansion see Mikael Hörnquist, *Machiavelli and Empire* (Cambridge: Cambridge University Press, 2004).

and always will be, that great and rare men in a republic are neglected in peaceful times; for through the envy that has accompanied the reputation that their virtue has given them, one finds in such times many citizens who wish, not only to be their equals, but to be their superiors."[59] That such is not the immediate object of Machiavelli's concern should be readily apparent in light of his understanding, which I articulated in the previous chapter, of the non-superiority of the great in relation to the people. In short, there is no natural foundation for the esteemed position of the grandees within society, their social elevation being entirely conventional.

The social division between the great and the people in a newly instituted principality grounded in the great, for example, is the result of the will of the prince, not a non-identity of the being of citizens. Hence Machiavelli writes that "the prince always lives with the same people; but he can do well without the same grandees, being able to make and unmake them every day, and take away and give, of his accord, their reputation."[60] And within the context of his discussion of gentlemen in the *Discourses* he states that "where there is much equality, one who wishes to make a kingdom or a principality will never be able to do it if one does not draw from that equality many of ambitious and restless spirit and make them gentlemen in fact, and not in name, gifting them castles and possessions, and giving them favour through possessions and men."[61] Once again it is worth pointing out: the great do not have a fundamental nature distinct from the people. Rather, their differing humour is to be located in their attempt to actualize ambition through denying such actualization to others, such being a concrete possibility only to the extent that they occupy a contingent social or political place within the city. Being not concerned with the disjunction between the self-perceived superiority of a few and the extent of their social recognition in a community of ostensible equality, in the second paragraph of 3:16 Machiavelli reveals the true disorder at the heart of the chapter. It is that the grandees have an intuition of being not properly esteemed, this intuition intensifying their insolence: "That thing makes them indignant in two modes: the one, to see themselves lacking their rank; the other, to see made comrades and superiors unworthy men not as

---

59 Machiavelli, "Discorsi sopra la prima Deca di Tito Livio," bk. 3.16.
60 Machiavelli, "Il Principe," in *Tutte le opere*, chap. 9.
61 Machiavelli, "Discorsi sopra la prima Deca di Tito Livio," bk. 1.55.

sufficient as themselves."[62] Such insolence can be neutralized through one of the two modes already suggested, going to war so as to allow the great to vent their ambition, or deepening equality within the city, eliminating the great and the desire to oppress which gives rise to the very disorder.

Several chapters later in 3:25, Machiavelli elaborates on the relation between the establishment of equality and the extension of virtue. Here Machiavelli again affirms that "the most useful thing to order in a free city is to maintain the citizens poor."[63] The specified advantage of this order, of the institution of a general social and economic equality, is that there is thereby no artificial barrier erected preventing the actualization of *virtù* on the part of individuals, here represented in terms of the assumption of office and the achievement of distinction: "through experience one sees that four hundred years after Rome had been built there was a very great poverty; nor can one believe that any other greater order produced this effect than seeing that the way to any rank and any honour was not blocked to you because of poverty, and that one went to find virtue in any house that it occupied. That mode of living made riches undesirable."[64] Not only does the establishment of equality militate against the leveraging of wealth toward political ends by a few, allowing all to strive after virtue, but it also neutralizes the very desire for economic accumulation through allowing people an outlet for self-expression via political participation, through giving them a concrete stake in public life. For Machiavelli this lesson is expressed particularly well in the case of Lucius Quintius Cincinnatus. Fearing the loss of the consul Minucius and his army while battling the Aequi, Rome created Cincinnatus as dictator, who at this point was living a particularly modest life: "Cincinnatus was plowing his small villa, which did not exceed four *jugera*, when from Rome came the legates of the Senate to reveal to him his election to the dictatorship, to show in what danger the Roman republic found itself."[65] Not only was Cincinnatus able to actualize *virtù* through defeating his enemy and liberating Minucius, but after the termination of the crisis he demonstrated no desire to increase his estate through the appropriation of the spoils of

---

62 Ibid., bk. 3.16.
63 Ibid., bk. 3.25.
64 Ibid.
65 Ibid.

war. Hence, "One notes, as was said, the honour that was done in Rome to poverty, and how to a good and valiant man, which Cincinnatus was, four *jugera* of land was enough to nourish him."[66]

Contrary to figures like Cincinnatus, Machiavelli is ultimately highly sceptical that the majority of the great, given the orientation of their humour, will ever rest satisfied with their share of government or their institutional allotment within the city. To illustrate this point, in the *Florentine Histories* he calls attention to an episode in which the people and the nobles, after a period of negotiation, agreed on a specific distribution of positions that was intended to satisfy each group, the great ultimately being granted one-third of the Signoria and one half of the remaining offices. Needless to say, however, the nobles immediately worked to undermine the organization of the city through increasing their political share: "with this order, this government, the city would have settled, if the great had been content to live with that modesty that is required for civil life; but they operated in the contrary way, for as private individuals they did not want companions, and in the magistracies they wanted to be lords; and every day there emerged some example of their insolence and arrogance."[67] This recognition of the *grandi*'s perpetual tendency to resist the sharing of political authority should immediately lead us to question the earnestness of the ideal of the mixed regime, in which each social part is apportioned a political place and function, contributing toward the healthy reproduction of the city through the voluntary acceptance of its particular role.

On Machiavelli's account there is no grounds for thinking the great will ever be satisfied with their social position, and hence for thinking it possible for the people to establish a lasting conciliation with them. Especially relevant here is a discussion in book two of the *Histories*. After the self-exile of the Ghibellines Florence was reordered in an effort to create an institutional milieu that would be able to resist the type of civil purging that had been carried out by this faction. Specifically, "they elected twelve heads, who were to sit in the magistracy for two months, and they called these not Ancients, but Good Men; alongside these was a council of eighty citizens, which they called the *Credenza*; after this was one hundred and eighty from the people, thirty for each of the six [wards], which with the *Credenza* and twelve Good Men

---

66 Ibid.
67 Machiavelli, "Istorie fiorentine," bk. 2.39.

were called the General Council. They ordered yet another council of one hundred and twenty citizens, people and nobles, through which was rendered complete all the things determined in the other councils; and with that they distributed the offices of the republic."[68] The problem, however, was that as a consequence of reflection on the Ghibelline tyranny it was decided to invest the Guelfs specifically with more offices, authorities, and magistracies, with predictable results given what we know of noble desire: "Florence was then in a very bad condition, because the Guelf nobility had become insolent and did not fear the magistrates."[69]

What the Florentines forgot was that, Guelf or Ghibelline, "the few always act in the mode of the few."[70] In light of the former's insolence the people thought it prudent to invite back into the city the latter as a counter-force, producing a reordering in which the final result was an overall decline of noble influence, both Guelfs and Ghibellines agreeing to a form of mutual political exclusion out of fear that the other would gain power at the one's expense. The suppression of factional conflict, however, allowed for a clearer emergence of the primary division between the humours of the people and the great, the latter no longer being contaminated or blurred by internal factional difference. In the end the laws and orders were powerless to contain the elite persecution of the people, as was the institution of a Gonfalonier of justice.[71] Subsequently yet another reordering was carried out in light of this situation, this time stimulated by Giano della Bella – "of very noble lineage, but lover of the freedom of the city" – who lobbied to create laws to deny the *grandi* certain offices and privileges.[72] After accidents conspired to compel Giano to voluntarily leave the city the nobles took the opportunity to reassert themselves, which they were able to do through further neutralizing their internal divisions. Just before the *grandi* and the

---

68 Ibid., bk. 2.10.
69 Ibid., bk. 2.11.
70 Machiavelli, "Discorsi sopra la prima Deca di Tito Livio," bk. 1.7. Indeed, this phrase is situated in a passage in which Machiavelli highlights the noble tendency to disrespect ordinary modes, such disrespect being a concrete manifestation of their sense of exceptionality. Their willingness to subvert legal orders for their own good is a sign of their belief that the people should not possess a designated means for the satisfaction of their desire.
71 Machiavelli, "Istorie fiorentine," bk. 2.12.
72 Ibid., bk. 2.13.

people were to come to arms, certain prudent individuals intervened in order to try and prevent the emergence of bloodshed, reminding the great that the laws made to deny them authority were only instituted in light of their insolence. At the same time, however, they made an appeal to the opposite side: "The people, on the other hand, were reminded of how it was prudent to want always the final victory, and how it was never a wise choice to make men despair, because one who does not hope for the good does not fear the evil. They should think that the nobility was that which had in war honoured the city, and thus it was neither a good nor a just thing to persecute them with so much hatred; and as the nobles easily suffered not enjoying the supreme magistracy, they could not suffer that it should be in the power of everyone, through the orders made, to expel them from their homeland. Therefore it was good to mitigate them, and by this benefit lay down their arms; nor should they want to test the fortune of battle relying on their number, for many times it has been seen that the many have been overcome by the few."[73]

It may seem as if Machiavelli is here calling attention to the necessity of a conciliatory form of compromise in which each side of the conflict is willing to make concessions for the sake of a peaceable way of life. In fact, however, Machiavelli is simply advocating the replacement of extraordinary with ordinary modes to control and accuse elites. His ultimate conclusion is that the city should use laws in order to check the insolence of nobles, this being the most prudent position in social situations marked by, first, an already firmly established noble class, and second, an impossibility of denying this class political authority altogether. After the positive institutionalization of modes of accusation and the restriction of noble participation in government, the city lived in relative peace, Machiavelli concluding that "never was our city in a greater and more happy state than in these times, being filled with men, riches and reputation."[74] As demonstrated throughout the rest of the book, however, no established order is sufficient to quell the insatiable humour of the great for long. Hence the words that Machiavelli has Piero de' Medici speak in a lamenting speech chastising the mode of expression of the ambition of the few, Piero bemoaning his inability to

---

73 Ibid., bk. 2.14.
74 Ibid., bk. 2.15.

check the latter: "I know now how much I have deceived myself, as one that knew little of the natural ambition of all men, and less of yours: for it is not enough for you to be princes in such a city and for you few to have those honours, dignities, and benefits of which formerly many citizens were wont to be honoured; it is not enough for you to have divided between yourselves the goods of your enemies; it is not enough for you to be able to afflict all with public burdens, while you, free from those, have all the public advantage. You afflict everyone with every type of injury. You despoil your neighbour of his goods, you sell justice, you avoid civil judgments, you oppress peaceful men, and you exalt the insolent."[75]

Machiavelli's Unrealized Ideal:
The Elimination of the Noble Humour

Machiavelli's normative ideal is the establishment of a city in which all citizens are capable of expressing their political will, democratic partici-pation in public affairs being the primary mode by which individuals externalize their ambitious desire. Such a situation, however, would seem to necessitate the elimination of the *grandi*, to the extent that the latter always attempt, through the private deployment of their wealth and resources, to dominate others, an element of such domination being the exclusion of these others from participatory modes. Again, the few always act in the mode of the few. There certainly seem to be cases where Machiavelli suggests that it is possible to purge from the city the desire to oppress, at least inasmuch as this desire is concretely articulated in the formation of a political humour identified with a determinate group of individuals united in their end. Putting aside the question of whether the following examples reveal to us the specificity of Machiavellian *virtù* as I attempted to define it in chapter 3, they nev-ertheless no doubt reveal the practical possibility of eliminating the *grandi* within a city. Clearchus of Heraclea, for example, was raised to the position of tyrant by the city's aristocrats in their effort to strengthen their own position relative to the people. Finding himself stuck between a people who had been deprived of its freedom and an insolent aristoc-racy, however, Clearchus correctly realized that his own security depended on grounding his authority in the popular element, which

---

75 Ibid., bk. 7.23.

would be most effectively achieved through completely purging the city of the desire for domination. Hence, recognizing "a convenient occasion for this, he cut to pieces all the aristocrats, to the extreme satisfaction of the people."[76] Agathocles the Sicilian, meanwhile, followed the same pattern: "he gathered together one morning the people and the Senate of Syracuse, as if he had to decide things pertaining to the republic; and, with a signal he arranged, he made his soldiers kill all the senators and the richest of the people; they being dead, he occupied and held the principality of that city without any civil controversy."[77]

Machiavelli is highly sceptical, however, of the efficacy of relying on singular individuals or princes in order to eliminate the *grandi*. There remains the potential for such individuals to become tyrants, thus generating a new internal social hierarchy that equally militates against the popular venting of desire.[78] Hence the identification of the error of the Roman plebs' support of Appius when it appeared to them that he would improve their standing relative to the nobility: "when a people is led to make this error – to give reputation to one – because he beats down those that it hates, and if that one is wise, he always will become tyrant of that city. For he will wait, together with the favour of the people, to eliminate the nobility; and he will never turn to the oppression of the people until he has eliminated [the nobles]; at that time, when the people recognize itself as servile, it has nowhere to take refuge. This mode has held for all those who have founded tyrannies in republics."[79] This establishment of a singular concentration of authority was doubly injurious in that it took place in a republican context in which the people were already in possession of certain popular modes and orders for

---

76 Machiavelli, "Discorsi sopra la prima Deca di Tito Livio," bk. 1.16.

77 Machiavelli, "Il Principe," chap. 8. For the suggestion that Machiavelli is a champion of Greek tyrants like Clearchus and Agathocles to the extent that they reform corrupted states and defend the people from those who would oppress them, see John P. McCormick, "Of Tribunes and Tyrants: Machiavelli's Legal and Extra-Legal Modes for Controlling Elites," *Ratio Juris* 28, no. 2 (2015): 252–66; John P. McCormick, "Machiavelli's Greek Tyrant as Republican Reformer," in *The Radical Machiavelli: Politics, Philosophy, and Language*, ed. Filippo Del Lucchese, Fabio Frosini, and Vittorio Morfino (Leiden: Brill, 2015), 337–48.

78 For an account of Machiavelli as a radical critic of tyranny in all its forms see Giovanni Giorgini, "The Place of the Tyrant in Machiavelli's Political Thought and the Literary Genre of the *Prince*," *History of Political Thought* 29, no. 2 (2008): 230–56.

79 Machiavelli, "Discorsi sopra la prima Deca di Tito Livio," bk. 1.40.

regulating the trajectory of noble decision making: "where they ought to place a guard over [the magistrates] to keep them good, the Romans removed it, making [the Decemvirate] the only magistracy in Rome, annulling all the others due to the excessive wish (as said above) that the Senate had to eliminate the consuls. This blinded them in such a mode that they agreed to such a disorder."[80] Speaking more generally of the singular reordering of the social field via extraordinary means, Machiavelli posits the internally contradictory form of such a model of political transformation, seemingly invalidating thereby the logic of singular foundation: "the reordering of a city to a political life presupposes a good man, and becoming prince of a republic through violence presupposes an evil man; from this it will be found that it very rarely happens that a good person will want to become prince through evil ways, even if his end would be good, and that a wicked person who became prince wants to work well, as it will never cross his mind to use that authority well which he has acquired evilly."[81]

More notable than the examples of Clearchus and Agathocles, then, to the extent that the relevant purging of the great is carried out by the people themselves – with external assistance – as opposed to a prince acting in their name, is the account of the civil war in Corcyra during the Peloponnesian War. The internal division in Corcyra mirrored that between Athens and Sparta, there emerging groups supportive of each of these powers, with the nobles looking to appropriate authority for their faction exclusively. However, "having occurred in that city that the nobles prevailed, and took away the freedom of the people, the popular [group] regained its power by means of the Athenians, and laying their hands on the whole nobility, locked them in a prison capable of holding them all, from which they drew out eight or ten at a time, under pretence of sending them into exile in different places, and had them put to death with many examples of cruelty."[82] The fact, furthermore, that the people are commonly such oriented toward the attempt to establish freedom via the elimination of the nobles and their desire to oppress is revealed in Machiavelli's observation that "it is no wonder, then, that peoples take extraordinary revenges against those who have taken their freedom."[83]

---

80 Ibid.
81 Ibid., bk. 1.18.
82 Ibid., bk. 2.2.
83 Ibid.

If the possibility of eliminating the nobility is a real one, what should we make of Machiavelli's critique of the people's desire for such an elimination, or at least a noble exclusion from institutions of rule, in the Florentine context? The universal participatory form of popular desire is once again affirmed in the *Histories*, Machiavelli noting, however, the different form it took in Florence as opposed to in Rome. Whereas "the people of Rome desired to enjoy the supreme honours together with the nobility," in Florence the people "fought to be alone in the government, without the nobles participating."[84] It was this effort to exclude the nobility altogether from rule, which Machiavelli calls "unfair and unjust," that intensified the noble desire to oppress, instigating the latter's violent reaction in Florence.[85] As always, however, we must be sensitive to the historical specificity of the narration. Machiavelli is affirming that the people have not yet transcended their status as unshackled, that they have not yet been fully socialized to exclusive rule, as evidenced in their wish to immediately express their political will without having undertaken a transformative learning process via participation in shared deliberative activities. This is made explicit when Machiavelli claims that in Rome it was by governing with the nobles, that is to say, those who had prior experience in political life, that the people actualized their deliberative potential: "in the victories of the people the city of Rome became more virtuous; for as the people could administer the magistracies, the armies, and the high offices along with the nobles, they were filled with the same virtue as the latter were, and that city, growing in virtue, grew in power."[86] Contrary to the Roman experience, in Florence the exact opposite movement occurred, for there, when "the people overcame [the nobles], the nobles remained deprived of magistracies; and if they wanted to reacquire them it was necessary – in conduct, in spirit, and in mode of living – not only to be but to appear similar to the people."[87] This non-concern with popular political education, and the nobles' abandonment of their virtue as expressed in the orientation toward the transmission of political knowledge, made it impossible to institute good orders looking toward

---

84 Machiavelli, "Istorie fiorentine," bk. 3.1.
85 Ibid.
86 Ibid.
87 Ibid.

political socialization: "So the virtue of arms and generosity of spirit that was eliminated in the nobility – and in the people, where it never was – could not be rekindled; thus Florence became more and more meek and abject."[88] There is thus a concrete trajectory of democratic socialization that can be read in terms of Machiavelli's recognition of the transformative potential of dialogical learning, such as was detailed in the previous chapter. Despite the fact that the political education of the people takes place in an institutional world that it occupies with the nobles, it is still a self-education, one that takes place through shared rule.[89]

My suggestion has been that we can read the ultimate end of such self-education in terms of the abolition of the *grandi*. As we have already seen, in the "Discourse on Florentine Affairs" Machiavelli contends that each of the main social groups within the city must have access to political institutions that allow these groups' members to vent their ambition. As we have also seen, however, Machiavelli here suggests as well both the possibility of constructing a city in which the nobility have been eliminated, and that his proposed reconstitution of Florence would be characterized by an increasing empowerment of the people, who are invested with more and more authority as they increasingly educate themselves regarding political things. The acquisition of political knowledge tends toward increasing democratization and wealth equalization that would ideally lead to the elimination of the great as an organized class. Machiavelli, though, is not so utopian as to imagine that such an elimination might result in the harmonization of the interests of the city and the concomitant eradication of all impulses to domination. It is not possible to structure a regime that will produce citizens whose desire is incapable of taking the form of a will to oppress. For example, in *Discourses* 3:17 he maintains, despite an earlier claim that healthy republics will not allow for the emergence of corrupt citizens,

---

88 Ibid.

89 Hence Dante Germino writes that "Machiavelli's critical study of politics, then, far from shoring up the position of the political elite and providing them with esoteric 'secrets of rule,' has the effect, if seriously pursued, of democratizing politics through the spread of political knowledge to elites and non-elites alike." Dante Germino, "Machiavelli's Thoughts on the Psyche and Society," in *The Political Calculus: Essays on Machiavelli's Political Philosophy*, ed. Anthony Parel (Toronto: University of Toronto Press, 1972), 76.

that it is always possible for insolent individuals to arise.[90] Given this concession, we must once more remind ourselves of how we specified the definition of the *grandi* in Machiavelli's work.

Machiavelli seems to define the great in term of the orientation of their humour: the fact that they have a desire to oppress. This simple definition is complicated by the fact that in many places Machiavelli identifies members of the people as also possessing such a desire. The matter becomes clearer when we identify a second component of the noble humour, that is, its class characteristic. Machiavelli's use of the term *umore* refers not to the orientation of individual wills, but of social groupings, the range of which far exceed the typical bifurcation of humours into the categories of the people and the great. In the *Florentine Histories* Machiavell expands upon the possibility of a city containing a plurality of humours, thus engendering a diversity of enmities. For example, after the failures of Niccolao da Prato to eliminate the tumults in Florence, "full of disdain he went back to the Pontiff, and left Florence full of confusion and interdicted. And not was that city disrupted by one humour, *but by many*; it contained hostilities between the people and the great, the Ghibellines and the Guelfs, the Whites and the Blacks."[91] Thus only insolent individuals constitute grandees, representatives of one specific humour, when enough of them simultaneously emerge and are able to succeed in organizing themselves into a class self-conscious of its generally unified end, acquiring sufficient economic resources to work toward the actualization of this end.

Although the political community is powerless to prevent the appearance of wills to domination, it is not inevitable that these wills will be

---

90 Machiavelli, "Discorsi sopra la prima Deca di Tito Livio," bk. 3.17. On the former claim, for example, see *Discourses* 3:12, where Machiavelli writes that the potential for conspiracy is neutralized in the healthy republic, for the thought of privately subverting established institutional norms would not occur to citizens socialized in such a context. Only the corrupt republic thus need worry about conspiratorial threats. Ibid., bk. 3.12.

91 Machiavelli, "Istorie fiorentine," bk. 2.21. Emphasis added. There are other places in which Machiavelli notes that the variety of humours in a city may exceed those of the people and the great. Most obviously, for example, see his discussion of the humour of the soldiers in Machiavelli, "Il Principe," chap. 19. For a recent example of an argument grounded in the presumption of the existence of this third humour see Paul A. Rahe, "Machiavelli and the Modern Tyrant," in *Machiavelli on Liberty and Conflict*, ed. David Johnston, Nadia Urbinati, and Camila Vergara (Chicago: University of Chicago Press, 2017), 207–31.

consolidated into a humour that is perpetually opposed to that to live freely. On the contrary, the community must be vigilant in repressing such urges to oppress when they manifest themselves precisely so that they do not organize themselves into a shared humour, that is, into the *grandi*, through for example, excluding such individuals from accessing major office.[92] As we have seen, the people do not possess any intrinsic nature that is specific to them and that would provide a natural ground for psychologically distinguishing them from the great. It is thus not surprising that Machiavelli should provide many examples of insolent individuals emerging from within the body of the people. Such is impossible to overcome. However, it is not impossible to institutionally structure the political regime such that these individual wills are not immediately capable of concentrating themselves into an organized class that can actualize the particular form of appearance of their desire. Hence in the *Florentine Histories* Machaivelli notes that "evil humours" do not necessarily appear naturally with a city, but only when there do not exist social conditions that act as checks preventing their appearance.[93] A city can overcome the formation of organized class humours, which is what Machiavelli's democratic theory would ultimately seem to demand. As I have suggested in this chapter, one of the most essential mechanisms in this respect is the equalization of economic conditions, as the leveraging and deployment of wealth is the key instrument by which the humour to oppress expresses itself. Not only can an *umore* be neutralized, then, as in those cases of institutional pacification of the *grandi* that are detailed in the *Discourses*, but the city can be so structured so as to militate against its very appearance. Although the *Florentine Histories* provide us with some examples of the people eliminating the nobility, as we will see later, new enmities perpetually emerged in Florence not because the antagonistic opposition of humours is inherent to social being, but because Florence failed to create institutional modes and orders that would be able to productively stabilize conflict so as prevent the re-emergence of separate class interests.

Machiavelli's concession of the impossibility of eradicating insolence within a city also allows us to grasp a further political consequence

---

92 Machiavelli, "Discorsi sopra la prima Deca di Tito Livio," bk. 3.17.
93 Machiavelli, "Istorie fiorentine," bk. 4.28.

of the potential elimination of the *grandi*. Specifically, it demonstrates that this movement is not characterized by a homogenization of the social field that would render individual desires identical, thereby instaurating a regime of consensus that effaces social conflict. As I specified in chapter 2, human difference greatly exceeds that difference that characterizes the opposition of the noble and the popular humours. Although Machiavelli often suggests that the enmities between the people and the great are the "cause of all the evils that emerge in cities,"[94] he does not maintain that this precise form of social division exhausts all possible forms, nor even that it is naturally instrinsic to cities. Human multiplicity is an ineradicable feature of human life, and thus conflict a perpetual dimension of human co-relation.[95] The key political issue is not whether conflict can be eliminated, but rather the form that conflict takes and the modes by which it is negotiated. What must be distinguished is the contingent conflict between the desire to oppress and the desire not to oppress, and the more generalized and universal conflict grounded in the very fact of human multiplicity. It is no doubt the case that Machiavelli concerns himself most with detailing the manifestation of the former expression of conflict. Such results not as a consequence of a belief in its naturalness or inevitability, but of Machiavelli's own precise social-historical situation. It is not the case that the overcoming of inequality, represented in the overcoming of the division of humours, leads to an elimination of conflict, for conflict is irreducible to this division, grounded as it is in natural human difference. Equality, however, can be affirmed in difference through the equal participation of all in institutionalized agonistic conflict over the direction of the political community. The conflictual confrontation between always non-identical wills in the public sphere, proceeding non-antagonistically and being inclusive of all citizens, is the ground upon which democratic determinations are formulated and the principles of freedom and equality

---

94 Ibid., bk. 3.1.

95 Although Alfredo Bonadeo, for example, recognizes that the realization of the Machiavellian political ideal involves the elimination of the nobility, he is incorrect in presuming that this would entail a correlative elimination of social conflict with the city. Alfredo Bonadeo, "Machiavelli on Civic Equality and Republican Government," *Romance Notes* 11, no. 1 (1969): 163.

concretely expressed and affirmed. In short, the key issue is not whether conflict exists, but the quality of the conflict and the mode by which the energies structuring it are expressed. I will outline some of the productive and democratic of such modes in what remains of the present study.

Chapter Six

Institutionalizing Ambitious Expression: The Republic as the Self-Overcoming Regime

In the previous two chapters I highlighted select passages from Machiavelli's *Florentine Histories* and "Discourse on Florentine Affairs" that suggest 1) the existence of a popular desire for political participation, 2) the existence of a popular capacity for autonomous self-organization, and 3) a critique of economic inequality that ultimately points toward the elimination of the *grandi* as a determinate social class. In emphasizing this content I position myself in opposition to that "now nearly hegemonic interpretation" that identifies a fundamental transition or break in Machiavelli's work.[1] For these latter readers Machiavelli's later Florentine writings are marked by a general conservative turn that repudiates the earlier defence of the people's productive role in civil life.[2] I argue, on the contrary, that there remains in this later work a clear democratic content, and indeed, a somewhat unique democratic

---

1 John P. McCormick, "On the Myth of the Conservative Turn in Machiavelli's *Florentine Histories*," in *Machiavelli on Liberty and Conflict*, ed. David Johnston, Nadia Urbinati, and Camila Vergara (Chicago: University of Chicago Press, 2017), 204.

2 In his own contribution to this tendency, Mauricio Suchowlansky sums up the position concisely: "It has been argued that the Machiavelli of the tracts from the 1520s no longer endows the people with an instrumental role as guardians of liberty; that Machiavelli is critical of the tumultuous form of popular republicanism as quintessentially represented by ancient Rome; and finally that the Machiavelli of the 1520s no longer sees in the figure of the princely individual a solution to a republic's difficulties." Mauricio Suchowlansky, "Machiavelli's *Summary of the Affairs of the City of Lucca*: Venice as *buon governo*," *Intellectual History Review* 26, no. 4 (2016): 429. For a critique of this interpretation of the Florentine writings see McCormick, "On the Myth of the Conservative Turn in Machiavelli's Florentine Histories."

content relative to the earlier republican writings, in that the issue of the potential for the equalization of material conditions of life is considered to be more of a realistic historical possibility. To the extent that the mode of political being detailed in the *Discourses on Livy* continues to assume the existence of the *grandi*, it cannot be identified as embodying Machiavelli's democratic ideal, for there still exists an organized humour to oppress as a concrete form of appearance of the desire for ambitious self-expression.

Such is not at all to suggest, however, that the *Discourses* is thereby irrelevant to Machiavelli's normative defence of popular political self-activity, or even that it is more distant from the Machiavellian ideal than the image presented in the *Florentine Histories*.[3] On the contrary, the complete revelation of a Machiavellian form of democratic life as a normative political goal is achieved only through a combination of various of the lessons contained within these texts. Although the texts do emphasize differing elements of democratic life, these emphases are not mutually incompatible, thereby necessitating our thinking the form of relation between them in terms of break or transition. On the one hand, in the Florentine writings Machiavelli highlights the fact that the equalization of economic conditions is a possibility that may be concretely actualized. This possibility was closed off in the republican Rome of the *Discourses* as a result of the continued existence of the great as a separate social class. On the other hand, in the *Discourses* Machiavelli highlights the fact that the non-antagonistic expression of human ambition is possible only if there exist political forms that can productively channel it. This possibility was closed off in the Florence of the *Florentine Histories* as a result of the lack of stable institutional orders respected by all citizens. What unites both the republican writings of the *Discourses* and the later Florentine writings is the affirmation of an ambitious popular desire for self-expression. In the former text

---

3 Distinguishing between the form of conflict in Rome as opposed to Florence, Filippo Del Lucchese, for example, maintains that democratic life is ultimately not possible in the former given its reproduction of inequality. Filippo Del Lucchese, "La città divisa: esperieza del conflitto e novità politica in Machiavelli," in *Machiavelli: immaginazione e contingenza*, ed. Filippo Del Lucchese, Luca Sartorello, and Stefano Visentin (Pisa: Edizioni Ets, 2006), 23–4. If the *Florentine Histories* is Machiavelli's most democratic text, however, its radically democratic potential can nevertheless be gleaned in certain other scattered places through the Machiavellian oeuvre. Ibid., 24.

Machiavelli theorizes the institutional conditions for the socially productive sublimation of this popular desire, while in the latter texts Machiavelli theorizes the possibility of the establishment of a general economic equality via the abolition of the *grandi* and the self-education of the people. The synthesis of these two accounts, never undertaken systematically by Machiavelli, generates a more complete and coherent democratic constellation.

Even though Rome failed to institute conditions of social and economic equality, the presentation of republican life in the *Discourses* nevertheless allows us to grasp the main contours of Machiavelli's democratic thought. Specifically, the existence of the *grandi* in Rome does not obscure the recognition of the need for all citizens to have an assured political outlet for the venting of their desire. Reconstructing the constellation that aims to articulate the image of a regime in which the capacity for political self-expression is universalized allows us to go well beyond those readings that locate in Machiavelli only "the germs of a theory of democracy."[4] At the same time,

---

4 David Held, *Models of Democracy* (Cambridge: Polity Press, 1999), 54. Needless to say, the vast majority of readers of Machiavelli do not even identify this germinal potential. An exhaustive list of the readings that posit Machiavelli as an anti-democratic thinker would be impossible to construct, although some representative ones – primarily from republican and Straussian perspectives – may be noted. Those who attempt to assimilate Machiavelli to a classical republican tradition argue that the actualization of the common good cannot be grounded in the equal participation of all citizens, the aristocratic structure of the republic being a consequence of the fact that it is the virtuous few alone who are competent to enact policies that can ensure such an actualization. See, for example, Colish, "The Idea of Liberty in Machiavelli," 347; de Grazia, *Machiavelli in Hell*, 180; Werner Maihoffer, "The Ethos of the Republic and the Reality of Politics," in *Machiavelli and Republicanism*, ed. Gisela Bock, Quentin Skinner, and Maurizio Viroli (Cambridge: Cambridge University Press, 1990), 287; Maurizio Viroli, "Machiavelli and the Republican Idea of Politics," in *Machiavelli and Republicanism*, ed. Gisela Bock, Quentin Skinner, and Maurizio Viroli (Cambridge: Cambridge University Press, 1990), 155; Pettit, *Republicanism: A Theory of Freedom and Government*, 11; Maddox, "The Secular Reformation and the Influence of Machiavelli," 555; Maihoffer, "The Ethos of the Republic and the Reality of Politics," 287. Similarly affirming an inequality of capacity between the people and political elites, readers influenced by Strauss tend to jettison concern with any conception of a common human good, emphasizing elite manipulation of the people and the tyrannical elements of Machiavelli's republicanism. See, for example, Thomas Pangle, *The Ennobling of Democracy: The Challenge of the Postmodern Age* (Baltimore: Johns Hopkins University Press, 1992), 135; Vickie B. Sullivan, *Machiavelli's Three Romes: Religion,*

recognizing the explicitly institutional form of the democratic republic – specifically, that it is through institutional life that the people
express their creative energies – allows us to go beyond those radical
democratic readings that posit an unbridgeable chasm between the
instituted form of the political regime and the instituting power of
popular self-activity. I argue that through theorizing the possibility
of creating institutions open to their own perpetual self-interrogation,
Machiavelli provides the means to think the simultaneous affirmation of the instituted and the instituting in one democratic form.[5]
Machiavelli's discovery lies in his conception of a political regime that
is able to affirm, through its institutional structure, the negative
desire of the citizens of the polity, the democratic form of the positive
structure being ethically grounded in the universality of the negative desire. After detailing the key elements of Machiavelli's theorization of democratic institutionalization and how it functions so as to
give an expression to the form of ambitious desire that was detailed
in chapter 3, in the final section of the chapter I will re-examine the
centrality of the question of the institution negatively through a brief
account of the democratic deficiencies of the historical episodes
detailed by Machiavelli in the *Florentine Histories*, reiterating why it is
a mistake to identify this text as Machiavelli's main democratic
contribution.

Human Liberty, and Politics Reformed (DeKalb: Northern Illinois University Press,
1996), 178; Harvey C. Mansfield, *Machiavelli's Virtue* (Chicago: University of Chicago
Press, 1996), 307; Harvey C. Mansfield, "Bruni and Machiavelli on Civic Humanism," in *Renaissance Civic Humanism: Reappraisals and Reflections*, ed. James Hankins
(Cambridge: Cambridge University Press, 2000), 239; J. Patrick Coby, *Machiavelli's
Romans: Liberty and Greatness in the Discourses* (Lanham: Lexington, 1999), 256; Daniel
Schillinger, "Luck and Character in Machiavelli's Political Thought," *History of Politi-
cal Thought* 37, no. 4 (2016): 619–20. It should be noted that it is perhaps the case that
whereas contemporary Straussian readers tend to cover up Machiavelli's democratic
commitments and read him as an aristocratic critic of the people, Strauss himself
seems to recognize these commitments, they in fact being the source of his distaste for
Machiavelli. On this point see Benedetto Fontana, "Reason and Politics: Philosophy
Confronts the People," *Boundary 2* 33, no. 1 (2006): 35. For a Strauss-influenced reading that in fact understands Machiavelli's goal to be the foundation of a democratic
republic see Zuckert, *Machiavelli's Politics*.

5 Bernard Flynn notes that Machiavelli's Rome can be seen as both an instituting and
   instituted society. Flynn, *The Philosophy of Claude Lefort*, 57.

The Republican Multiplication of Virtuous
Self-Expression

Machiavelli's participatory demand is given an expression as early as *Discourses* 1:2. This chapter is often read as evidence that Machiavelli appropriated the theory of cyclical historical movement posited by Polybius. For Polybius there is "a regular cycle of constitutional revolutions, and the natural order in which constitutions change, are transformed, and return again to their original stage."[6] Such changes are the result of "an undeviating law of nature."[7] Every unmixed form of government is unstable to the extent that it contains within itself its negative malignity, which will eventually pervert it into its opposite. It is often assumed on the part of readers that Machiavelli's defence of the mixed regime is the means by which he attempts to overcome the instability of the political realm and stabilize the being of the polity. As Lefort points out, however, it is highly doubtful that Machiavelli intends to read Polybius literally, as there is no reference to the cyclical theory of regimes after the very beginning of the *Discourses*, and the ideal of the mixed regime is quickly abandoned.[8] Already in the chapter dealing with the cyclical theory is Machiavelli undermining the traditional image of the harmonious mixed regime by emphasizing Rome's affirmation of the disunion between the plebs and the nobles, thus contradicting the classical position that the virtue of the mixed regime lay in the establishment of a proportioned unity in which each part through performing its social role contributes to the overall concord of the society. By the end of the book it has become clear that the very goal of social stability has been rejected as a normative end, Machiavelli instead theorizing the republic in terms of a political regime that is open to the necessity of being continually restructured so as to adapt to the contingent indeterminacy of history.

---

6 Polybius, *The Histories of Polybius*, vol. 1, ed. and trans. Evelyn S. Shuckburgh (Cambridge: Cambridge University Press, 2012), bk. 6.9.

7 Ibid., bk. 6.10.

8 Lefort, *Machiavelli in the Making*, 224. Needless to say, however, Lefort is not the only commentator to question the literalness of Machiavelli's engagement with Polybius. See also, for example, Salvatore di Maria, "Machiavelli's Ironic View of History: The *Istorie Fiorentine*," *Renaissance Quarterly* 45, no. 2 (1992): 251–2.

The purpose of *Discourses* 1:2 is not to articulate a philosophy of history grounded in a determinate principle of movement, but rather to call attention to the necessity of generalizing public participation within the republican polity. Machiavelli begins by noting that he will concern himself specifically with states that have been free with respect to their institution, he not being interested in servile principalities or republics. Importantly, the contingency of such institution, the independence of political foundation from a fixed logic of creation, is immediately affirmed through the recognition of the multiplicity of free states, which "have had, like diverse beginnings, diverse laws and orders."[9] Machiavelli will recapitulate the traditional taxonomy of regimes, distinguishing between the principality, the aristocracy, and the popular form, along with their corrupted opposites. Already Machiavelli will depart from Polybius in suggesting that the cycle's monarchical origin is not a natural phenomenon, but rather emerges by chance. In any case, what is clear is that the corruption of each political form stimulating the movement to the next is identified with a principle of exclusive authority: degeneracy is in each moment grounded in the failure of the regime to incorporate all of its citizens into the participatory life of the city. This is the case even in the so-called democratic regime, where the people themselves take responsibility for the ordering of the polity, but so as to deny any authority to those who had previously excluded them: "the memory of the prince and of the injuries received from him still being fresh, and having unmade the state of the few and not wanting to remake that of the prince, [the people] turned to the popular state; and they ordered it in a way that neither the powerful few nor a prince would have any authority."[10] In other words, the people cannot order a popular republic in a city in which there is an established class of *grandi* in such a way as they could if there were not. The potential democratic form leans upon the realities of the historical matter, placing limits on the institutional possibility germinating within the social field. Again, the essential point is that all citizens have a place in government so as to vent their ambition, including the great in republican contexts in which they are an organized social class. This then is the virtue of the mixed regime identified with Rome. It is not that the distribution of political roles generates a social stability through giving an expression to an organically or naturally differentiated set of class elements, but

---

9 Machiavelli, "Discorsi sopra la prima Deca di Tito Livio," in *Tutte le opere*, bk. 1.2.
10 Ibid.

rather that it provides the concrete conditions, in a contingent historical environment, for the generalization of political participation. It was only after the creation of the tribunes of the plebs that each element in the city had a legal place, and even as it oscillated between kingly government and noble government and popular government, "nevertheless it never took away, to give authority to the aristocrats, all the authority of a kingly quality; nor did it diminish wholly the authority of the aristocrats, in order to give it to the people; but remaining mixed, it made a perfect republic: and that perfection came through the disunion of the plebs and the Senate."[11]

I have already suggested that Machiavelli posits an ethical imperative to expand as widely as possible the fields that allow for the expression of individual *virtù*, an imperative that is grounded in his perception of both the universality of human ambition, and the universality of the capacity of individuals to autonomously externalize or vent this ambition through creative self-activity.[12] Such an imperative was affirmed in a partial form already in *The Prince*, specifically in chapter 21, where Machiavelli maintains that the prince should make it a policy to encourage the development of citizens' creative and critical capacities in all spheres of human activity: "A prince furthermore ought to show himself a lover of virtue, giving recognition to virtuous men, and honour the excellent in an art. Alongside this, he ought to encourage his citizens to exercise their powers peacefully, in trade and in commerce and in every other activity of men."[13] Even if virtuous self-expression is politically denied in the new principality, there nevertheless remain outlets for the expulsion of creative desire, and the prince should work to honour those citizens who distinguish themselves in their endeavours in these fields: "he ought to prepare rewards for whoever wants to do these things."[14] Indeed, in his very

---

11 Ibid.

12 Given that the majority of Machiavelli's readers insist on conceptually differentiating between civic and princely *virtù*, it is perhaps not surprising that this process of generalization is not often recognized. One commentator who does come close to using this language, however, is Eugene Garver, who suggestively writes that in the *Discourses* Machiavelli is attempting to think the possibility of instituting a political community in which all citizens have acquired *virtù* in a sort of "movement of universalization." Garver, *Machiavelli and the History of Prudence*, 124.

13 Machiavelli, "Il Principe," in *Tutte le opere*, chap. 21.

14 Ibid.

celebration of the capacity for virtuous innovation the prince renders himself "an example of humanity."[15] Nevertheless, despite the princely imperative to encourage and reward virtue, it remains true that the generalization of the capacity is incapable of being actualized in the context of monarchical life. In *The Art of War* Machiavelli notes that where individuals are under the command of one or a few princes, not many citizens of virtue will emerge. It remains true, though, that "the world has been more virtuous where there have been more states that have favoured virtue, either by necessity or by another human passion."[16] To the extent that the achievement of political virtue is closed off to citizens in a principality as a consequence of the lack of participatory organs, Machiavelli notes that ultimately the republic is the necessary political form for the widespread actualization of *virtù*: "for from republics come more excellent men than in kingdoms, because while in the former virtue is honoured most of the time, in kingdoms it is feared; so it arises that in the one virtuous men are nourished, in the other they are eliminated."[17]

The republic is thus conceptualized by Machiavelli as that form of political regime that is capable of multiplying the spaces for virtuous self-expression, most notably through the institution of participatory modes and orders that open up the potential for the actualization of a specifically political form of such self-expression. And indeed, in *Discourses* 1:30 Machiavelli maintains that a republic must attempt to generalize virtue to the greatest degree possible, such as happened in Rome: "Because the whole city, both the nobles and the ignobles, was participating through war, there emerged in Rome in every age so many virtuous men, adorned from manifold victories, that the people had no reason to doubt any of them, as they were many, and one guarded the other."[18] Not only was this increasingly large group of individuals satisfied with its positive role in the city, to the extent that it allowed for an externalization of the desire for virtue, but each particular one acted as a check against those whose ambition might lead to an attempt to privately appropriate authority. Such orders were so well-instituted "that, coming to the dictatorship, one brought back from it

---

15 Ibid.
16 Machiavelli, "Dell'Arte della guerra," in *Tutte le opere*, 332.
17 Ibid.
18 Machiavelli, "Discorsi sopra la prima Deca di Tito Livio," bk. 1.30.

greater glory the sooner one laid it down. And so, not being able to generate suspicion, such modes did not generate ingratitude."[19]

What is more, the association of virtuous self-expression with the type of creative innovation that is articulated in *The Prince* is detailed in the next chapter, where Machiavelli speaks of the need for the city to cultivate and nurture a spirit of experimentation. This need is manifested in a particularly notable way in the fact that the Romans were more hesitant than most when it came to punishing captains who erred. If the error was made not through malice, but honestly through ignorance, the captain would not only not be punished, but in fact be rewarded. For Machiavelli "this mode of proceeding was well considered by them: for they judged that it should be so important to those who governed their armies that they have a free and expeditious spirit, without other extrinsic considerations in taking resolutions, that they did not want to add to a thing – in itself difficult and dangerous – new difficulties and dangers, thinking that if they added them, nobody would ever be able to work virtuously."[20] The elimination of the fear of punishment allows actors to more consistently affirm risk through the development of innovative and hence necessarily unproven strategies, unsullied by considerations that would limit in advance the range of their action.

We must not think, however, that the only medium for the expression of virtue is that of civic participation in activities associated with war. In 3:34, for example, Machiavelli maintains that one of the greatest sources of social recognition is to be found in the active doing of virtuous public works. Such a mode of acquiring reputation is contrasted with those that depend upon pedigree or association. Although the latter two speak to the significance of positive socialization, of the fact that one may be educated to good modes through exposure to the examples of others, such socialization is sufficient only for the production of the conditions of good action, but not that action itself. The actual doing of the deed is thus a superior criterion when making judgment on virtue, and all citizens in the republic should strive to not only demonstrate their virtue through such self-activity, but perpetually expand the scope of this action. As Machiavelli says, judgment grounded in action, "having been begun and founded on the deed and on your work, gives you

---

19 Ibid.
20 Ibid., bk. 1.31.

so much name at the beginning that afterwards you need to do many things contrary to this if you want to annul it. Men born in a republic ought, therefore, to take this route, and strive, with some extraordinary action, to begin to become notable."[21] Machiavelli gives as examples of such notable things "promulgating a law that was for the common benefit," "accusing some powerful citizen as a transgressor of the laws," or any "similar notable and new things, of which one would have to speak."[22] The expression of virtue is thus explicitly identified with participatory political activity that is oriented to the creation of the new, to the alteration of the structure of the political form in such a way as to benefit public life. Machiavelli is adamant in this chapter, though, that it is not sufficient to simply act virtuously in an instant. Rather, the political actor must strive to continue to extend the process through perpetually renewing creative virtue in expansive action: "Not only are such things necessary to give oneself reputation but are likewise necessary to maintain and increase it. And if one wants to do this, one needs to renew them."[23]

The imperative is further elaborated within the context of a discussion of Spurius Maelius in 3:28, where Machiavelli raises the topic of the distribution of reputation, locating the republican degeneration into tyranny in the improper deployment of high honours. The question is how to order a city so that reputation can be used only for the sake of the good of the city, as opposed to the good of the individual who has the reputation alone. Machiavelli argues that to achieve such a condition – the mutual actualization of individual and collective good in the distribution – reputation should be founded on specifically public service: "one ought to examine the modes with which they get reputation. There are in effect two: either public or private. The public modes are when one individual, counselling well and acting better, for the common benefit, acquires reputation."[24] Private modes of achieving reputation, in opposition, are those that look toward the exclusive benefit of the private person. Such benefit can be achieved "by lending [others] money, marrying off their daughters, defending them against the magistrates, and doing for them similar private favours, which

---

21 Ibid., bk. 3.34.
22 Ibid.
23 Ibid.
24 Ibid., bk. 3.28.

make men partisans, and give spirit to whoever is so favoured to be able to corrupt the public and break the laws."[25] If public modes are to be privileged over private ones then the city must provide the conditions for a generalization of the capacity to benefit the public, providing outlets for citizens to achieve civic distinction. Such a project of extension constitutes an essential moment in the goal of generalizing virtue, the city opening the path to reputation to as many citizens as possible. Hence Machiavelli's celebration of the Roman mode: "for as reward to whoever worked well for the public, it ordered triumphs, and all the other honours that it gave to its citizens; and as punishment to whoever searched under various colours to make themselves great through private ways, it ordered accusations."[26]

What Machiavelli details is a dialectic between individual and collective virtue, demonstrating how the generalization of the former provides the condition for the actualization of the latter. This movement is most explicitly articulated in *Discourses* 3:31. Here Machiavelli reasserts the nature of the virtue of the individual, locating it not in the ability to replicate precise patterns of behaviour, nor in the actualization of a concrete end, but rather in a certain type of spiritual resolve that proves itself in the encounter with the world: "one sees how great men are always the same in every fortune; and if it varies, now by exalting them, now by oppressing them, they do not vary, but always keep their spirit firm, and united with their mode of living, so that one easily knows for each that fortune does not have power over them."[27] Weak individuals, on the contrary, are those who mistake their good fortune for their own virtue, not recognizing the dialectic – mediated through the occasion – that exists between the two terms.[28] After recapitulating this dialectic of *fortuna* and *virtù*, more systematically developed in *The Prince*, and the differing characters resulting from its recognition or non-recognition,

25 Ibid.

26 Machiavelli, "Discorsi sopra la prima Deca di Tito Livio," bk. 3.28.

27 Ibid., bk. 3.31.

28 In the *Discourses* the dialectical form of the relation between *virtù* and *fortuna*, mediated through the appearance of the *occassione*, is represented in chapter 2:29, where Machiavelli again interprets *virtù* in terms of the capacity to recognize the spaces of action opened up by *fortuna*. Indeed, here the relationship between the two terms is taken to be so obvious as to not even warrant specific examples. Ibid., bk. 2.29. Machiavelli does, of course, provide many examples of the dialectic of virtue and fortune as manifested in the Roman case. See, for example, ibid., bk. 2.1.

Machiavelli goes on to argue that these latter orientations are always observable among republics. In Rome, for example, no bad fortune ever rendered them abject, nor did any good fortune generate in them insolence, whereas the Venetians, because they interpreted their worldly condition to be an exclusive product of their non-existent virtue, did become insolent, and as their condition changed over time they were of necessity ruined.[29] Stressing the extent to which virtue as opposed to insolence is grounded in a concrete knowledge of the historical specificity of existence, and the extent to which this knowledge is acquired through being subject to a productive form of socialization, Machiavelli writes: "For this becoming insolent in good fortune and abject in bad emerges from your mode of proceeding, and from the education in which you are nurtured: this, when it is weak and vain, renders you similar to itself; when it has been otherwise, it renders you also of another fate; and, making you a better knower of the world, it makes you rejoice less in the good, and be saddened less in the bad."[30]

The virtuous city is thus defined in terms of its production of virtuous citizens, who themselves collectively constitute the essential substance of the virtuous city. The manifestation of the collective virtue of the republic is realized through the generalization of the individual virtue of the citizens that compose it. Although the structure of the action of the prince represents the Machiavellian ideal, a city "founded on good laws and good orders has no necessity of the virtue of one man, as have the others, to maintain it."[31] This is because in the democratic republican city all citizens take responsibility for the maintenance of the polity through a collective exercise of their virtue. The specifically creative nature of such virtuous self-expression is revealed through Machiavelli's continual emphasis on the necessity of perpetual innovation and reinstitutionalization for the reproduction of the polity through time. Under such conditions, not a single individual, but all, are princes. This formulation is given its best-known expression in *Discourses* 2.2, where the generalization of virtue is seen as one element of a more expansive generalization of social goods characteristic of republican life. Machiavelli here thinks the co-determination of economic, social, and political freedom: "all the towns and the provinces that live freely

---

29 Machiavelli, "Discorsi sopra la prima Deca di Tito Livio," bk. 3.31.
30 Ibid.
31 Machiavelli, "Istorie fiorentine," in *Tutte le opere*, bk. 4.1.

in every part, as said above, make very great gains. For there one sees more people, because marriages are freer and more desirable to men, since each one willingly procreates those children that he believes he can nurture, and he does not worry that his patrimony will be taken; and he knows not only that they are born free and not slaves, but that they can, by means of their virtue, become princes. One sees riches multiply in greater number, both those that come from cultivation, and those that come from the arts."[32] This possibility, of citizens becoming princes through the exercise of their capacity for virtuous self-expression – or better, the association of the image of the prince with this capacity – is further suggested elsewhere, such as in the *Florentine Histories,* where Machiavelli speaks of "the whole multitude" of Milan becoming "almost as princes of the city."[33]

In the chapter that follows *Discourses* 2:2 Machiavelli expands on what is there suggested: that the enrichment of life in the various human spheres is intensified through the demographic multiplication of free citizens, which necessarily implies a further deepening of human multiplicity.[34] The generalization of virtue must not be read in terms of a process of homogenization that reduces individuals to the same generic content as simple members of an organic community. On the contrary, human plurality is preserved and affirmed through the expression of the collective virtue of the republic, which is rooted in the conflictual expression of the individual virtues of the always multiple citizens that constitute this republic. Machiavelli claims that the common good is capable of being actualized only in republican contexts, writing: "And without doubt, this common good is not observed except in republics, for all that looks toward its goal is executed; and although it may damage this or that private individual, there are so many benefited by that spoken of that they can go forward against the disposition of the few suppressed by it."[35] Machiavelli is here explicit that the actualization of the common good is not a universal actualization of every individual good, such a coalescence of individual and general interest being possible only in a social environment in which the human will has been sufficiently homogenized. Although he will differentiate

---

32 Machiavelli, "Discorsi sopra la prima Deca di Tito Livio," bk. 2.2.
33 Machiavelli, "Istorie fiorentine," bk. 6.24.
34 Machiavelli, "Discorsi sopra la prima Deca di Tito Livio," bk. 2.3.
35 Ibid., bk. 2.2.

between different forms of articulation of social division – particularly those that are accompanied by sects and partisans and those that are not – Machiavelli will be adamant that there is no possibility of instituting a republic that is internally unified: "those who hope that a republic can be united are very deceived in this hope."[36] What characterizes republican life cannot thus be the imposition of a singular social identity on all individuals such that their desire tends toward the same end. Human multiplicity remains an essential fact of life, this multiplicity foreclosing the possibility of a universality of satisfaction. The generalization of the capacity for virtuous self-expression does not refer to a social situation in which all individuals are capable of equally realizing their desire, but one in which all are equally capable of expressing their will, that is, articulating the form of their desire. It is facilitated through the appearance of social conflicts rooted in the ineradicable fact of human multiplicity.[37] This conflict is in fact the ground for the determination of political trajectories of action, the latter's democratic formulation being articulated through the perpetual confrontation of particulars via dialogue, debate, discussion, and so on, the significance of which for Machiavelli I detailed in chapter 4.

To further illustrate this conjunction of internal conflict and creative instituting power we can again return briefly to Machiavelli's account of accusation as a political mode. Machiavelli's most systematic treatment of the function of accusation to republican life is undertaken in *Discourses* 1:7. The centrality of this mode is asserted through his contention that "to those who in a city are responsible for guarding its freedom, one cannot give a more useful and necessary authority than that to be able to accuse citizens to the people, or to some magistrate or council, when they sin in anything against the free state."[38] This centrality, however, should not be reduced to the reactive principle that interprets the accusatory activity of the people as simply functioning to

---

36 Machiavelli, "Istorie fiorentine," bk. 7.1.
37 This emphasis on the conflictual basis of political generation is obscured, for example, in the reading of Negri, who despite seeing the democratic city as collectively expressing the constituent power of *The Prince*, interprets this power in terms of a singular will. Negri, *Insurgencies*, 74. For a critique of this position see Filippo Del Lucchese, "Machiavelli and Constituent Power: The Revolutionary Foundation of Modern Political Thought," *European Journal of Political Theory* 16, no. 1 (2017): 3–23. On Machiavelli and constituent power see also Vatter, *Between Form and Event*, 223.
38 Machiavelli, "Discorsi sopra la prima Deca di Tito Livio," bk. 1.7.

restrict or repel the encroachments of the great. On the contrary, Machiavelli identifies two beneficial results of the practice. Interpreters tend to focus primarily on the former, the fact that as a result of the potential for accusation citizens are dissuaded from attempting to privately appropriate power, and even if they do make such an attempt, they are capable of being thwarted in their effort. The more significant from the standpoint of my reading, however, is the second benefit, the fact that in constructing an institutional space for accusation a political field for the expulsion of the creative energy of the people is generated. That is, there "is given an outlet to vent those humours that grow in cities, in some mode, against some citizen; and when these humours do not have an outlet for being vented ordinarily, they have recourse to extraordinary modes that bring to ruin an entire republic. And therefore there is nothing that makes a republic so stable and firm as to order it in a mode so that those changing humours that agitate it can be vented in a way ordered by the laws."[39]

The co-determination of the two benefits is revealed through the example of Coriolanus, whose transgressions against the people are stimulated by his belief that only the nobles should have the opportunity to politically express their will. In an effort to pacify the plebs Coriolanus suggested withholding from the city badly needed grain, believing that through this action the nobility "could punish the plebs, and take away that authority that had been the prejudice of the nobility."[40] The subsequent tribunal movement against Coriolanus had the effect not only of resisting his indiscretion, but also of expressing in an institutional form that popular desire for participation that motivated the indiscretion in the first place. The extent of accusation as a mode for the expression of popular energy, furthermore, exceeds the persecution of insolent nobles who voice that will to domination that characterizes their social class. In 1:50 Machiavelli maintains that the object of accusatorial activity may be individuals belonging to either the *grandi* or the people: "one has to note, first, the benefit of the tribunate, which was not only useful to restrain the ambition that the powerful used against the plebs, but also that which they used among themselves."[41] What this suggests is that the institution is capable of being productively

---

39 Ibid.
40 Ibid.
41 Ibid., bk. 1.50.

deployed in democratic contexts marked by social equality as a general mechanism for the agonistic expulsion of ambitious energy. It is one of the orders that can be established to productively manage social conflict between individual elements within the city, providing institutional space for the venting of human ambition. There is of course nothing necessary or permanent about the structure of such orders. As will be further elaborated on below, the impossibility of instituting a fixed constitutional configuration capable of indefinitely regulating social life is a consequence of the perpetual fact of human difference, the multiplicity of ideal forms of being, doing, and thinking ultimately foreclosing the establishment of a firm consensus over the normative ends to be affirmed by the political community. Although the republic can institutionalize conflict through, for example, modes of accusation that allow desires to express themselves relative to one other, the dynamism of desire precludes the possibility of a permanently stable negotiation or mediation between particulars.[42]

The Mechanics of Popular Rule

The orientation of accusatory activity toward the venting of energy reveals the extent to which it transcends the merely instrumental and reactive persecution of those that might attempt to deny the people their security or negative liberty. On the contrary, accusation is one of the means facilitating the expulsion of an always surplus plebeian desire. Given that human ambition is primarily directed toward value creation, it should not be surprising that Machiavelli considers as the most politically appropriate media for such expression explicitly legislative modes and orders.[43] Machiavelli affirms the creative legislative

---

42 In this sense, in the words of Neal Wood, "politics is a kind of dialectical process characterized by a clash of opposites, their temporary reconciliation in a rather tenuous social balance, and then the need to readjust the equilibrium because of new causes of conflict." Neal Wood, "The Value of Asocial Sociability: Contributions of Machiavelli, Sidney, and Montesquieu," *Bucknell Review* 16, no. 3 (1966): 8.

43 It is not the case, as suggested by Hélène Landemore for example, that Machiavelli's defence of popular judgment is purely negative, limited to the ability to mediate between pre-formulated policy options: "This ability to make good judgments is, in Machiavelli's account, passive and reactive. The people do not initiate a view; they simply respond to those voiced in the public forum." Hélène Landemore, *Democratic Reason: Politics, Collective Intelligence, and the Rule of the Many* (Princeton: Princeton University Press, 2013), 66.

capacity of the people, for example, in 1:18. He notes that, so long as a city is healthy – such health being largely associated with the continuing inculcation of civic-mindedness among the citizen body – the people's active participation in the formulation of and deliberation over the law is a good to be affirmed: "A tribune or any other citizen could propose a law to the people, on which every citizen could speak, either in favour or against, before it was decided. This order was good when the citizens were good, because it was always good that everyone who intends a benefit for the public can propose it; and it is good that everyone can speak their opinion on it, so that the people, having heard everyone, could then choose the best."[44]

Machiavelli's language of the selection of "the best" here should not however lead us to question his commitment to political equality. Although clearly recognizing the impossibility of the institution of a political system that is capable of guaranteeing a literal universality of participation at all moments, in 3:19 Machiavelli provides a gesture toward the problem of the democratic distribution of functions in large and complex societies. The topic is approached through the question of whether one should tend toward cruelty or humaneness when commanding or ruling. Ultimately the tendency to be affirmed, which is not at all to say the universal technique, is dependent upon the historical situation, specifically on the establishment or non-establishment of equality as a social condition of human life. Punishment and severity as educative modes are potentially appropriate apparently only when one is engaging with those with whom one does not share an equal status, such as pre-political or corrupt populations. Such, however, did not define republican Rome, Machiavelli here positing a strong participatory equality between the people and the nobles: "I say, you have to rule men that are ordinarily partners with you, or men that are always subjects. When they are partners, one cannot fully use punishment, nor that severity on which Cornelius reasons; and because the Roman plebs had in Rome *equal* rule with the nobility, one who became a prince *for a time*, could not manage with cruelty and coarseness."[45] Implicit in this quotation is a recognition of democratic life as embodying a principle of ruling and being ruled in turn, individuals temporarily occupying particular offices for determinate periods, and in this

---

44 Machiavelli, "Discorsi sopra la prima Deca di Tito Livio," bk. 1.18.
45 Ibid., bk. 3.19. Emphases added.

capacity achieving the status of prince, that is to say, of a virtuous and creative actor.[46]

The defence of an ideal of ruling and being ruled in turn as a mechanism for the generalization of legislative power is perhaps most clearly discernible in Machiavelli's advocacy of lottery as a political mode for filling office.[47] Such an advocacy represents "the closest possible institutional realization of the demos's desire to rule themselves; more specifically, its desire to be ruled intermittently by random citizens who wished to serve politically but were not sufficiently rich or renowned to gain office through elections."[48] In the "Discourse on Florentine Affairs," as we have seen, Machiavelli proposes a lottery-selected office of magistrates that productively integrates common citizens into the constitutional order, which is otherwise grounded in election and appointment. This office has the double function of not only checking the insolence and ambition of the great, but also of generalizing participation through providing a space within which the people can express their desire and further their political education. In the *Florentine Histories*, meanwhile,

---

46 For Mary Dietz the principle of ruling and being ruled in turn is not only actualized in the context of free republican life. It can also be seen to operate in a different form in princely contexts, Machiavelli in fact refusing the categorical distinction between ruling and ruled, seeing the identification with one or the other term as a merely temporary product of political struggle between active participants. Mary G. Dietz, *Turning Operations: Feminism, Arendt, and Politics* (New York: Routledge, 2002), 150–1.

47 For a brief account of Machiavelli's proposal for remodelling the government of Florence in the context of the wider potential for the institution of lottery as a mode for filling political offices, see Oliver Dowlen, *The Political Potential of Sortition: A Study on the Random Selection of Citizens for Public Office* (Exeter: Imprint Academic, 2008), 117–20.

48 McCormick, "Defending the People from the Professors." Despite his emphasis on the capacity of the people to articulate their political demands independent of representative expression, McCormick sometimes seems to nevertheless neutralize the concept of self-rule through reading the popular desire not to be ruled partly in terms of a desire to be ruled well: "Machiavelli clearly distinguishes between oppression, on the one hand, which the people rightfully resist, and government or command, on the other, which they tolerate and even welcome, when performed well." John P. McCormick, "Subdue the Senate: Machiavelli's 'Way of Freedom' or Path to Tyranny," *Political Theory* 40, no. 6 (2012): 722. This being ruled well seems to be a moment independent of ruling themselves, and is perhaps an expression of McCormick's belief that any democratic regime will need to accommodate elites in some significant way (as opposed to eliminating any distinction between the common and the elite via an equalization of social and political conditions). Ibid.

Machiavelli identifies the concrete actualization of participatory freedom with the institution of lottery as a mode for creating magistrates. He notes in particular how the people themselves perceive that such a mode is most appropriate for a free city in which all are able to potentially share in government through joint deliberation and decision making: "The city thus having returned to creating magistrates by lot, it appeared to the generality of citizens that they had recovered their liberty, and that the magistrates were judging, not according to the will of the powerful, but according to their own judgment."[49] This and other similar reforms, in particular the reinstitution of the *catasto*, "where the taxes were assessed not by men, but by the laws," horrified the great, who recognized they had "become equal to those whom they were long accustomed to see as inferior."[50]

Although Machiavelli shows a preference for distributing political offices through the democratic mode of sortition, he also clearly advocates election in those instances in which the demands of the position require a particular knowledge or ability that it would not be reasonable to expect all citizens to possess immediately.[51] Nevertheless, if the differentiation of political tasks necessitates that decisions be made by select persons or groups who hold office, there need to be institutional guards in place in order to ensure that such decisions map onto public will.[52] In the context of a discussion of the consuls Quintius Cincinnatus and Gnaeus Julius Mentus, who as a consequence of internal disagreements ground the republic to a halt through their inaction, Machiavelli writes: "For example, if you give an authority to a council to make a distribution of honours and uses, or to a magistrate to administer a matter, one must either impose a necessity so that he has to do it in any mode, or, if he does not want to, order that another can and ought to do it; otherwise, this order would be defective and dangerous, as would

---

49 Machiavelli, "Istorie fiorentine," bk. 7.2.

50 Ibid.

51 On the fact that certain positions or offices do require a specialized technical skill or knowledge, and that this justifies the autonomy of the office holders from those who are lacking in this capacity, see, for example, Machiavelli, "Discorsi sopra la prima Deca di Tito Livio," bk. 2.33.

52 Again, however, such will cannot be interpreted as unified and homogeneous. Indeed, Arlene Saxonhouse notes how the strong emphasis on voting as a key element of democratic practice tends to mask or cover up the conflictual core of politics. Saxonhouse, "Do We Need the Vote?," 176.

have been seen in Rome, if to the obstinacy of those councils could not be opposed the authority of the tribunes."[53] Indeed, in *Discourses* 1:35 Machiavelli makes a sustained effort to highlight the fact that the distribution of authority through the deployment of "free and public votes" may generate harmful consequences within the republic if not used carefully, and that its use is thus appropriate only if certain limiting conditions attach.

The extent to which the form of election – to the degree that through its internal principle of distinction it operates to construct a necessary political inequality – may be harnessed for non-democratic ends is revealed through the example of the Roman Decemvirate. The Decemvirate acquired authority via "free and public votes," but was ultimately able to transgress the limits of this authority through leveraging its newly exalted political position toward the further acquisition and consolidation of power. To guard against such potential the utilization of election should be subject to certain limits. Specifically, "one ought to consider the modes of giving authority and the time for which it is given."[54] With respect to the latter, "if free authority is given for a long time, calling a long time one year or more, it will always be dangerous, and will make the effects either good or bad, in accordance with whether those to whom it was given are bad or good."[55] Indeed, in 3:24 the prolongation of commands is identified as one of the two primary causes of the dissolution of the Roman republic, Machiavelli noting that wise citizens recognized the corrupting nature of such prolongation. For example, after the plebs prolonged the command of the tribunes, thinking they were especially well suited to checking the ambition of the *grandi*, the Senate offered to prolong Lucius Quintius's consulate in response. However, he "altogether refused this decision, saying that he wanted to try and eliminate bad examples, not to increase them with another worse example; and he wanted new consuls made."[56] As commands in Rome were increasingly prolonged, the starting point given being Publius Philo's ascension to the rank of the first proconsul, there resulted both a degeneralization of participation – fewer and fewer individuals having the opportunity to actively participate in the

---

53 Machiavelli, "Discorsi sopra la prima Deca di Tito Livio," bk. 1.50.
54 Ibid., bk. 1.35.
55 Ibid.
56 Ibid., bk. 3.24.

life of the city – as well as an increase in private authority. As Machiavelli writes: "This thing produced two inconveniences: one, that a lesser number of men exercised rule, and through this they came to restrict reputation to a few; the other, that when a citizen remained for a long time commander of an army, he would win it to himself and make it partisan to him, for that army in time forgot the Senate and recognized him as head."[57]

With respect to the former limit, there must be concrete restrictions regarding the parameters and quality of the authority acquired through election. In 1:35 this principle is expressed through Machiavelli's observance of the inability of the dictator to encroach upon the prerogative of the tribunes, consuls, and Senate. In this way "the Senate, the consuls, the tribunes, remaining with their authority, came to be like his guard, making him not exit from the right way."[58] Precisely the opposite occurred after the election of the Ten, however, the latter acting to abolish the consuls and tribunes, political corruption necessarily resulting as a consequence: "So, finding themselves alone, without consuls, without tribunes, without appeal to the people, and because of this not coming to have anyone observe them, they could, in the second year, motivated by the ambition of Appius, become insolent."[59] Machiavelli concludes by noting that to say that positions given by free votes is never hurtful to a republic is to assume such votes are given under the proper conditions, that is, that the offices subject to election are limited in duration and have a definitive scope of authority. Authority must be given "in the proper circumstances and for the proper times."[60] What authority must never be is absolute, "for an absolute authority very quickly corrupts the matter, and makes itself friends and partisans."[61] As Machiavelli notes in 1:49, "And although many times, through public and free votes, for the power to reform it, extensive authority will be given to a few citizens, they have not thereafter ever ordered it for the common benefit, but always to the goal of their party; this has made, not order, but greater disorder in that city."[62]

---

57 Ibid.
58 Ibid., bk. 1.35.
59 Ibid.
60 Ibid.
61 Ibid.
62 Ibid., bk. 1.49.

It is significant that the chapter immediately following his critical investigation into the nature of election as a mode for filling certain offices in 1:35 is one in which Machiavelli defends rotation, a much more essentially democratic mode, as a scheme of political distribution. There is again something of a principle of ruling and being ruled in turn implicit in Machiavelli's observation that "although the Romans were great lovers of glory, nevertheless they did not esteem it a dishonourable thing to obey now someone whom they had commanded another time, and to find themselves serving in the army of which they had been princes. This custom is contrary to the opinion, orders, and modes of citizens of our times."[63] Citizens should not be ashamed to follow a high rank with occupation of a lower one, and indeed, Machiavelli will partially locate the health of the city precisely in citizens' willingness to voluntary accept such a movement: "For a republic ought to have more hope in, and rely more on, a citizen that descends from a high office to govern a lesser one, than one who rises from a lesser one to govern a higher one. For one cannot reasonably believe in the latter, unless one sees around him men of so much reverence or so much virtue that the novelty of him can be, through their counsel and authority, moderated."[64] And notably, with respect to the latter part of the quoted passage, it is not any lack of intrinsic ability that should generate scepticism with respect to the movement from lower to higher rank, but simply unfamiliarity with the political role, an unfamiliarity that is easily corrected through political collaboration. In any case, rotation – like lottery – concretely affirms equality through the presumption of an equivalent ability of many or more than a few to carry out political tasks, the willingness of citizens to oscillate between positions of higher and lower rank functioning as a sign of the popular recognition and affirmation of this equality.

In sum, as a general principle Machiavelli maintains that those determinations having to do with the maintenance of the republic should lay in the hands of all whenever possible. Machiavelli affirms a principle of isonomy, political equality being irreducible to an equal status before the law, but including as well an equal ability to participate in the active formulation of the law through concrete participation in legislative

---

63 Ibid., bk. 1.36.
64 Ibid.

activities.[65] Machiavelli's preference for the distributive modes of sortition and rotation over election – the former being two means for the realization of the goal of generalizing participation – is one of the most prominent manifestations of his rejection of aristocracy in the name of democracy and isonomy.[66] Election, as is often noted, is an aristocratic mode to the degree that it is grounded in the recognition of a "principle of distinction," the fact that the elected are in some sense dissimilar and unique from the body of electors.[67] What Machiavelli recognizes is that elected office holders constitute, in short, a few, and are thus predisposed to act in the interests of those other few of perceived distinction.

The Form of Political Decision

In the *Discourses* Machiavelli attempts to think the possibility of a generalization of individual *virtù*, such a generalization producing a new collective *virtù* whose subject is the city as a whole, and whose

---

65 Readers who fail to recognize the isonomic form of Machiavelli's democratic thought, focusing only on a principle of negative liberty or equal status before the law, tend to reduce him to a proto-liberal thinker who merely anticipates modern representative forms of government. For different manifestations of this tendency see, for example, Julia Conaway Bondanella, "*The Discourses on Livy*: Preserving a Free Way of Life," in *Seeking Real Truths: Multidisciplinary Perspectives on Machiavelli*, ed. Patricia Vilches and Gerald Seaman (Leiden: Brill, 2007), 82; Kocis, *Machiavelli Redeemed*, 17; Clifford Orwin, "Machiavelli's Unchristian Charity," *American Political Science Review* 72, no. 4 (1978): 1227; Philippe Van Parijs, *Just Democracy: The Rawls-Machiavelli Programme* (Colchester: ECPR Press, 2011); Dragica Vujadinovic, "Machiavelli's Republican Political Theory," *Philosophy and Social Criticism* 40, no. 1 (2014): 60. Garver, "After *Virtù*: Rhetoric, Prudence, and Moral Pluralism in Machiavelli," 195–6; Edward Burns, "The Liberalism of Machiavelli," *Antioch Review* 8, no. 3 (1948): 321–30.

66 The isonomic character of Machiavellian equality has been noted by Miguel Vatter: "Republican freedom means that the citizens can become princes, that freedom is not only negative liberty (i.e. the knowledge that one is born free and not a slave) but also isonomy, understood as the equal freedom to make and unmake laws, and not simply as the equality of everyone before these laws." Vatter, *Between Form and Event*, 293.

67 The term "principle of distinction" is drawn from the work of Bernard Manin, who notes that "representative government was instituted in full awareness that elected representatives would and should be distinguished citizens, socially different from those who elected them. We shall call this the 'principle of distinction.'" Bernard Manin, *The Principles of Representative Government* (Cambridge: Cambridge University Press, 1997), 94.

trajectory of decision making is stimulated by the conflictual interaction of the multiplicity of social fragments within the republic. As we recall from chapter 3, Machiavellian creation is highly specified, and is thus significant that the features of princely self-activity that are presented in *The Prince* reappear in a new context in the *Discourses*, the dynamics of creative determination re-emerging in a specifically republican context. This, for example, can be seen in the extent to which political creation is mediated by worldly indeterminacy, the latter in fact providing the objective conditions for the expulsion of ambitious desire. Such a mediation is most clearly revealed in Machiavelli's account of the function of the dictator.

Machiavelli's defence of the institution of the dictator is meant to reveal the human potential to negotiate and manage – if not master – worldly contingency, it being one of the Roman remedies to the immediate and indeterminate dangers that often accompany those accidents produced as a consequence of the non-identity of objects. The institution involves "giving power to one man, who could decide without any consultation, and could execute his decisions without any appeal."[68] Machiavelli argues that it is not true, as claimed by some, that the establishment of tyranny in Rome can be traced to the creation of the order of the dictator, but rather the name of the order was conceptually appropriated by those who attempted to usurp public authority.[69] Machiavelli calls attention to the distance between concept and object, and the consequent potential for the continual reconstruction of the form of the idea, when he writes that "if in Rome the dictatorial name

68 Machiavelli, "Discorsi sopra la prima Deca di Tito Livio," bk. 1.33. Despite Machiavelli's language here, Marco Geuna suggests that the dictator in fact need not be one person, but that the institution could be a council composed of several or more people, the important issue being simply the possession of a prerogative to act and decide swiftly in the face of the extraordinary situation. Marco Geuna, "Machiavelli and the Problem of Dictatorship," *Ratio Juris* 28, no. 2 (2015): 234–5; Marco Geuna, "Extraordinary Accidents in the Life of Republics," in *Machiavelli on Liberty and Conflict*, ed. David Johnston, Nadia Urbinati, and Camila Vergara (Chicago: Chicago University Press, 2017), 293.

69 Hence Carl Schmitt writes that for Machiavelli "the dictator was not a tyrant and dictatorship was not a form of absolute government but rather an instrument to guarantee freedom, which was in the spirit of the Republican constitution." Carl Schmitt, *Dictatorship: From the Origin of the Modern Concept of Sovereignty to the Proletarian Class Struggle*, trans. Michael Hoelzl and Graham Ward (Cambridge: Polity, 2014), 4.

had been lacking, they would have taken another; for it is forces that easily acquire names, not names forces."[70] In reality, however, never did the dictator do harm to the city so long as it remained subject to public control: "it is seen that the dictator, while he was instituted according to public orders, and not by his own authority, always did good to the city. For the magistrates that are made and the authorities that are given through public ways, not those that come through ordinary ways, harm republics: such one sees follow in Rome, where through a long period of time no dictator did anything if not good to the republic."[71]

There were several reasons why this was the case. First, if a citizen desired to seize power extraordinarily and for his own benefit he must be in possession of "qualities that in a republic that is not corrupt he can never have."[72] Specifically, he will not have the required wealth nor the willing partisans that such wealth can buy, the conditions for the acquisition of such being lacking in a well-ordered state. What is implied here is the power of socialization to shape human desire, a socialization that, when combined with the establishment of a general economic equality – itself implied through the claim regarding the non-sufficiency of financial resources – seems to point again toward the elimination of the apparently originary division between the great and the people. That is, the existence of a desire to oppress as an organized social humour is not a feature of a well-ordered republic that has achieved a general equality. Second, the appointment to the office was temporary in nature, not intended to extend beyond the actuality of the emergency. And third, there were determinable limits on the legitimate range of dictatorial activity, Machiavelli arguing that the legislative capacity to reinstitute the social was constitutionally precluded. Specifically, "his authority extended to the power to decide for himself about the remedies for that urgent danger, and to do everything without consultation, and punish everyone without appeal; but he could not do things that might diminish the state, as would have been done through taking away the authority of the Senate or of the people, unmaking the old orders of the city, and making new ones."[73] When all of these facts are

---

70 Machiavelli, "Discorsi sopra la prima Deca di Tito Livio," bk. 1.34.
71 Ibid.
72 Ibid.
73 Ibid. As Filippo Del Lucchese points out, however, this should not lead us to obscure the constitutive dimension of dictatorial power. Situating Machiavelli's theorization

combined, "it was impossible that he transcend its limits, and harm the city; and through experience ones sees that he always worked to benefit it."[74] In the final instance Machiavelli concludes that the dictator was one of the most useful of Roman orders, allowing the city to respond to the emergence of accidents which it might otherwise have been too slow to, for as is reaffirmed again in this chapter, time drives all things forward. When such orders are lacking, where there is no publicly sanctioned mode for engaging with the emergency situation, cities must resort to extraordinary modes, which are of their essence always dangerous.[75]

Most readers of Machiavelli recognize that the dictator represents a statement regarding the necessity of exceptional action, a concrete attempt to institutionalize such action through legal means, or rather, the attempt to legalize extra-legality. Hence Nomi Claire Lazar, for example, writes that "the constitution itself allows for its own suspension, for the suspension of quotidian norms in exceptional cases."[76] For Lazar as for others, though, the dictator is also a representation of Machiavelli's bifurcated ethics: it or the political founder can act in a way that the people cannot. The exercise of the exception must be by one who is necessarily exceptional: "The state must be continually maintained by one who is beyond the reach of everyday norms. The exceptional figure, but only the exceptional figure, acts according to existential ethics because his aim is the moral aim of establishing or preserving the worthy state."[77] But is this true? Can we instead use the

---

of the dictator within a discussion of the antinomies of constituent power, Del Lucchese writes that "dictatorship is precisely the tool – legal and constitutional – with which the republic recognizes its own incapacity to face the extraordinary with ordinary means." Del Lucchese, "Machiavelli and Constituent Power," 7. What is significant for Del Lucchese, and what is not recognized by commentators such as Carl Schmitt, is that Machiavelli's dictator reveals to us the fact that constituent power, here represented in the dictator's ability to creatively respond to the extraordinary situation irresolvable via existing norms, cannot be thought of as completely external to the already instituted social order: "Instead, constituent power lives in the institutional politics of the republic. Far from acrtically justifying the institutional moment, though, constituent power continuously transforms the actual institutional configuration." Ibid., 8.

74 Machiavelli, "Discorsi sopra la prima Deca di Tito Livio," bk. 1.34.
75 Ibid.
76 Lazar, "Must Exceptionalism Prove the Rule?," 256.
77 Ibid., 253.

dictator as an example of a self-interrogating political order, one that exists alongside others which might be potentially generalizable? Can the people themselves be seen as possessing the legal means to alter constitutional arrangements, reform legal orders, reinstitute the political sphere, and so on? Although the dictator is a useful example that reveals to us the fact of worldly indetermination and the necessity of virtuous adaptation to it, it certainly does not exhaust the modes of such adaptation.[78] The variability of the world is necessarily countered by a variable politics that affirms multiple forms of acting and reacting.

Before exploring the mechanics of popular reinstitutionalization, however, two further features of political determination as outlined in the *Discourses* – features that refer us back to Machiavelli's ontology of creation as developed in *The Prince* – should be mentioned. First, if the dictator represents an institutional example of the political imperative for action or decision in the face of worldly contingency, in the *Discourses* Machiavelli also stresses the extent to which the actualization of such a capacity for resolution must exceed mere voluntarism. That the efficacy of the decision requires transcending the immediacy of action is revealed in Machiavelli's long chapter on conspiracy, where potentially successful reordering is explicitly said to depend on the actor having the time for reflection and deliberation. The conspirator as actor generally lacks this time, and hence Machiavelli maintains that as a general rule he or she should not attempt to vary the stratagem: "I say, therefore, that there is not anything that makes so much disturbance or hindrance to all the actions of men, than in an instant, without having time, having to vary an order and distort it from that which had been ordered before."[79] Machiavelli is not rejecting here innovation itself, however, stringently affirming the necessity of obedience to the pre-formulated and fixed rule, for "this happens when one does not have the time to reorder; because, when one has the time, man can govern in his own mode."[80] The danger lay in the formulation of hasty

---

78 Such a possibility seems to be gestured toward by John McCormick, the dicta-
    tor being seen as potentially just one order among others that is deployed so as to
    engage the political exception. John P. McCormick, "Addressing the Political Excep-
    tion: Machiavelli's 'Accidents' and the Mixed Regime," *American Political Science
    Review* 87, no. 4 (1993): 888–900.
79 Machiavelli, "Discorsi sopra la prima Deca di Tito Livio," bk. 3.6.
80 Ibid.

determinations independently of deliberation, a danger reasserted in 3:44: "when one prince desires to obtain a thing from another, he ought, if the occasion allows, not give him space to deliberate, and make it so that he sees the necessity of a quick decision; this is when he who is asked sees that from refusing or from deferring emerges a sudden and dangerous indignation."[81] Indeed, the superiority of reflective to immediate decision is revealed in Machiavelli's own political engagements. Hence, for example, his frustration at his masters in Florence demanding that he produce knowledge of the intentions of Cesare Borgia, without having first had the opportunity to deliberate on the various particularities of the case, and their interrelation and meaning: "one who does not want to write fancies and dreams has to verify things, and in verifying them time passes."[82]

The key chapter on this topic of embedded determination, however, on the necessity of grounding decision in rational consideration of the particularity of the historical situation, is *Discourses* 2:15. The fact that one's action needs to be delimited by the realities of the concrete case is articulated at the very beginning of the chapter, Machiavelli noting that "in every consultation it is good to come to the particular of that which has to be deliberated on, and not remain always in ambiguity or uncertainty of the thing."[83] This understanding, though, is politically useless if it remains merely contemplative, the objects of rational consideration expressed through speech not being externalized via outward action in the world. As Piero de' Medici says to one of his conspirators in the *Florentine Histories*, who attempt to cover up the malignancy of their action through using a language of freedom dissociated from any substantive reality: "one ought to esteem deeds more than words."[84] The very rectification of the concept is made difficult if it is not formulated in light of the necessity of the situation. This dialectic, the construction of a relational order between concept and act, is given an expression in the statement of the Latin praetor Annius in a council with the Romans:

---

81 Ibid., bk. 3.44.
82 Machiavelli, "Legazione alla duca Valentino in Romagna," in *Tutte le opere*, sec. 42. On the extent to which Machiavelli's diplomatic activity both informs and is informed by his political philosophy see Greg Russell, "Machiavelli's Science of Statecraft: The Diplomacy and Politics of Disorder," *Diplomacy and Statecraft* 16, no. 2 (2005): 227–50.
83 Machiavelli, "Discorsi sopra la prima Deca di Tito Livio," bk. 2.15.
84 Machiavelli, "Istorie fiorentine," bk. 7.18.

"'I judge it to belong to the highest of our affairs for you to consider more what one ought to do than what is to be said. Once the counsels are made clear, it will be easy to accommodate words to things.' These words are, without doubt, very true, and ought to be savoured by every prince and by every republic."[85]

Although it is very easy to formulate the word when one has an understanding of the concrete political project one wants to undertake, the consistency of the word is degraded where the latter condition is lacking. One's understanding is structured by one's recognition of the specificity of the historical context, knowledge of the goals to which words are to be put: "for, in ambiguity and incertitude about what to do, they cannot accommodate words; but, once their spirit is firm, and what to be executed is decided, it is an easy thing to find the words."[86] What is essential, then, is the political moment, the actualization of the word through the making of a decision. The failure to act not only neutralizes political potential but degrades understanding through the production of ambiguity. Hence Machiavelli's example drawn from an event after the death of the tyrant Hieronymus, the Syracusans having to decide between supporting the Romans or Carthaginians in their war against one another: "And such was the ardour of the parties that the thing remained ambiguous, nor was any resolution taken until Apollonides, one of the highest in Syracuse, with an oration full of prudence, showed how those were not to blame who held the opinion that they should adhere to the Romans, nor those who wanted to follow the Carthaginian party; but it was good to detest that ambiguity and indolence in making a resolution, for he saw the whole ruin of the republic in such ambiguity; but if the resolution was taken, whatever it might be, one could hope for some good."[87] Again, Machiavelli is not celebrating decision for the sake of decision. On the contrary, there was a long process of discussion between the deliberative participants over the preferred mode. Such deliberation, though, is impossible of being productive of universal consensus. To the extent that the deliberative process is incapable of producing such an outcome – that is, to the extent that there will always be ineradicable differences grounded in human

---

85 Machiavelli, "Discorsi sopra la prima Deca di Tito Livio," bk. 2.15. Latin translation taken from Machiavelli, *Discourses on Livy*, bk. 2.15.1.
86 Machiavelli, "Discorsi sopra la prima Deca di Tito Livio," bk. 2.15.
87 Ibid.

multiplicity – there always exists the need to will a decision. What is crucial is that the deliberation leading up to this decision be grounded in relevant factual content, both word and act being mutually implicated in the procedural mode.

In 2:23, where Machiavelli returns to the question of the decision, he maintains that there is a primary ethical substance that should guide the deliberation that precedes it. Once again the actor is cautioned to avoid the middle way. The initial context is Camillus's speech to the Senate regarding the fate of Latium, it being ultimately maintained that "subjects ought to be either benefited or eliminated."[88] The prudent actor must not temporize, but exercise virtue through the affirmation of the will to make a decision. The goal in this instance, the object to which the decision looks, is identified as security, which is here seen as being potentially actualized only through one of the two modes mentioned. Machiavelli immediately goes on, however, to proclaim that these modes are not equivalent in the sense of being of the same neutral moral value. On the contrary, as we have suggested, there is an essential ethical imperative to generalize human equality and virtue, and when this imperative is applied to the deliberation, Machiavelli clearly comes down on the side of assimilation rather than elimination. The ethical and instrumental elements of decision making are unified toward the end of the chapter, the former not being subordinate to, but rather structuring, the latter. This is revealed through Machiavelli's account of the Roman Senate's consideration of the action to take against the Privernates, who were recently defeated and subordinated to Roman authority. Several citizens of Privernum appealed before the Senate, during which one senator asked a representative of the city to articulate the punishment that he thought they deserved. Machiavelli writes: "To this the Privernate responded, 'That which they deserve who consider themselves worthy of freedom.' To this the consul replied, 'If we remit your punishment, what sort of peace can we hope to have with you?' To which he responded, 'If you give a good one, both faithful and perpetual; if a bad one, not long-lasting.'"[89] Recognizing and respecting the desire and will for freedom, the Privernates were granted citizenship, the Senate stating, "The voice of a free man had been heard, nor could it be believed that any people or indeed any man should

---

88 Ibid., bk. 2.23.
89 Machiavelli, *Discourses on Livy*, bk. 2.23.4.

remain in a condition that was painful longer than necessary. Peace is faithful where men are willingly pacified, nor could faith be hoped for in that place where they wished for freedom ... Only those who think of nothing but freedom are worthy to become Romans."[90] Eventually in the chapter, then, the strategic advice to avoid the middle way gives way to ethical advice guided by a universal human imperative: to respect the will to freedom through initiating processes of incorporative institutionalization.

The political lesson – that the virtuous actor must possess the will to make an informed decision in light of the particularities of *fortuna* – morphs into a democratic affirmation of the capacity for a people to live in freedom. This same logic can be seen to be at play with respect to our second consideration of the form of virtuous action. In *Discourses* 3:9 Machiavelli returns to a theme that he acknowledges he has "considered many times," that it is to say, "how the cause of the bad and good fortune of men is the matching of [the actor's] mode of proceeding with the times; for one sees in their works that some men proceed with impetuosity, some with care and with caution. And because in either of these modes they exceed appropriate limits, they cannot observe the true way, erring in both the one and the other. But one comes to err less, and to have prosperous fortune, if one matches, as I said, one's mode with the times, always proceeding as nature forces you."[91] We have already noted that Machiavelli associates *virtù* with the human capacity to deliberate on the shifting conditions of the being of the world, launching action in accord with one's knowledge of the form of the occasion. Hence Machiavelli's emphasis on the virtuous actor's oscillation between different personas or modes of proceeding. In this chapter, however, Machiavelli moves from the particular to the general, examining the issue of the correspondence of mode and world not from the standpoint of the singular actor, or even the political body where legislative authority is concentrated in the singular actor, but from the standpoint of the free collectivity, where action is grounded in the interplay of the diversity of desires within the city.

Once again it is affirmed that the existence of "diverse citizens and diverse humours" is an essential feature of republican life.[92] To the

---

90 Ibid.
91 Machiavelli, "Discorsi sopra la prima Deca di Tito Livio," bk. 3.9.
92 Ibid.

extent that the object of the analysis is the republican collectivity as political actor, interrogated in light of its capacity to adjust its mode to the times, the determination of political action must be grounded in this diversity. Determinations are not representative of an exteriorization of a homogeneous popular will that is simultaneously expressed in the particular will of each citizen. Rather, determinations are the result of conflictual political interaction between necessarily distinct and potentially opposed wills. It is precisely the diversity of republican will that renders the republic more adequate to respond to worldly contingency, and hence which makes the republic, as I will note again in the next section, a more properly historical regime than the principality. It is a regime more open, that is, to historical becoming: "Hence it arises that a republic has greater life, and has more sustained good fortune, than a principality; for it can better accommodate itself to temporal diversity – through the diversity of the citizens that are in it – than can one prince. For a man who is accustomed to proceed in one mode never changes, as was said; and it must be of necessity that, when the times change in disconformity with his mode, he is ruined."[93] Although Machiavelli will go on to give the examples of Piero Soderni and Julius II as being representative of the incapacity of the singular actor to reflectively alter his or her own mode, the fact that virtue itself is elsewhere identified with this ability must lead us to conclude only that Machiavelli is sceptical about the possibility of an actor being able to perform such an operation in every instant, not that individual nature is so fixed so as to preclude such alteration in particular cases. After all, even Cesare Borgia, the paradigm of the actor capable of oscillating between performative modes for the sake of political creation, himself erred in supporting the elevation of Giuliano della Rovere to the papacy, not adequately perceiving the nature of the latter's hostility.[94] Such a threat of mismanagement, however, is neutralized in the republic, not because individuals are any more virtuous or less likely to err than a figure like Borgia, but because authority is diffused through such a diverse body of citizens.

What is significant about Machiavelli's discussion in 3:9, which leads into my discussion in the following section, is that the necessity of republican openness to alteration in the face of worldly contingency is

93 Ibid.
94 Machiavelli, "Il Principe," chap. 7.

seen as referring not just to shifts in the content of decisions, but the very institutional form of the decision-making organs. If republics are to survive they must perpetually interrogate and modify their orders, as "The ruin of cities also stems from not varying the orders of republics with the times."[95] This necessity is revealed two chapters later in 3:11, where Machiavelli once again emphasizes the significance of the tribunes as an institutional means for restraining the expression of noble ambition. Here Machiavelli will be explicit, though, that the institutional form of the tribunes is incapable of becoming fixed in a determinate order that is capable of perpetually regulating the relations between the people and the Senate. On the contrary, like any other object or order, the tribunes are subject to the vicissitudes of time, and must therefore be open to the possibility of their own institutional alteration – which includes an alteration of their relation with other institutions, through for example the creation of new orders to counterpose them – in light of changing external circumstances. As Machiavelli writes, "because everything, as has been said other times, conceals some evil in itself that makes new accidents emerge, it is necessary to provide for this with new orders."[96] Political orders must thus be structured so as to be able to accommodate a self-interrogation of the legitimacy of their existing form. This renovation may be achieved through either the internal restructuring of the order or the creation of new orders that enter into a relation with the existing order in such a way as to fundamentally redefine the latter's mode of being.

In short, it is necessary to reflectively alter institutional forms in light of the indeterminacy of the social field. Indeed, Machiavelli goes on in this chapter to give one of his most significant statements on this indeterminacy and its root in the multiplicity of human being. In the Roman case, for example, Machiavelli notes how potential tribunal insolence came to be checked by the generation of a new mode demonstrated by Appius Claudius: "this was that they found always amongst themselves someone who was fearful, or corruptible, or a lover of the common good, so that they disposed him to oppose the will of those others who wanted to move forward some decision against the will of the Senate. This remedy was a great temporizer of so much authority, and many times worked

---

95 Machiavelli, "Discorsi sopra la prima Deca di Tito Livio," bk. 3.9.
96 Ibid., bk. 3.11.

to benefit Rome."[97] Machiavelli goes on to locate the potential for such a mode to succeed in the impossibility of social groups being perpetually homogenized, reduced to a coherent unity expressive of the same will or orientation. The advice is that one should always consider the single power of the greatest, even if in the immediate situation the many united powers are more dominant, and this precisely because there is nothing essential about this social unity. There is no means by which it is possible to permanently hold the many together, to perpetually impose unity on diversity: "any time there are many powers united against another power, even though all together are much more powerful than that one, nevertheless one ought always to expect more from that one alone, who is less strong, than from the many others, though very strong. For, leaving aside all those things in which one alone can prevail more than many (which are countless), this will always occur: that [the one] will be able to, using a bit of industry, disunite the many, and make weak that body which was strong."[98] The Senate was able to counter the power of the tribunes through fracturing popular identity, an identity that is always precarious to the extent that it is a manifestation of an always contingent unity of diverse and plural human beings. To the extent that the people are always multiple, there is no guaranteed method for keeping them united.[99] The democratic project, on the contrary, consists in attempting to think an institutional means for affirming difference in unity, which necessarily includes potential institutional reformation in response to the shifting contingency of human co-relation.

Machiavelli's Innovative Republic: On the Self-Overcoming Form of Republican Institutions

Several readers of Machiavelli have pointed out the unique character of his preferred republican institutions such as they are detailed in the *Discourses*: the fact that they are open to self-innovation or refinement.[100]

---

97 Ibid.
98 Ibid.
99 The fragility of the people as plurality is recognized, for example, by Stefano Visentin. Stefano Visentin, "The Different Faces of the People: On Machiavelli's Political Topography," in *The Radical Machiavelli: Politics, Philosophy, and Language*, ed. Filippo Del Lucchese, Fabio Frosini, and Vittorio Morfino (Leiden: Brill, 2015), 368.
100 See, for example, Shumer, "Machiavelli: Republican Politics and Its Corruption," 16; Benner, *Machiavelli's Ethics*, 385; Fleisher, "The Ways of Machiavelli and

My argument is that this specific form of institutional being is a reflection of Machiavelli's perception of the universality of the desire for virtuous self-expression. In the previous three sections I have attempted to demonstrate how the logic of *virtù* developed in *The Prince* re-emerges in the republican context. In particular, Machiavelli demonsrates how the republic multiplies the spaces for the expression of *virtù*, how *virtù* is associated with self-legislation, how such self-legislation is predicated on the contingent openness of the being of the world, how it must be rational and historically embedded, and how it necessitates a performative embodiment of a plurality of political modalities. In this section I will show how the realization of *virtù* in the republican context, to the extent that virtuous action is defined in terms of creative transgression and value formation and that in this context the people themselves are the subject of such action, is achieved through the ability of democratic institutions to perpetually call into question their own efficacy through a process of self-interrogation.

We must recall that Machiavelli's critique of positively defined models of the human essence – models grounded in the affirmation of determinate human drives or orientations that unduly circumscribe the possible range of human doing and being – is inseparable from his affirmation of a negative essence, a specifically indeterminate human capacity to create the new. The creation of the human world is coextensive with the creation of the human being to the extent that it is human beings themselves who are responsible for instituting those socializing objects and forces that lean on and structure their existence. For Machiavelli, to be human is to be both a being born of a particular social and cultural heritage, yet also one capable of contributing to the making, refinement, or transmission of this history. Machiavelli's project is to think the conditions for the possibility of actualizing this latter capacity, an actualization that depends upon the existence of a political world that is understood to be neither absolutely fixed nor completely indeterminate or accidental.[101] Humans, in other words, are both the subjects and objects of historical creation. The philosophical anthropology that Machiavelli develops structures his normative political theory. It is

---

the Ways of Politics," 341; Lefort, *Machiavelli in the Making*, 344; John Kennedy, "Machiavelli and Mandeville: Prophets of Radical Contingency," *Political Theology* 5, no. 1 (2004): 108.

101 See, for example, Viroli, "Machiavelli and the Republican Idea of Politics," 155.

not the case that the question of human nature is irrelevant to politics, or simply that human nature's fickleness or instability refers us to nothing more than the impossibility of instituting a form of regime that is foundationally stable and secure.[102] On the contrary, reflection on Machiavelli's radical destabilization of positive essences, and his interpretation of ambitious desire in terms of transgressive value formation, provides a means to deepen our understanding of his theorization of the ideal republic as a system of orders that is perpetually open to the possibility of its own institutional renovation or even transcendence. This openness is a necessity if the polity is to persist in its freedom and stave off ruin.[103] It is precisely because the human desire for creative expression is insatiable – that is, that the human is constantly redefining the nature of itself and its world through its self-activity – that the form of the political regime is never capable of becoming permanently fixed. Machiavelli's republic is singular in that it is oriented toward its own perpetual interrogation and possible overcoming.[104] The project is to think a system of institutions that is capable, through harnessing the creative energy of the people who constitute the society, of continually calling itself into question, and through reinstituting itself provide a means for the actualization of what is taken to be a fundamental creative human desire. The republic is thus a historical regime in a way that the new principality – even in relation to the hereditary and ecclesiastical principality – is not, the latter ultimately looking to stabilize political life through the homogenization of the social field, through singularly imposing an artificial unity on the fragmented elements of the city.

Whereas in *The Prince* Machiavelli is making the effort to highlight the political actor's perpetual need to be active in response to the shifting of *fortuna*, thus articulating the mode of being of a person open to time, in the *Discourses* he turns to the question of the form of political society that is capable of actualizing such an active mode of being in all individuals. Such a form would necessitate a temporality that rejects an

---

102 For one example of the latter position see Rebhorn, "Machiavelli's *Prince* in the Epic Tradition," 88.
103 Machiavelli, "Discorsi sopra la prima Deca di Tito Livio," bk. 3.9.
104 It is thus very misleading to suggest that Machiavelli's ideal of Rome "has all the charactersitics of a Platonic form." Stelio Cro, "Machiavelli e l'antiutopia," in *Machiavelli attuale / Machiavel actuel*, ed. Georges Barthouil (Ravenna: Longo Editore, 1982), 29.

ideal of political fixity, to the extent that the creation of political institutions is the primary mode of expression of virtuous self-activity. That the historical prince, the head of an actually existing principality, is not particularly well suited to embodying this ideal subjectivity is suggested in Machiavelli's poem "Of Ingratitude." Here Machiavelli not only highlights this particular quality of princes, but also links it to their hostility to temporal alteration, to their orientation toward social preservation as opposed to innovation:

> Search through all the world's shores; you will find few princes to be
>   grateful, if you read that which is written of them;
> and you will see how changers of states and givers of kingdoms are
>   always repaid with exile or death.
> For when you cause a state to change, the prince you have made doubts
>   that you will not take away that which you have given;
> and he does not observe faith nor compact with you, for more powerful
>   is the fear he has of you, than the obligation agreed to.
> And this dread lasts so long, that it sees your lineage extinguished, and
>   the burial of you and yours.
> Hence you struggle often in serving, and then for your good service are
>   repaid with miserable life and violent death.[105]

Princes, then, appear as doubly unsuited to initiate a project of reinstitutionalization for the sake of public benefit, the principality not being a regime open to the movement of time.

The particular temporality of the Machiavellian republic is initially approached through contrasting Rome with Sparta and Venice. Machiavelli notes that if the former were to remain as internally peaceful and unified as the latter, it would have needed to arrest historical time through reifying the being of the polity. This reification could have been achieved, for example, in different ways, such as: "either not deploy the plebs in war, like the Venetians; or not open the way to foreigners, like the Spartans."[106] The Romans, however, rejected both of these modes in favour of a principle of innovation, represented in this chapter in a

---

105 Machiavelli, "Dell'Ingratitudine," in *Tutte le opere*, 983. On the blindness of princes to historical time see also Niccolò Machiavelli, "Decennale secondo," in *Tutte le opere*, 954.
106 Machiavelli, "Discorsi sopra la prima Deca di Tito Livio," bk. 1.6.

dynamic expansion that, beyond merely functioning to externally redirect noble desire, was characterized in terms of the ability to harness the productive energies of the plebs. In 2:6, furthermore, Machiavelli will more explicitly locate the source of Roman virtue in the willingness to divert from established patterns of action, to be generally oriented toward reflective innovation in all endeavours: "in all their actions it will be seen with how much prudence they deviated from the universal modes of others, to facilitate the way to come to a supreme greatness."[107] Rome for Machiavelli is especially well suited to articulating the historical being of society to the extent that it is a city that does not attempt to cover up historical mutation through the affirmation of immutable constitutional laws, but rather is always open to its own self-transformation, grounding creative institutionalization in the play of forces that perpetually express themselves through the non-identity of desire.

In 1:18 Machiavelli provides perhaps his clearest statement on the necessity of institutional and legal reform in the face of the fluctuation of time. He writes that "the orders and the laws made in a republic at its origin, when men were good, are not afterwards to the purpose, when they have become bad."[108] Temporal variability is here grounded in the variability of the psyche, the indeterminacy of the human mind allowing for the possibility of the emergence of a disjuncture between the structure of the polity and the circumstances of human being. The distinction in this chapter between laws and orders is fundamental, Machiavelli writing that "if the laws vary according to the accidents in a city, its orders never vary, or rarely: this makes new laws insufficient, because the orders, which are durable, corrupt them."[109] The potential for renovating orders, however, is certainly not closed off. Indeed, such potential is significant enough that Machiavelli identifies as one of the seemingly few deficiencies of Roman republicanism its one-sided willingness to alter law, but not the more fundamental institutional substratum represented by the concept of order. He notes that "The order of the state was the authority of the people, of the Senate, of the tribunes, of the consuls, the mode of selecting and creating the magistrates, and the mode of making the laws."[110] Although as the nature of

---

107 Ibid., bk. 2.6.
108 Machiavelli, "Discorsi sopra la prima Deca di Tito Livio," bk. 1.18.
109 Ibid.
110 Ibid.

individuals changed specific laws were varied in an effort to accommodate such movement, this alteration could only have so much effect: "by holding firm the orders of the state, which in corruption were no longer good, those laws that were renewed were not enough to keep men good; but they would have assisted much if with the innovation of the laws, the orders had been retransformed."[111] Innovation must thus take as its object those elements that constitute the very core of the social order. Indeed, such institutional innovation would seem to be necessary if, as suggested by the key passages cited from the *Florentine Histories* and the "Discourse on Florentine Affairs," Machiavelli's end is the increasing entrenchment of democratic life, made possible through the actualization of a requisite civic orientation achieved through popular political education.

In any case, in the context of Rome Machiavelli provides two examples of this general movement: the selection of magistrates and the creation of laws. Initially in the republic high offices were distributed according to a principle of self-selection, this being an appropriate order when virtue was sufficiently generalized such that only those individuals who considered themselves most adequate for the position put themselves forward. However, in a corrupt city lacking such a generalization, where there is no fear of public exposure and derision in the case of a non-suitability to the office, only the already powerful would seek authority, other more apt candidates not nominating themselves out of fear. Machiavelli identifies such corruption in this instance as the end result of a gradual subduing of external threats, one that produced a passive sense of security among the population: "This security and this weakness of their enemies made the Roman people, in giving the consulate, no more regard virtue, but favour, putting in that office those who best knew how to entertain men, rather than those who best knew how to overcome enemies. Afterwards from those who had more favour, they descended to giving it to those who had more power; so the good, through the defect in that order, remained entirely excluded."[112] With respect to the creation of the laws, meanwhile, as we have already seen, initially the order was such that any citizen was empowered to propose a law to the people, and such that any citizen could interrogate and scrutinize this proposal publicly. Machiavelli

---

111 Ibid.
112 Ibid.

writes that "this order was good when the citizens were good; because it was always good that everyone who intends a benefit for the public can propose it; and it is good that everyone can speak their opinion on it, so that the people, having heard everyone, could then choose the best."[113] When citizens are corrupt, however, only the powerful propose laws, and only for the sake of their own private advantage. No citizen, meanwhile, would dare speak against such a process of privatization out of fear of retribution at the hands of the powerful. As a consequence of this dynamic "the people came to be deceived or forced to decide its ruin."[114]

The continuing reproduction of the freedom of Rome would have necessitated the latter's perpetual self-alteration of its orders: "It was necessary, therefore, if Rome wanted to in its corruption maintain itself free, that, just as in the course of its life it made new laws, it should have made new orders."[115] The fundamental principle is that unique social-historical circumstances demand unique modes and orders: "for one ought to order different orders and modes of life in a bad subject than in a good; nor can there be a similar form for an entirely different matter."[116] What this principle closes off in advance is the thought of the potential for the creation of any fixed system of institutions or terminal political form that is capable of stabilizing the social being of the city and indefinitely regulating human affairs. Such an impossibility is noted by Machiavelli in several places and in various contexts throughout the *Discourses*. In 3:17, for example, the impossibility is rooted specifically in the invariability of human desire, as revealed through the example of Claudius Nero. Claudius took foolish and rash action in a confrontation with the Carthaginians, believing that if he succeeded his honour would be restored, and if he failed the Roman people would be appropriately punished for the injustice that Claudius thought was perpetrated against him. On Machiavelli's account Claudius's passion interrupted his capacity for prudent decision making, overwhelming the rational understanding of the necessity to moderate desire for the sake of life in common. It is the possibility for the indeterminate expression and redirection of human desire that necessitates the perpetual renegotiation of those institutions necessary to channel it. Machiavelli

---

113 Ibid.
114 Ibid.
115 Ibid.
116 Ibid.

thus writes, "when these passions of such offences can do so much in a Roman citizen, and in those times when Rome was still uncorrupt, one ought to think of how much they can do in a citizen of another city that was not made as was [Rome] then. And because in similar disorders that arise in republics one cannot give a sure remedy, it follows that it is *impossible to order a perpetual republic*, because its ruin is caused through a thousand unexpected ways."[117]

Such an image of the perpetual republic is counterposed with that of the historical republic, the republic that affirms becoming through its openness to institutional innovation. In 1:49 Machiavelli claims that cities with free beginnings are capable of preserving themselves only through such openness, it being impossible to order a city such that all of the laws providing for freedom are given in advance. Continual refinement of the institutional form of the republic is needed as accidents arise. In the case of Rome, "always in managing that city new necessities were being discovered, and it was necessary to create new orders: such happened when they created the censors, which were one of those provisions that helped keep Rome free, that time that it lived in freedom."[118] What is perhaps suggested here by the juxtaposition of the notions of freedom and self-alteration, if not made explicit, is the extent to which the latter is not simply the means for the preservation of the latter, but the very mode through which the latter is actualized.

If human freedom lies in the expression of *virtù*, which as we have seen refers us to a creative activity of giving form, the republic's openness to its own alteration via popular reinstitution represents a generalization of this expression at the collective level. Recognizing this fact allows us to reconsider the place of *The Prince* in relation to the *Discourses*, according to the model of relation that I have proposed in this study. We may note again the specificity of the Machiavellian republic, the latter being distinguished from the principality in 1:58. Here Machiavelli notes that innovation in a popular republic is much more dynamic than in a principality, and thus more comprehensively affirms creation: "one sees, beyond this, that cities where the people are princes make extreme gains in a very brief time, and much greater than those that have always been under a prince."[119] There is not necessarily a

---

117 Ibid., bk. 3.17. Emphasis added.
118 Ibid., bk. 1.49.
119 Ibid., bk. 1.58.

contradiction in this chapter between the recognition of the intensity of popular innovation in a republic and the claim that whereas princes excel at creating initial laws and orders, people excel at maintaining them. Regarding the latter Machiavelli writes, "if princes are superior to peoples in ordering laws, forming civil existences, ordering new statutes and orders, peoples are so much superior in maintaining ordered things that they attain, without doubt, the glory of those who order."[120] This is because maintenance in the republic is a form of creation, it demanding the perpetual renovation of existing laws and orders in response to temporal variability. It is because of the republican openness to popular innovation, to the generalized expression of *virtù*, represented in the continual interrogation of existing institutional forms, "that those governments of peoples are better than those of princes."[121]

The freedom of the republic is thus manifested in the multiplication of creation, which is realized through the popular reinstitutionalization of the city. The *Discourses* demonstrates the extent to which the form of creative subjectivity articulated in *The Prince* is capable of being given a popular actualization through democratic activity. Hence the significance of a statement made by Machiavelli in *Discourses* 1:60, where he notes approvingly that Roman magistrates distributed according to the will of the plebs did not give "regard to age or to blood," but rather endeavoured always "to find virtue, whether it was in the young or in the old."[122] This is again one manifestation of the republic's superiority with respect to innovation, it being better equipped than the principality to harness the active vitality of youth: "when a young person is of so much virtue that he makes himself known in some notable thing, it would be a very injurious thing if the city could not then affirm it, and if it had to wait until that vigour of spirit and that readiness, which it could have affirmed at that time, had aged with him."[123] The republic is thus the regime of the young, which is to say, the regime of the bold and the innovative. In other words, it is the regime that is most appropriate to harness the particular political subjectivity detailed in *The Prince*, where Machiavelli famously identifies the capacity to productively engage with fortune with the spirit of youth, fortune being "the friend

---

120 Ibid.
121 Ibid.
122 Ibid., bk. 1.60.
123 Ibid.

of the young, because they are less cautious, more aggressive, and command it with more audacity."[124]

The Return to Beginnings and the Potential for Democratic Innovation

We can conclude our discussion of the self-overcoming form of republican institutions through reading within its context one of the most commented upon concepts in Machiavelli's oeuvre: that of the republican return to beginnings, which is most systematically developed in *Discourses* 3:1. For a long time the traditional way of interpreting Machiavelli's theorization of the return to beginnings as a mode for the rejuvenation of the spirit of the republic was to assimilate it to a cyclical or self-identical philosophy of history that emphasized the historical recurrence that results from the invariability of human doing and being. Such a reading, though, is certainly inconsistent with the repeated emphasis placed on the new and on the diversity of forms and modes of human existence. On the contrary, what we ultimately see is that the account of the return to beginnings is in no way indicative of a conservative belief in the necessity of a literal reproduction of the existent, but rather one element of Machiavelli's stress on creativity and innovation. This is because what returns in this movement is nothing but creative virtue itself. The return to beginnings is thus an essential expression of Machiavelli's revolutionary emphasis on the human potential to upset the order of things and reinstitute the political community.[125]

Machiavelli begins 3:1 by once again calling attention to the fleetingness of the objects of the temporal world, writing that "It is a very true

---

124 Machiavelli, "Il Principe," chap. 25.
125 Indeed, Miguel Vatter claims that through his emphasis on historical repetition as a return to innovation, and specifically an innovation considered as the overcoming of form grounded in the popular desire for freedom, Machiavelli initiates the tradition of modern revolutionary thinking. Vatter, *Between Form and Event*, 219. Arendt also suggests that Machiavelli is the first modern thinker of revolution and foundation in the Western tradition of political thought, even if he did not utilize this precise vocabulary. Arendt, "What Is Authority?," 136. Unlike Vatter, though, Arendt emphasizes the necessarily institutional ground of Machiavelli's revolutionary thought: he is "the spiritual father of revolution," because "he was the first to think about the possibility of founding a permanent, lasting, enduring body politic." Hannah Arendt, *On Revolution* (New York: Viking Press, 1965), 27, 26.

thing, that all the things of the world have a limit to their life."[126] The fact of historical flux necessitates human intervention in the order of things, objects having to be purposefully altered if their being is to be preserved through time. The condition of the object's being, in other words, must be adapted to the perpetually changing condition of the being of the world. In this chapter Machiavelli is concerned with outlining the form of activity which is capable of altering the republican political object, which is just as susceptible to the vicissitudes of history as any other. In the case of republics, preservation through alteration depends upon a return to beginnings: "And because I am speaking of mixed bodies, such as republics and sects, I say that those alterations are healthy that take them back to their beginnings. And therefore those are better ordered, and have a longer life, that by means of their orders can frequently renew themselves, or that, by some accident external to that order come to said renewal. And it is a thing clearer than light that, if not renewing themselves, these bodies do not last."[127] This explicitly self-renewal through a return to beginnings is seen as necessarily embodying a certain intrinsic virtue: "For all beginnings of sects, and of republics and of kingdoms, must have some internal goodness, by means of which they recapture their first reputation and their first growth."[128] The question then becomes, what is this internal goodness in beginnings? Clearly it cannot simply be associated with the reproduction of a stable or fixed pattern or order, for we know that the invariability of historical movement forecloses the possibility of the institution across time of identical forms. The answer can only lie in the very capacity that makes possible the initiation of the process of beginning itself: to return to the beginning is to return to, to reactivate, the specifically human capacity for creation. To affirm the return to beginnings is to affirm, not a specific organization of things, but the uniquely human ability to begin.[129]

---

126 Machiavelli, "Discorsi sopra la prima Deca di Tito Livio," bk. 3.1.

127 Ibid.

128 Ibid.

129 Such is often pointed out. See, for example, Shumer, "Machiavelli: Republican Politics and Its Corruption," 23; Lefort, *Machiavelli in the Making*, 343; Vatter, *Between Form and Event*, 250–1; Nomi Claire Lazar, *States of Emergency in Liberal Democracies* (Cambridge: Cambridge University Press, 2009), 26; Roberto Esposito, *Ordine e conflitto: Machiavelli e la letteratura politica del Rinascimento italiano* (Napoli: Liguori Editore, 1984), 200–1; Esposito, *Living Thought*, 51; Sebastián Torres, "Tempo e politica: una lettura materialista di Machiavelli," in *The Radical Machiavelli: Politics, Philosophy, and Language*, ed. Filippo Del Lucchese, Fabio Frosini, and Vittorio Morfino (Leiden: Brill, 2015), 186.

Now, as suggested by the quotation above, this return can be stimulated through either "extrinsic accident or intrinsic prudence."[130] Extrinsic accidents, as in for example the loss of Rome to the French, produce a political crisis significant enough to starkly reveal the corruption at the heart of the body politic, the neglect of those previously virtuous institutions that provided the foundation for a civil and free way of life. The external crisis is thus a manifestation of internal degeneracy so profound as to stimulate a will to reform: "This extrinsic beating thus came, so that all the orders of that city might be revived, and it might be shown to the people that it was not only necessary to maintain religion and justice, but also to esteem its good citizens, and to take more account of their virtue than of those conveniences that it appeared to them that they were missing through their works."[131] Intrinsically stimulated renewal, however, does not refer us to a fundamental crisis of the political order, but rather the civic recognition of the perpetual need to refine institutional life in the face of contingent temporality. This renewal, furthermore, can take one of two forms: it "must stem either from a law, which often examines the account of the men who are in that body; or indeed by a good man who is born among them, who with his examples and with his virtuous works produces the same effect as the order."[132]

Machiavelli is here suggesting that there are two modes for institutional alteration aimed at the preservation of the social order. One is a princely type of reordering in which a single great individual who, in possession of a unique skill or intelligence and acting seemingly independently of institutional authority, assumes responsibility for altering orders so as to bring them into line with the times. The second, however, is a form of alteration that is mediated precisely through institutional authority, through existing orders that are somehow or other structured such that they are capable of providing a ground for their own self-interrogation. According to this second model, the creative source for the renewal of the polity is to be located in the motion of existing laws and institutions themselves, as they, as Alfredo Bonadeo observes, are "so constituted that a constant and self-generating renovation occurs."[133] Contrary to most examples in Book One, in which

---

130 Machiavelli, "Discorsi sopra la prima Deca di Tito Livio," bk. 3.1.
131 Ibid.
132 Ibid.
133 Bonadeo, *Corruption, Conflict, and Power*, 95.

renewal is stimulated through the shock of an event that reveals the necessity of constitutional reform, in Book Three reform measures are primarily preventive in nature, demonstrating the degree to which the polity is capable of self-correcting without going through a process of total corruption.[134] Hence Machiavelli will call attention to several instances in which a tendency to institutional self-innovation can be perceived in the Roman case, one such being the tribunes of the plebs, but also the censors and "all the other laws that were against the ambition and the insolence of men."[135]

Even here, however, we see a manifestation of that tension within Machiavelli's thought, between the potential for democratic self-actualization and the necessity of single-person elite foundation and renovation, this latter moment appearing in the form of a guiding hand that takes leading responsibility for the renewal. Machiavelli writes that "such orders have need of being made to live through the virtue of one citizen, who spiritedly conduces to execute them against the power of those who transgress them."[136] Democratic self-alteration is thus apparently subsumed by a princely type of reordering, here manifested through purging from the city those insolent elements that would threaten to violate civic norms. Such executions should be carried out no less than every ten years, "for, after this time, men begin to vary in their customs and to transgress the laws."[137] The return to beginnings thus becomes a return to the origin of foundation, a reinstallation in the potentially insolent of the original fear that accompanied the institution of republican life. It is the *grandi*, in other words, who must be made to fear the authority of the collectivity. Following Florentine practice, Machiavelli calls "recapturing the state, putting that terror and that fear in men that had been put there in taking it, since they had at that time beaten down those who had, according to that mode of living, worked for evil. But as the memory of that beating is extinguished, men have the audacity to test new ways of asserting evil; and so it is necessary to provide for this, returning [the state] back toward its beginnings."[138]

The overall movement of the chapter at this point can be summed up through the isolation of the following moments: 1) political orders

---

134 Ibid., 96.
135 Machiavelli, "Discorsi sopra la prima Deca di Tito Livio," bk. 3.1.
136 Ibid.
137 Ibid.
138 Ibid.

become no longer appropriate for the times; 2) political corruption sets in as a consequence; 3) exploiting this corruption, certain insolent individuals attempt to privately appropriate power to advance their particular interest; 4) a purging of this insolence occurs through a reform of institutions of public accusation; 5) such reform reproduces the republic's initial generation of fear and terror among the *grandi*. Although the return to beginnings is here associated with a return to the popular power of the people and the execution of those who attempt to privately appropriate authority for themselves or their faction, there are two ambiguities in the narrative from a democratic perspective. The first is that which we have encountered numerous times throughout the study: the fact that republican institutionalization is realized not through the self-activity of the people, but through the action of a single princely individual who reforms in the name of the common good. The second is the persistence of inequality, as represented in the perseverance of a will to domination. The *grandi* continues to exist as an organized class, as that which is eliminated through the return to beginnings is not the organized humour to oppress, but rather just particular individuals who are seen as representative of this will, and whose execution is intended to serve as a symbolic communication to the *grandi* regarding the necessity of civil obedience.

These two ambiguities are not unrelated to each other. That the violence potentially accompanying the return to beginnings is specifically a violence against social elites – grandees who would attempt to privately appropriate surplus political authority for themselves at the expense of the people – is confirmed in 3:22. If it is possible, as I suggested it is, that Machiavelli is willing to think the non-existence of the *grandi* as a whole, then the necessity of elite initiated violence as a response to social corruption is eliminated, and noble insolence is thus no longer able to short-circuit the process of renovation. Institutional alteration in the face of worldly temporality can then proceed according to the internal logic of the political orders, the people democratically recreating these orders on the basis of their own rational understanding of the historical situation. If Machiavelli's original distinction between a prudent return to beginnings mediated by individuals versus one by institutions is collapsed through his affirmation of the necessity of singular reordering, this is as a consequence of his perception of the reality of the continuing existence of a *grandi* with a humour to oppress. A genuinely democratic regime requires not only the type of major institutional overhaul every ten years or so as suggested above, but a perpetual openness to self-alteration, a self-alteration that is realized through the everday collective activity of a participatory people.

Machiavelli closes chapter 3:1 by in fact returning to the distinction between two conceptually distinct forms of renewal, that generated by individuals who are external to political orders, and that internally mediated by political orders themselves: "one concludes, therefore, that there is not a thing more necessary in a common life, whether it is a sect or a kingdom or a republic, than to restore it to that reputation that it had at its beginning, and to strive that it be either good orders or good men that make this effect, and not to have it be made by an extrinsic force."[139] And Machiavelli throughout the *Discourses*, in fact, provides several examples of this institutional self-renewal, a self-renewal that can be thought of as a return to beginnings – to the extent that it is a concrete expression of the creativity of political foundation – despite it not being accompanied by the seeming terror and violence that Machiavelli associates with extraordinary or extra-institutional reform by individuals.[140] The possibility of such non-violent renewal is notably expressed, for example, in 3:7, where he writes: "One will perhaps doubt from whence it arises that of many changes that are made from free life to tyrannical, and to the contrary, some are made with blood, some without; for, as one understands through the histories, in similar variations sometimes countless men have died, sometimes no one is injured."[141] In fact, when violence is used as a technique for instituting the new regime, it will always generate additional violence later in time when crises arise and those who were injured previously attempt to avenge themselves. Machiavelli goes on to suggest that the more democratic the foundation, the greater the possibility for avoiding this cycle of violent retribution. This is because there is a lack of aggrieved individuals in instances in which regimes are founded through "common

---

139 Ibid.
140 Compare this to the reading of Strauss. Although Strauss correctly identifies the return to beginnings with the return to a mode of political creation, this mode belongs only to elite founders. Indeed, the return of political creation is necessarily accompanied by the return of a primordial terror, the fear that founders need to instil in the people in order to create. Strauss, *Thoughts on Machiavelli*, 167. See also Paul A. Rahe, *Republics Ancient and Modern: New Modes and Orders in Early Modern Political Thought* (Chapel Hill: University of North Carolina Press, 1994), 36.
141 Machiavelli, "Discorsi sopra la prima Deca di Tito Livio," bk. 3.7.

consent," that is, through a universal act of popular constitution.[142] In the final instance the return to beginnings, then, can be read as one key manifestation of Machiavelli's recognition of the necessity of perpetual institutional innovation, this innovation being demanded by the fact of worldly contingency and temporal flux, and being representative of the essential human desire for creative expression. This necessity is summed up most notably and with special clarity in the title of the concluding chapter to the text, which reads in part, "A republic, if one wishes to maintain it free, has each day need of new acts of foresight." Machiavelli here affirms that accidents arise in cities "every day," and that the maintenance of polities requires that these be corrected through specific modes and reorderings.[143]

Factional Activity and the Depoliticization of Republican Life

What I have attempted to demonstrate in the previous two sections, and which I believe is obscured by most radical democratic readers of Machiavelli, is the role of the institution as essential to democratic self-expression. It is the institution, albeit the institution as conceived in a very specific way, that productively expels human ambition, sublimating desire in non-antagonistic (which is not to say non-agonistic) and public ways.[144] This essentiality seems to be explicitly confirmed in various passages within the *Discourses* and the *Florentine Histories* in which Machiavelli contrasts the form of institutional life in republican Rome with that in contemporary Florence. It must be stressed, however, that Machiavelli's critique of Florence is certainly not one-sided, but grounded in a specific philosophical anthropology and theory of political change that recognizes the potential for the transformation and improvement of the city.[145] Such a redemptive critique is explicitly contrasted by Machiavelli with that of Dante, "who in every part

---

142 Ibid.
143 Ibid., bk. 3.49.
144 Mark Wenman argues that not only in Machiavelli can we "trace the first explicit formulation in western political thought of the agonistic idea of the positive value of conflict," but that Machiavelli also conceptually distinguishes his agonism from antagonism, as represented in the distinction between conflicts between *umori* and conflicts between *sette*. Wenman, *Agonistic Democracy*, 52, 53.
145 On this point see especially Jurdjevic, *A Great and Wretched City: Promise and Failure in Machiavelli's Florentine Political Thought*.

showed himself to be, through his genius, through his teaching, and through his judgment, an excellent man, except where he had to reason about his homeland, which, outside of all humanity and philosophical foundation, he persecuted with every type of injury. And he was not able to do other than defame it, accuse it of every vice, damn its people, speak badly of its customs and of its laws; and this he did not only in a part of his Cantica, but all of it, and differently and in diverse modes."[146]

What Florence was seen by Machiavelli to lack was a regime of institutionalization capable of mediating the diversity of desire that characterizes life in an internally divided city. The necessity of expressing human energy, and in particular plebeian energy, through institutional forms is articulated early in the *Discourses*, and is notably expressed in Machiavelli's account of the opposition of the people to Coriolanus. Although, upon learning of Coriolanus's attempt to persuade the Senate to withhold provisions as a stratagem for reversing plebeian political gains in the city, the people initially in their indignation confronted him upon his exit from the Senate with the threat of extra-legal violence, he was ultimately legally apprehended in order to be put before the tribunes. Tribunal prosecution would have the effect not only of releasing the energy of the people, but also of doing so in a controlled and mediated form, through its directed channelling via a publicly recognized order. Indiscriminate and potentially unlimited modes of private retribution, on the other hand, would have the effect of multiplying offence and generalizing illegality. Machiavelli thus concludes that in considering this episode "one notes that which was said above, how it is useful and necessary that republics, with their laws, give outlets to vent the anger that the generality conceives against one citizen: for when these ordinary modes are not there, one resorts to extraordinary ones; and without doubt, the latter produce much worse effects than the former."[147] Little disorder results in the city when insolent citizens are constrained via ordinary modes, for there is no necessity for

---

146 Machiavelli, "Discorso o dialogo intorno alla nostra lingua," in *Tutte le opere*, ed. Mario Martelli (Firenze: Sansoni Editore, 1971), 925. For a study of Machiavelli's critique of Dante in this text see Susan Meld Shell, "Machiavelli's Discourse on Language," in *The Comedy and Tragedy of Machiavelli: Essays on the Literary Works*, ed. Vickie B. Sullivan (New Haven: Yale University Press, 2000), 78–101.

147 Machiavelli, "Discorsi sopra la prima Deca di Tito Livio," bk. 1.7.

the intervention of private or foreign forces, "which are those that ruin the free way of life."[148]

Unlike private forces, for example, public ones have determinable limits that are generally known and acknowledged as legitimate, if not seen as beyond question and scrutiny, ensuring that sanctions and punishments do not multiply in a cycle of retribution. Indeed, in this chapter Machiavelli notes that much harm has been done in modern Florence precisely as a result of the lack of those institutions that are capable of mediating popular desire and allowing the people to vent in ordinary as opposed to extraordinary ways. Given as an example of such harm is the case of Francesco Valori, who after consolidating authority in the city increasingly offended against the people through violating civic modes. Such violation was undertaken reflectively and as a consequence of his perception of the lack of ordinary modes for accusation. Those who would attempt to resist him had no choice but to develop extraordinary strategies, which Valori guarded against through the recruitment of partisans. Conflict was reduced to the confrontation of private forces, and as a consequence there resulted a generalization of violence, harm ultimately coming to many.[149] Contrary to this and many other examples in Florence, then, "these modes were in Rome so well ordered that, in many dissensions of the plebs and the Senate, never did either the Senate or the plebs or any particular citizen design to make use of external forces; for, having the remedy at home, to go outside for it was not necessitated."[150]

In the subsequent chapter the distinction between ordinary and extraordinary modes of expulsion is more clearly mapped onto a distinction between public and private. Although both public and private action refer to the same economy of desire, they differ in their relation to the law, in the fact or non-fact of institutionalization. Specifically, public institutions function to give a legitimate expression to the inevitable discord that arises as a necessary consequence of social division, of a society's internal differentiation of desire. The distinction between the concepts of accusation and calumny is one of the most significant manifestations of the distinction between ordinary and extraordinary modes of action. In short, whereas accusations are public, calumnies

148 Ibid.
149 Ibid.
150 Ibid.

are private: "Men are accused to magistrates, to peoples, to councils; they are calumniated in the piazzas and in the loggias."[151] The problem with calumnies is their extra-legal form, no witnesses or corroboration being a prerequisite for the determination of guilt, such that every individual is capable of being calumniated by anyone else without discretion. On the contrary, "not [everyone] can be accused, accusations having the need of real evidence and circumstances that show the truth of the accusation."[152] Again, on this subject Rome is contrasted with Florence, the lack of orders allowing for legal forms of accusations leading to a multitude of calumnies in the latter. In Florence citizens would slander others indiscriminately and for the sake of private ambition, this further generating and intensifying existing hatreds, divisions, and sects. Indeed, "if there had been in Florence orders for accusing citizens, and punishing calumniators, the endless scandals that followed would not have followed; for those citizens, whether they were convicted or absolved, would not have been able to harm the city, and much fewer would have been accused than were calumniated."[153] Machiavelli concludes that the most effective method for avoiding calumnies is in fact to increase the number of accusational outlets, and that "an orderer of a republic ought to order that one can in it accuse every citizen, without any fear or without any respect; and this being done, and well observed, he ought to harshly punish calumniators."[154]

It is in the *Florentine Histories*, of course, that Machiavelli most systematically distinguishes between modes of ordinary and extraordinary political expression on the basis of this expression's relation or non-relation to the fact of institutionalization. This distinction accounts for the difference between the portrayals of conflictual civic practice in the *Histories* and the *Discourses*.[155] In the preface to the *Histories*

---

151 Ibid., bk. 1.8.
152 Ibid.
153 Ibid.
154 Ibid.
155 Such is noted by many readers. On the differing forms of conflictual practice in these texts see, for example, Gisela Bock, "Civil Discord in Machiavelli's *Istorie Fiorentine*," in *Machiavelli and Republicanism*, ed. Gisela Bock, Quentin Skinner, and Maurizio Viroli (Cambridge: Cambridge University Press, 1990), 181–201; Kent M. Brudney, "Machiavelli on Social Class and Class Conflict," *Political Theory* 12, no. 4 (1984): 507–19; Anna Maria Cabrini, "Machiavelli's *Florentine Histories*," in *The Cambrige Companion to Machiavelli*, ed. John M. Najemy (Cambridge: Cambridge University Press, 2010), 128–43; Nicolai Rubenstein, "Machiavelli and the World of

Machiavelli is adamant that the form of social division – the particular mode of appearance of human difference – that was most predominant in Florence must be qualitatively differentiated from that which was most predominant in Rome. As opposed to the productive division between noble and pleb, a division incorporating into the positive orders of the city both groups, in Florence one observes an unproductive multiplicity of divisions internal to these social groups, the victorious parties splintering among themselves after the establishment of their superiority relative to the others: "In Florence first the nobles were divided among themselves, then the nobles and the people, and finally the people and the plebs; and many times it occurred that one of these parts, remaining superior, divided into two."[156] This perpetual multiplication of division through the internal fragmentation of the social groups results from the fact that each of the latter posits itself in a relation of antagonism with the other groups, seeking to monopolize political right for itself. In this way any movement toward the universalization of political participation is blocked. Factional division can never be eliminated in a city with partisans, to the extent that the latter act only for an individual good that is relationally articulated: when one opponent is defeated the victorious party will necessarily itself be divided as its members attempt to further their private advantage relative to their peers.[157] In the final instance it is impossible for civic-minded citizens to flourish in a city that is divided into factions, where social difference becomes ossified into antagonistic poles that preclude mutual understanding and co-operation: "If it is a republic that governs it, there is no finer mode to make your citizens evil and to make your city divided, than to have a divided city to govern; for each part searches to obtain favours, and each makes friends through various corruptions. So then arise two very great inconveniences; the one, that you never make them your friends through being able to govern them well, the government varying often, now with one, now with the other humour; the other, that such concern with parties of necessity divides your republic."[158]

Florentine Politics," in *Studies on Machiavelli*, ed. Myron P. Gilmore (Firenze: G.C. Sansoni, 1979), 3–28; Marco Geuna, "Machiavelli ed il ruolo dei conflitti nella vita politica," in *Conflitti*, ed. Alessandro Arienzo and Dario Caruso (Napoli: Libreria Dante & Descartes, 2005), 19–57.
156 Machiavelli, "Istorie fiorentine," bk. proem.
157 Ibid., bk. 7.1.
158 Machiavelli, "Discorsi sopra la prima Deca di Tito Livio," 3.27.

The degeneracy of the Florentine regime lay in the fact that the actualization of ambitious desire on the part of some was seen to be exclusive of the actualization of it with respect to others. Particular good, in other words, was not perceived to be a constitutive element of a public good of which other particular goods were essential parts. To the extent that there did not exist a means for a generalized venting of desire, human ambition, precisely because grounded in a psychic desire to be which cannot be eradicated, was necessarily desublimated.[159] Hence the various private and direct modes of satisfaction that Machiavelli exhaustively details throughout the text. Such activity is differentiated from that detailed in the *Discourses* with respect to its object and its mode. First, the object of the activity is an invidious private good whose satisfaction is dependent upon closing off the potential for others' satisfaction. This fact is articulated by an anonymous citizen in the *Histories*, who identifies participation in factional parties with the quest for the actualization of a private ambition that is always realized at the expense of someone else, not to the degree that the other parties are incapable of achieving a mutual and identical satisfaction (impossible given the always divided nature of the city), but to the degree that the other parties are not even recognized as having a legitimate right to pursue their satisfaction through participation in civic modes: "For the prize they desire from victory is, not the glory of having liberated the city, but the satisfaction of having overcome the other, and of having usurped the principality. Where carried out, there is nothing so unjust, so cruel or avaricious, that they do not dare to do it. Hence they make orders and laws, not for the public, but for their own benefit; hence wars, peaces, friendships are decided not for the common glory, but for the satisfaction of the few."[160]

Second, the identification of personal utility with factionalism refers us to the form of the activity, which is associated with partisanship, private modes being the appropriate method for the acquisition of private objects: "citizens in cities acquire reputation in two modes: through

---

159 On such a form of expression as a necessary consequence of the inability of energy to be legitimately vented see, for example, Wood, "The Value of Asocial Sociability," 7; Honig, *Political Theory and the Displacement of Politics*, 71. On the concept of desublimation more generally see Herbert Marcuse, *One-Dimensional Man: Studies in the Ideology of Advanced Industrial Society* (Boston: Beacon Press, 1969), 74–9.

160 Machiavelli, "Istorie fiorentine," bk. 3.5.

public ways or through private modes. Publicly they acquire by winning a battle, acquiring a town, carrying out a legation with solicitude
and with prudence, advising the republic wisely and happily; through
private modes they acquire by benefiting this or that citizen, defending
them from the magistrates, helping them with money, getting them
unmerited honours, and gratifying the plebs with games and public
gifts."[161] Although it is impossible to eliminate social difference and
even "very great hatreds" given the divided nature of the city, which is
ontologically rooted in the diversity and multiplicity of human psyche,
such difference is not destructive of the civil order when human ambition is prevented from receiving a direct expression via partisan activity: rather, "they work to benefit it, because it is necessary to overcome
their obstacles for them to attempt to exalt [the republic] and observe
each other particularly, so that civil limits are not transgressed."[162]

The key political question is not how to eliminate conflict, but rather
how it is to be expressed, specifically, whether it will be legitimately
expressed ordinarily through public modes, or illegitimately expressed
extraordinarily through private ones. The failure to appreciate the distinction between these two general modes of ambitious expression is
what produces that confusion marked by the conceptual collapsing of
the categories of freedom and licence. Machiavelli locates the gap
between these notions in the willingness or unwillingness on the part
of social actors to undertake a project of self-limitation on the basis of
their consideration of the good and desire of others. Genuine freedom
depends upon obedience to institutional orders that have been collectively generated, Machiavelli affirming autonomy in the etymological
sense as the self-generation of and obedience to one's own law.[163]
Hence, for example, in *Discourses* 2:27 he stresses the extent to which
individuals must understand the necessity and the means to autonomously place limits on their desires and on actions looking toward
actualizing these desires: "men make this error, who do not know how
to put limits on their hopes; and by relying on these, without otherwise
measuring themselves, they are ruined."[164] The range of human action

---

161 Ibid., bk. 7.1.
162 Ibid.
163 This has been noted by Erica Benner, who in her reading of Machiavelli's ethics of
     self-legislation interprets *virtù* in terms of autonomy, the human being's capacity to
     reflectively give itself its own laws. Benner, *Machiavelli's Ethics*, 163.
164 Machiavelli, "Discorsi sopra la prima Deca di Tito Livio," bk. 2.27.

is clearly not limited only by the range of human desire. In 3:47 the need for such autonomous self-limitation is again affirmed, Machiavelli maintaining that civically minded citizens must not allow certain of their particular passions to interfere with publics modes, being willing instead to subordinate consideration of their private injuries for the sake of the good of the city.[165] Such a conception is entirely opposite to the so-called and false freedom that one sees in licentious republics, which are marked by the complete absence of internal limitation.[166] Hence, "Cities, and chiefly those not well ordered that are administered under the name of republic, often change their governments and states, not between freedom and servitude, as many believe, but between servitude and licence."[167] In the latter instance the language of freedom is exploited by those who possess the means to extract most private benefit from licentious behaviour, the *grandi* playing on that popular desire for liberty that Machiavelli, again in the *Histories*, maintains can never be effaced, even when individuals lack any past experience of the conditions of freedom. Wanting "to be subject to neither the laws nor to men,"[168] social elites perpetuate the myth that freedom is licence, thus seeking to legitimate a condition in which their ambition can be directly expressed through the utilization of techniques of violence.

As noted by several readers, the emergence of factional activity and the generalization of extraordinary modes of action constitute a process of privatization of the political, the expulsion of ambition being detached from public projects and offices, expressed instead in the egoistic quest for personal gain and profit.[169] The political is defined in terms of the popular sublimation of human ambition through public

---

165 Ibid., bk. 3.47.

166 We are thus justified in being sceptical that Florence, to the extent that it does not look to the generalization of participation, may even be classified as a republic. See, for example, Johann Gottlieb Fichte, "On Machiavelli, as an Author, and Passages from His Writings," trans. Ian Alexander Moore and Christopher Turner, *Philosophy Today* 60, no. 3 (2016): 767; Nicolai Rubenstein, "Machiavelli and Florentine Republican Experience," in *Machiavelli and Republicanism*, ed. Gisela Bock, Quentin Skinner, and Maurizio Viroli (Cambridge: Cambridge University Press, 1990), 3; Najemy, "Baron's Machiavelli and Renaissance Republicanism," 126.

167 Machiavelli, "Istorie fiorentine," bk. 4.1.

168 Ibid.

169 On political corruption and privatization see Shumer, "Machiavelli: Republican Politics and Its Corruption," 9; Pitkin, *Fortune Is a Woman*, 321; Najemy, "Society, Class, and State in Machiavelli's *Discourses on Livy*," 106–10.

modes and orders, or the institutional mediation of desire. The linking of factional activity is then associated with depoliticization, as is revealed with special clarity in the "Discourse on Florentine Affairs." Here the lack of institutional spaces allowing the people to share in government is identified as a fundamental perversion of republican life, one that leads to "countless disorders."[170] Such could be seen in the failed attempt of Maso degli Albizzi to order a republic governed by aristocrats. On the one hand, such a government had no institutional means to restrain and check the domineering ambition of the nobles, which was consolidated through the creation of factional parties: "there was not established a dread in the grandees so that they could not make sects, which are the ruin of a state."[171] On the other hand, faction was additionally encouraged to the extent that "private men" were often granted prominent roles in public deliberations, there emerging as a result a widespread drive toward the gain of private status as a means to acquiring authority. Such "maintained the reputation of private men, and removed it from public ones, and it took away authority and reputation from the magistrates: something that is contrary to every civil order."[172] Far from constituting an obstacle to the expression of human desire through fixing the being of the city and individual places and functions within it, the institution is that medium through which the universal ambitious desire that all individuals possess is channelled. As the case of Florence illustrates, no political or civil way of life is thus possible when cities fail to provide such media.

If the institution is to perform its role in expressing human desire, which we recall is a negative desire for creative value formation, than it must be an institution of a very particular kind. Far from reifying the institutional form of the polity and neutralizing individual self-expression, Machiavelli's orders affirm the creative potential through being perpetually open to their own interrogation and self-alteration, functioning as modes for the expulsion or venting of human ambition. Although Machiavelli often uses the language of necessity in describing institutional

---

170 Machiavelli, "Discursus florentinarum rerum post mortem iunioris Laurentii Medices," in *Tutte le opere*, 24.
171 Ibid.
172 Ibid.

innovation, we must not be misled into interpreting the latter in terms of a merely strategic technique for countering worldly contingency. The impossibility of the republic ever coming to rest in a fixed terminal form is grounded in the non-determination of being, a fact that is often pointed out. My argument, however, is that there is a further normative dimension to Machiavelli's positing of the openness of republican institutional orders. Not only does such openness allow for swift accommodation to objective changes caused by temporal flux, but it also provides an outlet for the expulsion of that essential human desire for creative expression that is revealed through the concept of ambition. The potentially self-overcoming republic can thus be read as that form of political regime that is capable of providing media for the actualization of the negative human essence as creative becoming. One's social context certainly leans on, yet does not determine, one's being. What the existence of ambition speaks to is the specifically human capacity to self-generate the conditions of its existence. The necessity of varying the laws and orders of the polity in order to stay in accord with the times transcends the realm of mere instrumental consideration and assumes a new ethical content in light of what Machiavelli takes to be the essentiality of human ambition and the desire for innovation and novelty. Machiavelli defends democratic participatory modes not only because they most effectively engage with the diversity of situations, but more importantly, because they allow for the actualization of an intrinsic human potential shared by all. Democracy is ethically grounded in the recognition of the essentiality of creative desire, and the recognition of the equal capacity of all to virtuously express this desire through political activity.

Works Cited

Abensour, Miguel. *Democracy against the State: Marx and the Machiavellian Moment*. Translated by Max Blechman and Martin Breaugh. London: Polity Press, 2011.

– "Machiavel: le grand penseur du désordre." *Le monde*, 11 April 2006.

– "'Savage Democracy' and the 'Principle of Anarchy.'" In *Democracy against the State: Marx and the Machiavellian Moment*, by Miguel Abensour, translated by Max Blechman and Martin Breaugh. London: Polity Press, 2011.

Adams, Robert M. "Machiavelli Now and Here: An Essay for the First World." *American Scholar* 44, no. 3 (1975): 365–81.

Adorno, Theodor. *Negative Dialectics*. Translated by E.B. Ashton. New York: Continuum, 1973.

Alighieri, Dante. *Inferno*. Edited by Giuseppe Mazzotta. Translated by Michael Palma. New York: W.W. Norton, 2008.

Althusser, Louis. "Is It Simple to Be a Marxist in Philosophy?" In *Essays in Self-Criticism*, translated by Grahame Lock. London: New Left Books, 1976.

– *Machiavelli and Us*. Edited by François Matheron. Translated by Gregory Elliott. London: Verso, 1999.

– "The Facts." In *The Future Lasts Forever: A Memoir*, edited by Olivier Corpet and Yann Moulier Boutang, translated by Richard Veasey, 288–364. New York: New Press, 1992.

– "The Underground Current of the Materialism of the Encounter." In *Philosophy of the Encounter: Later Writings, 1978–87*, edited by François Matheron and Oliver Corpet, translated by G.M. Goshgarian, 163–207. London: Verso, 2006.

Alvarez, Leo Paul S. de. *The Machiavellian Enterprise: A Commentary on The Prince*. DeKalb: Northern Illinois University Press, 1999.

Ardito, Alissa M. *Machiavelli and the Modern State: The Prince, the Discourses on Livy, and the Extended Territorial Republic*. Cambridge: Cambridge University Press, 2015.

Arendt, Hannah. *On Revolution*. New York: Viking Press, 1965.
– "Some Questions of Moral Philosophy." In *Responsibility and Judgment*, edited by Jerome Kohn, 49–146. New York: Schocken, 2003.
– *The Human Condition*. Chicago: University of Chicago Press, 1998.
– "What Is Authority?" In *Between Past and Future: Eight Exercises in Political Thought*, 91–141. New York: Penguin, 1993.
– "What Is Freedom?" In *Between Past and Future: Eight Exercises in Political Thought*, 143–71. New York: Penguin, 2006.
Arieti, James A. "The Machiavellian Chiron: Appearance and Reality in *The Prince*." *CLIO* 24, no. 4 (1995): 381–97.
Aron, Raymond. *Machiavel et les tyrannies modernes*. Edited by Rémy Freymond. Paris: Éditions de Fallois, 1993.
– "Machiavelli and Marx." In *Politics and History*, edited and translated by Miriam Bernheim, 87–101. New York: Free Press, 1978.
Baccelli, Luca. "Political Imagination, Conflict, and Democracy." In *Machiavelli on Liberty and Conflict*, edited by David Johnston, Nadia Urbinati, and Camila Vergara, 352–72. Chicago: University of Chicago Press, 2017.
Bacon, Francis. "The Advancement of Learning." In *Bacon's Advancement of Learning and the New Atlantis*, 1–234. Oxford: Benediction Classics, 2008.
Balakrishnan, Gopal. "Future Unknown: Machiavelli for the Twenty-First Century." *New Left Review* 32 (April 2005): 5–21.
Balibar, Étienne. "*Essere Principe, Essere Populare*: The Principle of Antagonism in Machiavelli's Epistemology." In *The Radical Machiavelli: Politics, Philosophy, and Language*, edited by Filippo Del Lucchese, Fabio Frosini, and Vittorio Morfino, 349–67. Leiden: Brill, 2015.
Ball, Terrence. "The Picaresque Prince: Reflections on Machiavelli and Moral Change." *Political Theory* 12, no. 4 (1984): 521–36.
Balot, Ryan, and Stephen Trochimchuk. "The Many and the Few: On Machiavelli's 'Democratic Moment.'" *Review of Politics* 74, no. 4 (2012): 559–88.
Baluch, Faisal. "Arendt's Machiavellian Moment." *European Journal of Political Theory* 13, no. 2 (2014): 154–77.
Banerjee, Kiran, and Mauricio Suchowlansky. "Citizens, Subjects or Tyrants? Relocating the People in Pocock's *The Machiavellian Moment*." *History of European Ideas* 43, no. 2 (2017): 184–97.
Bárcenas, Alejandro. *Machiavelli's Art of Politics*. Leiden: Brill, 2015.
Bargu, Banu. "Machiavelli after Althusser." In *The Radical Machiavelli: Politics, Philosophy, and Language*, edited by Filippo Del Lucchese, Fabio Frosini, and Vittorio Morfino, 420–39. Leiden: Brill, 2015.
Barlow, J.J. "The Fox and the Lion: Machiavelli Replies to Cicero." *History of Political Thought* 20, no. 4 (1999): 627–45.

Baron, Hans. *In Search of Florentine Civic Humanism: Essays on the Transition from Medieval to Modern Thought*, vol. 1. Princeton: Princeton University Press, 1988.

Barthas, Jérémie. "Machiavelli in Political Thought from the Age of Revolutions to the Present." In *The Cambridge Companion to Machiavelli*, edited by John M. Najemy, 256–73. Cambridge: Cambridge University Press, 2010.

– "Machiavelli, Public Debt, and the Origins of Political Economy." In *The Radical Machiavelli: Politics, Philosophy, and Language*, edited by Filippo Del Lucchese, Fabio Frosini, and Vittorio Morfino, 273–305. Leiden: Brill, 2015.

Basu, Sammy. "In a Crazy Time the Crazy Come out Well: Machiavelli and the Cosmology of His Day." *History of Political Thought* 2, no. 2 (1990): 213–39.

Beiner, Ronald. "Machiavelli, Hobbes, and Rousseau on Civil Religion." *Review of Politics* 55, no. 4 (1993): 617–38.

Benjamin, Walter. *The Origin of German Tragic Drama*. Translated by John Osborne. London: Verso, 1998.

– "Theses on the Philosophy of History." In *Illuminations: Essays and Reflections*, edited by Hannah Arendt, translated by Harry Zohn, 253–64. New York: Schocken, 1968.

Benner, Erica. *Machiavelli's Ethics*. Princeton: Princeton University Press, 2009.

– *Machiavelli's Prince: A New Reading*. Oxford: Oxford University Press, 2013.

– "The Necessity to Be Not-Good: Machiavelli's Two Realisms." In *Machiavelli on Liberty and Conflict*, edited by David Johnston, Nadia Urbinati, and Camila Vergara, 164–85. Chicago: University of Chicago Press, 2017.

Berlin, Isaiah. "The Originality of Machiavelli." In *Against the Current: Essays in the History of Ideas*, 25–79. New York: Viking Press, 1980.

Bernard, John. *Why Machiavelli Matters: A Guide to Citizenship in a Democracy*. Westport: Praeger, 2009.

Berns, Thomas. "Le retour à l'origine de l'état." *Archives de philosophie*, no. 59 (1996): 219–48.

– "Prophetic Efficacy: The Relationship between Force and Belief." In *The Radical Machiavelli: Politics, Philosophy, and Language*, edited by Filippo Del Lucchese, Fabio Frosini, and Vittorio Morfino, 207–18. Leiden: Brill, 2015.

Blair, Brook Montgomery. "Post-Metaphysical and Radical Humanist Thought." *History of European Ideas* 27, no. 3 (2001): 199–238.

Blanchard, Jr, Kenneth C. "Being, Seeing, and Touching: Machiavelli's Modification of Platonic Epistemology." *Review of Metaphysics* 49, no. 3 (1996): 577–607.

Bock, Gisela. "Civil Discord in Machiavelli's *Istorie Fiorentine*." In *Machiavelli and Republicanism*, edited by Gisela Bock, Quentin Skinner, and Maurizio Viroli, 181–201. Cambridge: Cambridge University Press, 1990.

Boethius. *The Consolation of Philosophy*. Translated by V.E. Watts. London: Folio Society, 1998.

Bonadeo, Alfredo. *Corruption, Conflict, and Power in the Works and Times of Niccolò Machiavelli*. Berkeley: University of California Press, 1973.

– "Machiavelli on Civic Equality and Republican Government." *Romance Notes* 11, no. 1 (1969): 160–6.

– "The Role of the 'Grandi' in the Political World of Machiavelli." *Studies in the Renaissance* 16 (1969): 9–30.

– "The Role of the People in the Works and Times of Machiavelli." *Bibliothèque d'Humanisme et Renaissance* 32, no. 2 (1970): 351–77.

Breaugh, Martin. *The Plebeian Experience: A Discontinuous History of Political Freedom*. Translated by Lazer Lederhendler. New York: Columbia University Press, 2013.

Breckman, Warren. "The Power and the Void: Radical Democracy, Post-Marxism, and the Machiavellian Moment." In *Radical Intellectuals and the Subversion of Progressive Politics*, edited by Gregory Smulewicz-Zucker and Michael J. Thompson, 237–54. New York: Palgrave Macmillan, 2015.

Breiner, Peter. "Machiavelli's 'New Prince' and the Primordial Moment of Acquisition." *Political Theory* 36, no. 1 (2008): 66–92.

Brown, Alison. "Lucretian Naturalism and the Evolution of Machiavelli's Ethics." In *The Radical Machiavelli: Politics, Philosophy, and Language*, edited by Filippo Del Lucchese, Fabio Frosini, and Vittorio Morfino, 105–27. Leiden: Brill, 2015.

– *The Return of Lucretius to Renaissance Florence*. Cambridge: Cambridge University Press, 2010.

Brown, Wendy. *Manhood and Politics: A Feminist Reading of Political Theory*. Totowa: Rowman and Littlefield, 1988.

Brudney, Kent M. "Machiavelli on Social Class and Class Conflict." *Political Theory* 12, no. 4 (1984): 507–19.

Burnham, James. *The Machiavellians: The Defenders of Freedom*. New York: John Day, 1943.

Burns, Edward. "The Liberalism of Machiavelli." *Antioch Review* 8, no. 3 (1948): 321–30.

Butterfield, H. *The Statecraft of Machiavelli*. London: G. Bell and Sons, 1960.

Cabrini, Anna Maria. "Machiavelli's *Florentine Histories*." In *The Cambrige Companion to Machiavelli*, edited by John M. Najemy, 128–43. Cambridge: Cambridge University Press, 2010.

Cadoni, Giorgio. *Crisi della mediazione politica e conflitti sociali: Niccolò Machiavelli, Francesco Guicciardini e Donato Giannotti di fronte al tramonto della Fiorentina libertas*. Rome: Jouvence, 1994.

– "Machiavelli teorico dei conflitti sociali." In *Machiavelli attuale / Machiavel actuel*, edited by Georges Barthouil, 17–22. Ravenna: Longo Editore, 1982.

Castoriadis, Cornelius. "Time and Creation." In *World in Fragments*, edited and translated by David Ames Curtis, 374–401. Stanford: Stanford University Press, 1997.

Cavallo, Jo Ann. "On Political Power and Personal Liberty in *The Prince* and *The Discourses*." *Social Research* 81, no. 1 (2014): 107–32.

Chabod, Federico. "An Introduction to *The Prince*." In *Machiavelli and the Renaissance*, translated by David Moore, 1–29. Londons: Bowes and Bowes, 1960.

– "Machiavelli's Method and Style." In *Machiavelli and the Renaissance*, translated by David Moore, 126–48. London: Bowes and Bowes, 1960.

– "*The Prince*: Myth and Reality." In *Machiavelli and the Renaissance*, translated by David Moore, 30–125. London: Bowes and Bowes, 1960.

Chiappelli, Fredi. "Machiavelli as Secretary." *Italian Quarterly* 14, no. 3 (1970): 27–44.

Chollet, Antoine. *Les temps de la démocratie*. Paris: Dalloz, 2011.

Christoforatou, Christina. "Ontologies of Power in the Sovereign Politics of Pindar and Machiavelli." *Italian Culture* 33, no. 2 (2015): 87–104.

Cicero. *On Duties*. Edited by M.T. Griffin and E.M. Atkins. Cambridge: Cambridge University Press, 1991.

– "On the Commonwealth." In *On the Commonwealth and On the Laws*, edited by James E.G. Zetzel, 1–103. Cambridge: Cambridge University Press, 1999.

Clarke, Michelle T. "Machiavelli and the Imagined Rome of Renaissance Humanism." *History of Political Thought* 36, no. 3 (2015): 452–70.

Coby, Patrick. "Machiavelli's Philanthropy." *History of Political Thought* 20, no. 4 (1999): 604–26.

– *Machiavelli's Romans: Liberty and Greatness in the Discourses*. Lanham: Lexington, 1999.

Coleman, Janet. *A History of Political Thought: From the Middle Ages to the Renaissance*. Oxford: Blackwell, 2000.

Colish, Marcia L. "The Idea of Liberty in Machiavelli." *Journal of the History of Ideas* 32, no. 3 (1971): 323–53.

Conaway Bondanella, Julia. "The *Discourses on Livy*: Preserving a Free Way of Life." In *Seeking Real Truths: Multidisciplinary Perspectives on Machiavelli*, edited by Patricia Vilches and Gerald Seaman, 69–102. Leiden: Brill, 2007.

Condé, J. "La sagesse machiavelique: politique et rhétorique." In *Umanesimo e scienza politica*, edited by E. Castelli. Milan: Marzorati, 1951.

Cox, Virginia. "Rhetoric and Ethics in Machiavelli." In *The Cambridge Companion to Machiavelli*, edited by John M. Najemy, 173–89. Cambridge: Cambridge University Press, 2010.

Cro, Stelio. "Machiavelli e l'antiutopia." In *Machiavelli attuale / Machiavel actuel*, edited by Georges Barthouil, 27–33. Ravenna: Longo Editore, 1982.

Cugno, Agnès. *Apprendre à philosopher avec Machiavel*. Paris: Ellipses, 2009.

– *Machiavel – Le Prince*. Paris: Ellipses, 2012.

– "Machiavel et le problème de l'être en politique." *Revue philosophique de la France et de l'étranger* 189, no. 1 (1999): 19–34.

D'Amico, Jack. "Machiavelli and Memory." *Modern Language Quarterly* 50, no. 2 (1989): 99–124.

Del Lucchese, Filippo. *Conflict, Power, and Multitude in Machiavelli and Spinoza*. London: Continuum, 2009.

– "Crisis and Power: Economics, Politics and Conflict in Machiavelli's Political Thought." *History of Political Thought* 30, no. 1 (2009): 75–96.

– "Freedom, Equality and Conflict: Rousseau on Machiavelli." *History of Political Thought* 35, no. 1 (2014): 29–49.

– "La città divisa: esperieza del conflitto e novità politica in Machiavelli." In *Machiavelli: immaginazione e contingenza*, edited by Filippo Del Lucchese, Luca Sartorello, and Stefano Visentin, 17–29. Pisa: Edizioni Ets, 2006.

– "Machiavelli and Constituent Power: The Revolutionary Foundation of Modern Political Thought." *European Journal of Political Theory* 16, no. 1 (2017): 3–23.

– "Machiavellian Democracy." *Historical Materialism* 20, no. 1 (2012): 232–46.

– "On the Emptiness of an Encounter: Althusser's Reading of Machiavelli." Translated by Warren Montag. *Décalages* 1, no. 1 (2010): 1–19.

– *The Political Philosophy of Niccolò Machiavelli*. Edinburgh: Edinburgh University Press, 2015.

Del Lucchese, Filippo, Fabio Frosini, and Vittorio Morfino, eds. *The Radical Machiavelli: Politics, Philosophy and Language*. Leiden: Brill, 2015.

Dietz, Mary G. "Trapping the Prince: Machiavelli and the Politics of Deception." *American Political Science Review* 80, no. 3 (1986): 777–99.

– *Turning Operations: Feminism, Arendt, and Politics*. New York: Routledge, 2002.

Dillon, Michael. "Lethal Freedom: Divine Violence and the Machiavellian Moment." *Theory and Event* 11, no. 2 (2008).

Dotti, Ugo. *Niccolò Machiavelli: la fenomenologia del potere*. Milano: Feltrinelli Editore, 1979.

Dowlen, Oliver. *The Political Potential of Sortition: A Study on the Random Selection of Citizens for Public Office*. Exeter: Imprint Academic, 2008.

Duff, Alexander F. "Republicanism and the Problem of Ambition: The Critique of Cicero in Machiavelli's *Discourses*." *Journal of Politics* 73, no. 4 (2011): 980–92.

Duhamel, Jérémie. "Machiavel et la vertu intellectuelle de prudence: étude du chapitre XXV du *Prince*." *Canadian Journal of Political Science* 46, no. 4 (2013): 821–40.

Dyer, Megan K., and Cary J. Nederman. "Machiavelli against Method: Paul Feyerabend's Anti-Rationalism and Machiavellian Political 'Science.'" *History of European Ideas* 42, no. 3 (2016): 430–45.

Ercole, Francesco. *La politica di Machiavelli*. Roma: Anonima Romana Editoriale, 1926.

Erfani, Farhang. "Fixing Marx with Machiavelli: Claude Lefort's Democratic Turn." *Journal of the British Society for Phenomenology* 39, no. 2 (2008): 200–14.

Esposito, Roberto. *Living Thought: The Origins and Actuality of Italian Philosophy*. Stanford: Stanford University Press, 2012.

– *Ordine e conflitto: Machiavelli e la letteratura politica del Rinascimento italiano*. Napoli: Liguori Editore, 1984.

Falvo, Joseph D. "Nature and Art in Machiavelli's *Prince*." *Italica* 66, no. 3 (1989): 323–32.

Femia, Joseph. "Machiavelli and Italian Fascism." *History of Political Thought* 25, no. 1 (2004): 1–15.

– *Machiavelli Revisited*. Cardiff: University of Wales Press, 2004.

Ferroni, Giulio. "'Transformation' and 'Adaptation' in Machiavelli's *Mandragola*." In *Machiavelli and the Discourse of Literature*, edited by Albert Russell Ascoli and Victoria Kahn, translated by Ronald L. Martinez, 81–116. Ithaca: Cornell University Press, 1993.

Fichte, Johann Gottlieb. "On Machiavelli, as an Author, and Passages from His Writings." Translated by Ian Alexander Moore and Christopher Turner. *Philosophy Today* 60, no. 3 (2016): 761–88.

Fischer, Markus. "Machiavelli's Political Psychology." *Review of Politics* 59, no. 4 (1997): 789–830.

– "Machiavelli's Rapacious Republicanism." In *Machiavelli's Liberal Republican Legacy*, edited by Paul A. Rahe, xxxi–lxii. Cambridge: Cambridge University Press, 2006.

Fleisher, Martin. "A Passion for Politics: The Vital Core of the World of Machiavelli." In *Machiavelli and the Nature of Political Thought*, edited by Martin Fleisher, 114–47. New York: Atheneum, 1972.

– "The Ways of Machiavelli and the Ways of Politics." *History of Political Thought* 16, no. 3 (1995): 330–55.

Fletcher, Angus. "The Comic Ethos of *Il Principe*." *Comparative Drama* 43, no. 3 (2009): 293–315.

Flynn, Bernard. *The Philosophy of Claude Lefort: Interpreting the Political*. Evanston: Northwestern University Press, 2005.

Fontana, Benedetto. *Hegemony and Power: On the Relation between Gramsci and Machiavelli*. Minneapolis: University of Minnesota Press, 1993.

– "Love of Country and Love of God: The Political Uses of Religion in Machiavelli." *Journal of the History of Ideas* 60, no. 4 (1999): 639–58.

– "Machiavelli and the Gracchi: Republican Liberty and Conflict." In *Machiavelli on Liberty and Conflict*, edited by David Johnston, Nadia Urbinati, and Camila Vergara, 235–56. Chicago: University of Chicago Press, 2017.

– "Reason and Politics: Philosophy Confronts the People." *Boundary 2* 33, no. 1 (2006): 7–35.

Fournel, Jean-Louis. "Is *The Prince* Really a Political Treatise? A Discussion of Machiavelli's Motivations for Writing *The Prince*." *Italian Culture* 32, no. 2 (2014): 85–97.

Frade, Carlos. "An Altogether New Prince Five Centuries On: Bringing Machiavelli to Bear on Our Present." *Situations* 5, no. 1 (2013): 35–60.

Francese, Joseph. "La meritocrazia di Machiavelli. Dagli scritti politici alla *Mandragola*." *Italica* 71, no. 2 (1994): 153–75.

Frazer, Elizabeth, and Kimberly Hutchings. "Virtuous Violence and the Politics of Statecraft in Machiavelli, Clausewitz and Weber." *Political Studies* 59, no. 1 (2011): 56–73.

Gaille, Marie. *Machiavel et la tradition philosophique*. Paris: Presses Universitaires de France, 2007.

Gaille-Nikodimov, Marie. "An Introduction to *The Prince*." In *Seeking Real Truths: Multidisciplinary Perspectives on Machiavelli*, edited by Patricia Vilches and Gerald Seaman, translated by Gerald Seaman, 21–42. Leiden: Brill, 2007.

– *Conflit civil et liberté: la politique machiavélienne entre histoire et médecine*. Paris: Honoré Champion, 2004.

Garver, Eugene. "After *Virtù*: Rhetoric, Prudence, and Moral Pluralism in Machiavelli." *History of Political Thought* 27, no. 2 (1996): 195–223.

– *Machiavelli and the History of Prudence*. Madison: University of Wisconsin Press, 1987.

– "Machiavelli and the Politics of Rhetorical Invention." *CLIO* 14, no. 2 (1985): 157–78.

– "Machiavelli's *The Prince*: A Neglected Rhetorical Classic." *Philosophy and Rhetoric* 13, no. 2 (1980): 99–120.

Gatti, Hilary. *Ideas of Liberty in Early Modern Europe: From Machiavelli to Milton*. Princeton: Princeton University Press, 2015.

Geerken, John H. "Elements of Natural Law Theory in Machiavelli." In *The Medieval Tradition of Natural Law*, edited by Harold J. Johnson, 37–65. Kalamazoo: Medieval Institute Publications, 1987.

– "Homer's Image of the Hero in Machiavelli." *Italian Quarterly* 14, no. 3 (1970): 45–91.
– "Machiavelli's Moses and Renaissance Politics." *Journal of the History of Ideas* 60, no. 4 (1999): 579–95.
Germino, Dante. *Machiavelli to Marx: Modern Western Political Thought*. Chicago: University of Chicago Press, 1979.
– "Machiavelli's Political Anthropology." In *Theorie und Politik: Festschrift zum 70. Geburstag für Carl Joachim Friedrich*, edited by Klaus von Beyme, 35–60. Haag: Martinus Nijhoff, 1971.
– "Machiavelli's Thoughts on the Psyche and Society." In *The Political Calculus: Essays on Machiavelli's Political Philosophy*, edited by Anthony Parel, 59–82. Toronto: University of Toronto Press, 1972.
– "Second Thoughts on Leo Strauss's Machiavelli." *Journal of Politics* 28, no. 4 (1966): 794–817.
Geuna, Marco. "Extraordinary Accidents in the Life of Republics." In *Machiavelli on Liberty and Conflict*, edited by David Johnston, Nadia Urbinati, and Camila Vergara, 280–306. Chicago: Chicago University Press, 2017.
– "Machiavelli and the Problem of Dictatorship." *Ratio Juris* 28, no. 2 (2015): 216–25.
– "Machiavelli ed il ruolo dei conflitti nella vita politica." In *Conflitti*, edited by Alessandro Arienzo and Dario Caruso, 19–57. Napoli: Libreria Dante & Descartes, 2005.
– "Skinner, Pre-Humanist Rhetorical Culture and Machiavelli." In *Rethinking the Foundations of Modern Political Thought*, edited by Annabel Brett, James Tully, and Holly Hamilton-Bleakley, 50–72. Cambridge: Cambridge University Press, 2006.
Gilbert, Felix. "Bernardo Rucellai and the Orti Oricellari: A Study on the Origin of Modern Political Thought." *Journal of the Warburg and Courtland Institutes* 12 (1949): 101–13.
– *Machiavelli and Guicciardini: Politics and History in Sixteenth-Century Florence*. New York: W.W. Norton, 1984.
– "Machiavelli in Modern Historical Scholarship." *Italian Quarterly* 14, no. 3 (1970): 9–26.
– "Machiavelli: The Renaissance of the Art of War." In *Makers of Modern Strategy: From Machiavelli to the Modern Age*, edited by Peter Paret, 11–31. Princeton: Princeton University Press, 1986.
– "Machiavelli's *Istorie Fiorentine*: An Essay in Interpretation." In *Studies on Machiavelli*, edited by Myron P. Gilmore, 75–99. Firenze: G.C. Sansoni, 1972.
– "The Concept of Nationalism in Machiavelli's *Prince*." *Studies in Renaissance* 1 (1954): 38–48.

– "The Humanist Concept of the Prince and *The Prince* of Machiavelli." In *History: Choice and Committment*, 91–114. Cambridge: Belknap Press of Harvard University Press, 1977.

Giorgini, Giovanni. "The Place of the Tyrant in Machiavelli's Political Thought and the Literary Genre of the *Prince*." *History of Political Thought* 29, no. 2 (2008): 230–56.

– "Five Hundred Years of Italian Scholarship on Machiavelli's *Prince*." *Review of Politics* 75, no. 4 (2013): 625–40.

Godorecci, Barbara J. *After Machiavelli: "Re-Writing" and the "Hermeneutic Attitude."* West Lafayette: Purdue University Press, 1993.

Gramsci, Antonio. "The Modern Prince." In *Selections from the Prison Notebooks*, edited and translated by Quintin Hoare and Geoffrey Nowell Smith, 123–205. New York: International Publishers, 1971.

Grant, Ruth W. *Hypocrisy and Integrity: Machiavelli, Rousseau, and the Ethics of Politics*. Chicago: University of Chicago Press, 1997.

Grazia, Sebastian de. *Machiavelli in Hell*. Princeton: Princeton University Press, 1989.

Guicciardini, Francesco. "Considerations on the *Discourses* of Niccolò Machiavelli." In *The Sweetness of Power: Machiavelli's Discourses and Guicciardini's Considerations*, translated by James B. Atkinson and David Sices, 387–438. DeKalb: Northern Illinois University Press, 2002.

– *Dialogue on the Government of Florence*. Edited and translated by Alison Brown. Cambridge: Cambridge University Press, 1994.

– *Maxims and Reflections of a Renaissance Statesman*. Translated by Mario Domandi. New York: Harper, 1965.

Hamilton, Lawrence. *Freedom Is Power: Liberty through Political Representation*. Cambridge: Cambridge University Press, 2014.

– "Real Modern Freedom." *Theoria* 60, no. 4 (2013): 1–28.

Harding, Brian. "Machiavelli's Politics and Critical Theory of Technology." *Argumentos de Razón Técnica*, no. 12 (2009): 37–57.

Harrington, James. "The Commonwealth of Oceana." In *The Commonwealth of Oceana and A System of Politics*, edited by J.G.A. Pocock, 1–266. Cambridge: Cambridge University Press, 1992.

Hegel, G.W.F. "The German Constitution." In *Political Writings*, edited by Lawrence Dickey and H.B. Nisbet, translated by H.B. Nisbet, 6–101. Cambridge: Cambridge University Press, 2004.

Held, David. *Models of Democracy*. Cambridge: Polity Press, 1999.

Held, Klaus. "Civic Prudence in Machiavelli: Toward the Paradigm Transformation in Philosophy in the Transition to Modernity." In *The Ancients and the Moderns*, edited by Reginald Lilly, translated by Anthony Steinbeck, 115–29. Bloomington: Indiana University Press, 1996.

Hochner, Nicole. "A Ritualist Approach to Machiavelli." *History of Political Thought* 30, no. 4 (2009): 575–95.

– "Machiavelli: Love and the Economy of the Emotions." *Italian Culture* 32, no. 2 (2014): 85–97.

Holman, Christopher. "Machiavelli and the Concept of Political Sublimation." *Italian Culture* 35, no. 1 (2017): 1–20.

– *Politics as Radical Creation: Herbert Marcuse and Hannah Arendt on Political Performativity*. Toronto: University of Toronto Press, 2013.

Honig, Bonnie. *Political Theory and the Displacement of Politics*. Ithaca: Cornell University Press, 1993.

Horkheimer, Max, and Theodor Adorno. *Dialectic of Enlightenment*. Translated by John Cumming. New York: Continuum, 2000.

Hörnquist, Mikael. *Machiavelli and Empire*. Cambridge: Cambridge University Press, 2004.

Howard, Dick. *The Primacy of the Political: A History of Political Thought from the Greeks to the French and American Revolutions*. New York: Columbia University Press, 2010.

Hulliung, Mark. *Citizen Machiavelli*. Princeton: Princeton University Press, 1983.

Jacobitti, Edmund E. "The Classical Heritage in Machiavelli's Histories: Symbol and Poetry as Historic Literature." In *The Comedy and Tragedy of Machiavelli: Essays on the Literary Works*, edited by Vickie B. Sullivan, 176–92. New Haven: Yale University Press, 2000.

Jacobson, Norman. *Pride and Solace: The Functions and Limits of Political Theory*. Berkeley: University of California Press, 1978.

Jacquette, Jane S. "Rethinking Machiavelli: Feminism and Citizenship." In *Feminist Interpretations of Machiavelli*, edited by Maria J. Falco, 337–66. University Park: Pennsylvania State University Press, 2004.

Janara, Laura. "Machiavelli, Elizabeth I and the Innovative Historical Self: A Politics of Action, not Identity." *History of Political Thought* 27, no. 3 (2006): 456–85.

Jay, Martin. *The Dialectical Imagination: A History of the Frankfurt School of Social Research, 1923–1950*. Berkeley: University of California Press, 1973.

Jurdjevic, Mark. *A Great and Wretched City: Promise and Failure in Machiavelli's Florentine Political Thought*. Cambridge: Harvard University Press, 2014.

– "Machiavelli's Hybrid Republicanism." *English Historical Review* 122, no. 499 (2007): 1228–57.

– "Virtue, Fortune, and Blame in Machiavelli's Life and *The Prince*." *Social Research* 81, no. 1 (2014): 1–30.

Kahn, Victoria. "Habermas, Machiavelli, and the Humanist Critique of Ideology." *PMLA* 105, no. 3 (1990): 464–76.

– *Machiavellian Rhetoric: From the Counter-Reformation to Milton*. Princeton: Princeton University Press, 1994.

– "Machiavelli's Afterlife and Reputation to the Eighteenth Century." In *The Cambridge Companion to Machiavelli*, edited by John M. Najemy, 239–55. Cambridge: Cambridge University Press, 2010.

– "Reduction and the Praise of Disunion in Machiavelli's *Discourses*." *Journal of Medieval and Renaissance Studies* 18, no. 1 (1988): 1–19.

– "Revisiting Agathocles." *Review of Politics* 75, no. 4 (2013): 557–72.

– *The Future of Illusion: Political Theology and Early Modern Texts*. Chicago: University of Chicago Press, 2014.

– "*Virtù* and the Example of Agathocles in Machiavelli's *Prince*." In *Machiavelli and the Discourse of Literature*, edited by Albert Russell Ascoli and Victoria Kahn, 195–217. Ithaca: Cornell University Press, 1993.

Kamenev, Lev. "Preface to Machiavelli." *New Left Review*, no. 1/15 (1962): 39–42.

Kapust, Daniel J. "Acting the Princely Style: Ethos and Pathos in Cicero's *On the Ideal Orator* and Machiavelli's *Prince*." *Political Studies* 58, no. 3 (2010): 590–608.

Kennedy, John. "Machiavelli and Mandeville: Prophets of Radical Contingency." *Political Theology* 5, no. 1 (2004): 102–20.

Khoury, Joseph. "Machiavelli Manufacturing Memory: Terrorizing History, Historicizing Terror." In *Ars Reminiscendi: Minds and Memory in Renaissance Culture*, edited by Donald Beecher and Grant Williams, 247–66. Toronto: Centre for Reformation and Renaissance Studies, 2009.

Kocis, Robert. *Machiavelli Redeemed: Retrieving His Humanist Perspectives on Equality, Power, and Glory*. Bethlehem: Lehigh University Press, 1998.

Kontos, Alkis. "Success and Knowledge in Machiavelli." In *The Political Calculus: Essays on Machiavelli's Political Philosophy*, edited by Anthony Parel, 83–100. Toronto: University of Toronto Press, 1972.

Lahtinen, Mikko. *Niccolò Machiavelli and Louis Althusser's Aleatory Materialism*. Translated by Gareth Griffiths and Kristina Kolhi. Leiden: Brill, 2009.

Landemore, Hélène. *Democratic Reason: Politics, Collective Intelligence, and the Rule of the Many*. Princeton: Princeton University Press, 2013.

Lazar, Nomi Claire. "Must Exceptionalism Prove the Rule? An Angle on Emergency Government in the History of Political Thought." *Politics and Society* 34, no. 2 (2006): 245–75.

– *States of Emergency in Liberal Democracies*. Cambridge: Cambridge University Press, 2009.

Lefort, Claude. *Le travail de l'oeuvre Machiavel*. Paris: Gallimard, 1986.

– "L'œuvre de pensée et l'histoire." In *Les formes de l'histoire: essais d'anthropologie politique*, 141–52. Paris: Gallimard, 1978.

– "Machiavel et les jeunes." In *Les formes de l'histoire: essais d'anthropologie politique*, 153–68. Paris: Gallimard, 1978.

– "Machiavel: la dimension économique du politique." In *Les formes de l'histoire: essais d'anthropologie politique*, 126–40. Paris: Gallimard, 1978.

– "Machiavelli: History, Politics, Discourse." In *The States of Theory: History, Art, and Critical Discourse*, 113–24. New York: Columbia University Press, 1990.

– "Machiavelli and the *Verità Effetuale*." In *Writing: The Political Test*, edited and translated by David Ames Curtis. Durham: Duke University Press, 2000.

– *Machiavelli in the Making*. Translated by Michael B. Smith. Evanston: Northwestern University Press, 2012.

– "Réflexions sociologiques sur Machiavel et marx: la politique et le réel." In *Les formes de l'histoire: essais d'anthropologie politique*, 169–94. Paris: Gallimard, 1978.

– "The Image of the Body and Totalitarianism." In *The Political Forms of Modern Society: Bureaucracy, Democracy, Totalitarianism*, edited by John B. Thompson, 292–306. Cambridge: MIT Press, 1986.

– "The Logic of Totalitarianism." In *The Political Forms of Modern Society: Bureaucracy, Democracy, Totalitarianism*, edited by John B. Thompson. Cambridge: Cambridge University Press, 1986.

Leibovici, Martine. "From Fight to Debate: Machiavelli and the Revolt of the Ciompi." *Philosophy and Social Criticism* 28, no. 6 (2002): 647–60.

Litvin, Boris. "Mapping Rule and Subversion: Perspective and the Democratic Turn in Machiavelli Scholarship." *European Journal of Political Theory*. Advanced online publication (2015): 1–23. doi:10.177/1474885115599894.

Livy. *Rome and Italy: Books VI–X of The History of Rome from Its Foundation*. Translated by Betty Radice. London: Penguin, 1982.

– *The Early History of Rome: Books I–V of The History of Rome from Its Foundations*. Translated by Aubrey de Sélincourt. London: Penguin Books, 2002.

Lukes, Timothy J. "Descending to the Particulars: The Palazzo, the Piazza, and Machiavelli's Republican Modes and Orders." *Journal of Politics* 71, no. 2 (2009): 1–13.

– "Fortune Comes of Age." *Sixteenth Century Journal* 11, no. 4 (1980): 33–50.

– "Lionizing Machiavelli." *American Political Science Review* 95, no. 3 (2001): 561–75.

Lynch, Christopher. "The *ordine nuovo* of Machiavelli's *Arte della guerra*: Reforming Ancient Matter." *History of Political Thought* 31, no. 3 (2010): 407–25.

Machiavelli, Niccolò. "Allocuzione fatta ad magistrato." In *Tutte le opere*, 36–7.

– "Capitoli per una compagnia di piacere." In *Tutte le opere*, 930–2.

– "Decennale secondo." In *Tutte le opere*, 950–4.
– "Del modo di trattare i popoli della Valdichiana ribellati." In *Tutte le opere*, 13–16.
– "Dell'Ambizione." In *Tutte le opere*, 984–7.
– "Dell'Arte della guerra." In *Tutte le opere*, 299–398.
– "Dell'Ingratitudine." In *Tutte le opere*, 980–3.
– "Di Fortuna." In *Tutte le opere*, 976–9.
– "Discorsi sopra la prima Deca di Tito Livio." In *Tutte le opere*, 73–254.
– "Discorso o dialogo intorno alla nostra lingua." In *Tutte le opere*, 923–30.
– *Discourses on Livy*. Translated by Harvey C. Mansfield and Nathan Tarcov. Chicago: University of Chicago Press, 1996.
– "Discursus florentinarum rerum post mortem iunioris Laurentii Medices." In *Tutte le opere*, 24–31.
– "Exortatione alla penitenza." In *Tutte le opere*, 932–4.
– *Florentine Histories*. Translated by Harvey C. Mansfield and Laura F. Banfield. Princeton: Princeton University Press, 1988.
– "Il Principe." In *Tutte le opere*, 255–98.
– "Istorie fiorentine." In *Tutte le opere*, 629–844.
– "La vita di Castruccio Castracani da Lucca." In *Tutte le opere*, 613–28.
– "L'Asino." In *Tutte le opere*, 954–76.
– "Legazione al duca Valentino in Romagna." In *Tutte le opere*, 401–96.
– "Lettere, 116, Niccolò Machiavelli a Giovan Battista Soderini." In *Tutte le opere*, 1082–3.
– "Lettere, 216, Niccolò Machiavelli a Francesco Vettori." In *Tutte le opere*, 1158–60.
– "Lettere, 239, Niccolò Machiavelli a Francesco Vettori." In *Tutte le opere*, 1190–2.
– "Lettere, 291, Niccolò Machiavelli a Francesco Guicciardini." In *Tutte le opere*, 1222–4.
– "Lettere, 296, Niccolò Machiavelli a Francesco Guicciardini." In *Tutte le opere*, 1228–30.
– *Machiavelli and His Friends: Their Personal Correspondence*. Edited and translated by James B. Atkinson and David Sices. DeKalb: Northern Illinois University Press, 1996.
– "Mandragola." In *Tutte le opere*, 868–90.
– "Parole da dirle sopra la provisione del danaio, facto un poco di proemio et di scusa." In *Tutte le opere*, 11–13.
– "Prima legazione alla corte di Roma." In *Tutte le opere*, 496–573.
– "Rapporto delle cose della Magna fatto questo di 17 giugna 1508." In *Tutte le opere*, 63–8.

– *The Art of War*. Translated by Christopher Lynch. Chicago: University of Chicago Press, 2003.

– *The Chief Works and Others*, vols 1–3. Translated by Allan Gilbert. Durham: Duke University Press, 1989.

– *The Prince*. Translated by Harvey C. Mansfield. Chicago: University of Chicago Press, 1998.

– *Tutte le opere*. Edited by Mario Martelli. Firenze: Sansoni Editore, 1971.

Maddox, Graham. "The Secular Reformation and the Influence of Machiavelli." *Journal of Religion* 82, no. 4 (2002): 539–62.

Maher, Amanda. "The Power of 'Wealth, Nobility and Men': Inequality and Corruption in Machiavelli's *Florentine Histories*." *European Journal of Political Theory*. Advanced online publication (2017): 1–20. doi:10.177/147885117730673.

– "What Skinner Misses about Machiavelli's Freedom: Inequality, Corruption, and the Institutional Origins of Civic Virtue." *Journal of Politics* 78, no. 4 (2016): 1003–15.

Maihoffer, Werner. "The Ethos of the Republic and the Reality of Politics." In *Machiavelli and Republicanism*, edited by Gisela Bock, Quentin Skinner, and Maurizio Viroli, 283–92. Cambridge: Cambridge University Press, 1990.

Major, Rafael. "A New Argument for Morality: Machiavelli and the Ancients." *Political Research Quarterly* 60, no. 2 (2007): 171–9.

Manent, Pierre. *An Intellectual History of Liberalism*. Translated by Rebecca Balinski. Princeton: Princeton University Press, 1995.

– *Naissances de la politique moderne*. Paris: Gallimard, 2007.

Manin, Bernard. *The Principles of Representative Government*. Cambridge: Cambridge University Press, 1997.

Mansfield, Harvey C. "Bruni and Machiavelli on Civic Humanism." In *Renaissance Civic Humanism: Reappraisals and Reflections*, edited by James Hankins, 223–46. Cambridge: Cambridge University Press, 2000.

– *Machiavelli's Virtue*. Chicago: University of Chicago Press, 1996.

– "Strauss's Machiavelli." *Political Theory* 3, no. 4 (1975): 372–84.

Marasco, Robyn. "Machiavelli Contra Governmentality." *Contemporary Political Theory* 11, no. 4 (2012): 339–61.

Marcuse, Herbert. *One-Dimensional Man: Studies in the Ideology of Advanced Industrial Society*. Boston: Beacon Press, 1969.

Maria, Salvatore di. "Machiavelli's Ironic View of History: The *Istorie Fiorentine*." *Renaissance Quarterly* 45, no. 2 (1992): 248–70.

Marx, Karl. *Capital: A Critique of Political Economy*, vol. 1. Translated by Ben Fowkes. London: Penguin, 1976.

– *The Eighteenth Brumaire of Louis Bonaparte*. Moscow: Progress Publishers, 1934.

Masters, Roger D. *Fortune Is a River: Leonardo Da Vinci and Niccolò Machiavelli's Magnificent Dream to Change the Course of Florentine History*. New York: Free Press, 1998.

Mazzeo, Joseph Anthony. *Renaissance and Revolution: The Remaking of European Thought*. New York: Pantheon, 1965.

– "The Poetry of Power: Machiavelli's Literary Vision." *Review of National Literatures* 1, no. 1 (1970): 38–62.

McCanles, Michael. *The Discourse of Il Principe*. Malibu: Undena, 1983.

McCormick, John P. "Addressing the Political Exception: Machiavelli's 'Accidents' and the Mixed Regime." *American Political Science Review* 87, no. 4 (1993): 888–900.

– "Defending the People from the Professors." Edited by John Swadley. *The Art of Theory*, 27 September 2010. www.artoftheory.com/mccormick -machiavellian-democracy (no longer available online).

– "'Keep the Public Rich, but the Citizens Poor': Economic and Political Inequality in Constitutions, Ancient and Modern." *Cardozo Law Review* 34, no. 3 (2013): 879–92.

– "Machiavelli and the Gracchi: Prudence, Violence, and Retribution." *Global Crime* 10, no. 4 (2009): 298–305.

– *Machiavellian Democracy*. Cambridge: Cambridge University Press, 2011.

– "Machiavelli's Agathocles: From Criminal Example to Princely Exemplum." In *Exemplarity and Singularity: Thinking through Particulars in Philosophy, Literature, and Law*, edited by Michèle Lowrie and Susanne Lüdemann, 123–39. London: Routledge, 2015.

– "Machiavelli's Greek Tyrant as Republican Reformer." In *The Radical Machiavelli: Politics, Philosophy, and Language*, edited by Filippo Del Lucchese, Fabio Frosini, and Vittorio Morfino, 337–48. Leiden: Brill, 2015.

– "Machiavelli's Inglorious Tyrants: On Agathocles, Scipio and Unmerited Glory." *History of Political Thought* 36, no. 1 (2015): 29–52.

– "Of Tribunes and Tyrants: Machiavelli's Legal and Extra-Legal Modes for Controlling Elites." *Ratio Juris* 28, no. 2 (2015): 252–66.

– "On the Myth of the Conservative Turn in Machiavelli's *Florentine Histories*." In *Machiavelli on Liberty and Conflict*, edited by David Johnston, Nadia Urbinati, and Camila Vergara, 330–51. Chicago: University of Chicago Press, 2017.

– "People and Elites in Republican Constitutions, Traditional and Modern." In *The Paradox of Constitutionalism: Constituent Power and Constitutional Form*, edited by Martin Loughlin and Neil Walker, 106–225. Oxford: Oxford University Press, 2007.

– "Pocock, Machiavelli and Political Contingency in Foreign Affairs: Republican Existentialism Outside (and within) the City." *History of European Ideas* 43, no. 2 (2017): 171–83.

– "Prophetic Statebuilding." *Representations* 115, no. 1 (2011): 1–19.

– "Subdue the Senate: Machiavelli's 'Way of Freedom' or Path to Tyranny." *Political Theory* 40, no. 6 (2012): 714–35.

– "The Enduring Ambiguity of Machiavellian Virtue: Cruelty, Crime, and Christianity in *The Prince*." *Social Research* 81, no. 1 (2014): 133–64.

McKenzie, Lionel A. "Rousseau's Debate with Machiavelli in the *Social Contract*." *Journal of the History of Ideas* 43, no. 2 (1982): 209–28.

Meinecke, Friedrich. *Machiavellism: The Doctrine of Raison d'État and Its Place in Modern History*. New Haven: Yale University Press, 1957.

Merleau-Ponty, Maurice. "A Note on Machiavelli." In *Signs*, translated by Richard C. McCleary, 211–23. Evanston: Northwestern University Press, 1964.

Minogue, K.R. "Theatricality and Politics: Machiavelli's Concept of *Fantasia*." In *The Morality of Politics*, edited by Bhikhu Parekh and R.N. Berki, 148–62. London: George Allen and Unwin, 1972.

Moggach, Douglas. "Fichte's Engagement with Machiavelli." *History of Political Thought* 14, no. 4 (1993): 573–89.

Mollat, Michel, and Philippe Wolff. *The Popular Revolutions of the Late Middle Ages*. Translated by A.L. Lytton-Sells. London: George Allen and Unwin, 1973.

Morfino, Vittorio. *Il tempo e l'occasione: l'incontro Spinoza Machiavelli*. Milano: LED, 2002.

– "Tra Lucrezio e Spinoza: la 'filosofia' di Machiavelli." In *Machiavelli: immaginazione e contingenza*, edited by Filippo Del Lucchese, Luca Sartorello, and Stefano Visentin, 67–110. Pisa: Edizioni Ets, 2006.

Moulfi, Mohamed. "Lectures machiavéliennes d'Althusser." In *The Radical Machiavelli: Politics, Philosophy, and Language*, edited by Filippo Del Lucchese, Fabio Frosini, and Vittorio Morfino, 406–19. Leiden: Brill, 2015.

Najemy, John M. *A History of Florence: 1200–1575*. Oxford: Blackwell, 2008.

– "Baron's Machiavelli and Renaissance Republicanism." *American Historical Review* 101, no. 1 (1996): 119–29.

– *Between Friends: Discourses of Power and Desire in the Machiavelli-Vettori Letters of 1513–1515*. Princeton: Princeton University Press, 1993.

– "Machiavelli and Cesare Borgia: A Reconsideration of Chapter 7 of *The Prince*." *Review of Politics* 75, no. 4 (2013): 539–56.

– "Papirus and the Chickens, or Machiavelli on the Necessity of Interpreting Religion." *Journal of the History of Ideas* 60, no. 4 (1999): 659–81.

– "Society, Class, and State in Machiavelli's *Discourses on Livy*." In *The Cambridge Companion to Machiavelli*, edited by John M. Najemy, 96–111. Cambridge: Cambridge University Press, 2010.

– "The 2013 Josephine Waters Bennett Lecture: Machiavelli and History." *Renaissance Quarterly* 67, no. 4 (2014): 1131–64.

Nederman, Cary J. "Rhetoric, Reason, and Republic: Republicanisms – Ancient, Medieval, and Modern." In *Renaissance Civic Humanism: Reappraisals and Reflections*, edited by James Hankins, 247–69. Cambridge: Cambridge University Press, 2000.

Negri, Antonio. *Insurgencies: Constituent Power and the Modern State*. Translated by Maurizia Boscagli. Minneapolis: University of Minnesota Press, 1999.

Nelson, Eric. *The Greek Tradition in Republican Thought*. Cambridge: Cambridge University Press, 2004.

Olschki, Leonardo. *Machiavelli: The Scientist*. Berkeley: Gillick Press, 1945.

Orr, Robert. "The Time Motif in Machiavelli." In *Machiavelli and the Nature of Political Thought*, edited by Martin Fleisher, 185–208. New York: Atheneum, 1972.

Orwin, Clifford. "Machiavelli's Unchristian Charity." *American Political Science Review* 72, no. 4 (1978): 1217–28.

Owen, David. "Machiavelli's *Il Principe* and the Politics of Glory." *European Journal of Political Theory* 16, no. 1 (2017): 41–60.

Palmer, Ada. *Reading Lucretius in the Renaissance*. Cambridge: Harvard University Press, 2014.

Panagia, Davide. *The Political Life of Sensation*. Durham: Duke University Press, 2009.

Pangle, Thomas. *The Ennobling of Democracy: The Challenge of the Postmodern Age*. Baltimore: Johns Hopkins University Press, 1992.

Parasher, Tejas. "Inequality and *Tumulti* in Machiavelli's Aristocratic Republics." *Polity* 49, no. 1 (2017): 42–68.

Parel, Anthony. "Farewell to Fortune." *Review of Politics* 75, no. 4 (2013): 587–604.

– *The Machiavellian Cosmos*. New Haven: Yale University Press, 1992.

– "Machiavelli's Method and His Interpreters." In *The Political Calculus: Essays on Machiavelli's Political Philosophy*, edited by Anthony Parel, 3–32. Toronto: University of Toronto Press, 1972.

– "Machiavelli's Notions of Justice: Text and Analysis." *Political Theory* 18, no. 4 (1990): 528–44.

– "Machiavelli's Use of *Umori* in *The Prince*." *Quaderni d'Italianistica* 11, no. 1 (1990): 91–101.

Parkin, John. "Dialogue in *The Prince*." In *Niccolò Machiavelli's The Prince: New Interdisciplinary Essays*, edited by Martin Coyle, 65–88. Manchester: Manchester University Press, 1995.

Parkinson, G.H.R. "Ethics and Politics in Machiavelli." *Philosophical Quarterly* 5, no. 18 (1955): 37–44.

Patapan, Haig. *Machiavelli in Love: The Modern Politics of Love and Fear*. Lanham: Rowman and Littlefield, 2006.

Peden, Knox. "Anti-Revolutionary Republicanism: Claude Lefort's Machiavelli." *Radical Philosophy*, no. 182 (2013): 29–39.

Pettit, Philip. *Republicanism: A Theory of Freedom and Government*. Oxford: Oxford University Press, 1997.

Pico della Mirandola, Giovanni. *On the Dignity of Man*. Translated by Glenn Wallis. Indianapolis: Hackett, 1965.

Pitkin, Hanna Fenichel. *Fortune Is a Woman: Gender and Politics in the Thought of Niccolò Machiavelli*. Berkeley: University of California Press, 1984.

Plamenatz, John. "In Search of Machiavellian *Virtù*." In *The Political Calculus: Essays on Machiavelli's Political Philosophy*, edited by Anthony Parel, 157–78. Toronto: University of Toronto Press, 1972.

– *Machiavelli, Hobbes, and Rousseau*. Edited by Mark Philp and Z.A. Pelczynski. Oxford: Oxford University Press, 2012.

Pocock, J.G.A. "Machiavelli and Rome: The Republic as Ideal and as History." In *Machiavelli and Republicanism*, edited by John M. Najemy, 144–56. Cambridge: Cambridge University Press, 2010.

– "Machiavelli in the Liberal Cosmos." *Political Theory* 13, no. 4 (1985): 559–74.

– *The Machiavellian Moment: Florentine Political Thought and the Atlantic Republican Tradition*. Princeton: Princeton University Press, 1975.

Polybius. *The Histories of Polybius*, vol. 1. Edited and translated by Evelyn S. Shuckburgh. Cambridge: Cambridge University Press, 2012.

Prezzolini, Giuseppe. "The Christian Roots of Machiavelli's Moral Pessimism." *Review of National Literatures* 1, no. 1 (1970): 26–37.

Quinet, Edgar. *Les révolutions d'Italie*, vol. 2. Paris: Germer-Baillière, 1874.

Qviller, Bjørn. "The Machiavellian Cosmos." *History of Political Thought* 27, no. 3 (1996): 326–53.

Rahe, Paul A. *Against Throne and Altar: Machiavelli and Political Theory under the English Republic*. Cambridge: Cambridge University Press, 2008.

– "In the Shadow of Lucretius: The Epicurean Foundations of Machiavelli's Political Thought." *History of Political Thought* 28, no. 1 (2007): 30–55.

– "Machiavelli and the Modern Tyrant." In *Machiavelli on Liberty and Conflict*, edited by David Johnston, Nadia Urbinati, and Camila Vergara, 207–31. Chicago: University of Chicago Press, 2017.

– *Republics Ancient and Modern: New Modes and Orders in Early Modern Political Thought*. Chapel Hill: University of North Carolina Press, 1994.

– "Situating Machiavelli." In *Renaissance Civic Humanism: Reappraisals and Reflections*, edited by James Hankins, 270–308. Cambridge: Cambridge University Press, 2000.

Rancière, Jacques. *Dis-Agreement: Politics and Philosophy*. Translated by Julie Rose. Minneapolis: University of Minnesota Press, 1999.

Rebhorn, Wayne A. *Foxes and Lions: Machiavelli's Confidence Men*. Ithaca: Cornell University Press, 1988.

– "Machiavelli's *Prince* in the Epic Tradition." In *The Cambridge Companion to Machiavelli*, edited by John M. Najemy, 80–95. Cambridge: Cambridge University Press, 2010.

Regent, Nikola. "Machiavelli, Empire, *Virtù* and the Final Downfall." *History of Political Thought* 32, no. 5 (2011): 751–72.

Regnault, François. "La pensée du prince." *Cahiers pour l'analyse* no. 6 (1967): 23–52.

Rélang, André. "La dialectique de la fortune et de la *virtù* chez Machiavel." *Archives de philosophie* 66, no. 4 (2003): 649–62.

Remer, Gary. "Rhetoric as a Balancing of Ends." *Philosophy and Rhetoric* 42, no. 1 (2009): 1–28.

Renaudet, Augustin. *Machiavel: étude d'histoire des doctrines politiques*. Paris: Gallimard, 1942.

Rinaldi, Rinaldo. "Appunti su utopia (tra Moro e Machiavelli)." *Forum Italicum* 21, no. 2 (1987): 217–25.

Rispoli, Tania. "Imitation and Animality: On the Relationship between Nature and History in Chapter XVIII of *The Prince*." In *The Radical Machiavelli: Politics, Philosophy, and Language*, edited by Filippo Del Lucchese, Fabio Frosini, and Vittorio Morfino, 190–203. Leiden: Brill, 2015.

Rodolico, Niccolò. *I Ciompi: una pagina di storia del proletariato operaio*. Firenze: G.C. Sansoni, 1945.

Roebuck, Carl. "A Search for Political Stability." *Phoenix* 6, no. 2 (1952): 52–65.

Roecklein, Robert J. *Machiavelli and Epicureanism: An Investigation into the Origins of Early Modern Political Thought*. Lanham: Lexington, 2012.

Rose, Julie L. "'Keep the Citizens Poor': Machiavelli's Prescription for Republican Poverty." *Political Studies* 64, no. 3 (2016): 734–47.

Roux, Emmanuel. *Machiavel, la vie libre*. Paris: Raisons d'agir, 2013.

Rubenstein, Nicolai. "Machiavelli and Florentine Republican Experience." In *Machiavelli and Republicanism*, edited by Gisela Bock, Quentin Skinner, and Maurizio Viroli, 3–16. Cambridge: Cambridge University Press, 1990.

– "Machiavelli and the World of Florentine Politics." In *Studies on Machiavelli*, edited by Myron P. Gilmore, 3–28. Firenze: G.C. Sansoni, 1979.

Ruggiero, Guido. *Machiavelli in Love: Sex, Self, and Society in the Italian Renaissance*. Baltimore: Johns Hopkins University Press, 2007.

Russell, Greg. "Machiavelli's Science of Statecraft: The Diplomacy and Politics of Disorder." *Diplomacy and Statecraft* 16, no. 2 (2005): 227–50.

Russo, Luigi. *Machiavelli*. Bari: Laterza, 1949.

Sartorello, Luca. "L'urna sanza fondo machiavelliana e l'origine' della politica." In *Machiavelli: immaginazione e contingenza*, edited by Filippo Del Lucchese, Luca Sartorello, and Stefano Visentin, 185–216. Pisa: Edizioni Ets, 2006.

Sasso, Gennaro. *Machiavelli e Cesare Borgia: storia di un giudizio*. Rome: Edizioni dell'Ateneo, 1966.

– *Niccolò Machiavelli: storia del suo pensiero politico*. Bologna: Società editrice il Mulino, 1980.

– "Problemi di critica machiavelliana." In *Studi su Machiavelli*, 13–74. Napoli: Morano, 1967.

Saxonhouse, Arlene W. "Comedy, Machiavelli's Letters, and His Imaginary Republics." In *The Comedy and Tragedy of Machiavelli: Essays on the Literary Works*, edited by Vickie B. Sullivan, 57–77. New Haven: Yale University Press, 2000.

– "Do We Need the Vote? Reflections on John McCormick's *Machiavellian Democracy*." *The Good Society* 20, no. 2 (2011): 170–83.

– "Machiavelli's Women." In *Machiavelli's Legacy: The Prince after Five Hundred Years*, edited by Timothy Fuller, 70–86. Philadelphia: University of Pennsylvania Press, 2016.

Schillinger, Daniel. "Luck and Character in Machiavelli's Political Thought." *History of Political Thought* 37, no. 4 (2016): 606–29.

Schmitt, Carl. *Dictatorship: From the Origin of the Modern Concept of Sovereignty to the Proletarian Class Struggle*. Translated by Michael Hoelzl and Graham Ward. Cambridge: Polity, 2014.

– *The Leviathan in the State Theory of Thomas Hobbes: Meaning and Failure of a Political Symbol*. Translated by George Schwab and Erna Hilfstein. Chicago: University of Chicago Press, 2008.

Sfez, Gérald. "Deciding on Evil." In *Radical Evil*, edited by Joan Copjec, translated by James Swenson, 126–49. London: Verso, 1996.

– *Machiavel, Le Prince sans qualités*. Paris: Editions Kimé, 1998.

Shaw, Carl K.Y. "Quentin Skinner on the Proper Meaning of Republican Liberty." *Politics* 23, no. 1 (2003): 46–56.

Shell, Susan Meld. "Machiavelli's Discourse on Language." In *The Comedy and Tragedy of Machiavelli: Essays on the Literary Works*, edited by Vickie B. Sullivan, 78–101. New Haven: Yale University Press, 2000.

Shumer, S.M. "Machiavelli: Republican Politics and Its Corruption." *Political Theory* 7, no. 1 (1979): 5–34.

Singleton, Charles S. "The Perspective of Art." *Kenyon Review* 15, no. 2 (1953): 169–89.

Skinner, Quentin. *Machiavelli*. Oxford: Oxford University Press, 1981.

– "Machiavelli on *Virtù* and the Maintenance of Liberty." In *Visions of Politics*, vol. 2: *Renaissance Visions*, 160–85. Cambridge: Cambridge University Press, 2002.

– *The Foundations of Modern Political Thought*, vol. 1: *The Renaissance*. Cambridge: Cambridge University Press, 1978.

– "The Republican Ideal of Political Liberty." In *Machiavelli and Republicanism*, edited by Gisela Bock, Quentin Skinner, and Maurizio Viroli, 293–309. Cambridge: Cambridge University Press, 1990.

Smith, Bruce James. *Politics and Remembrance: Republican Themes in Machiavelli, Burke and Tocqueville*. Princeton: Princeton University Press, 1985.

Snyder, R. Claire. "Machiavelli and the Citizenship of Civic Practices." In *Feminist Interpretations of Niccolò Machiavelli*, edited by Maria J. Falco, 213–46. University Park: Pennsylvania State University Press, 2004.

Speer, Ross. "The Machiavellian Marxism of Althusser and Gramsci." *Décalages* 2, no. 1 (2016): 1–15.

Strauss, Leo. "Machiavelli and Classical Literature." *Review of National Literatures* 1, no. 1 (1970): 7–25.

– *Thoughts on Machiavelli*. Seattle: University of Washington Press, 1969.

Suchowlansky, Mauricio. "Machiavelli's *Summary of the Affairs of the City of Lucca*: Venice as *buon governo*." *Intellectual History Review* 26, no. 4 (2016): 429–45.

– "Rhetoric and Violence in Machiavelli's *Florentine Histories*." *Shakespeare en devenir*, no. 5 (2011).

Sullivan, Vickie B. *Machiavelli, Hobbes, and the Formation of Liberal Republicanism in England*. Cambridge: Cambridge University Press, 2004.

– "Machiavelli's Momentary 'Machiavellian Moment': A Reconsideration of Pocock's Treatment of the *Discourses*." *Political Theory* 20, no. 2 (1992): 309–18.

– *Machiavelli's Three Romes: Religion, Human Liberty, and Politics Reformed*. DeKalb: Northern Illinois University Press, 1996.

Tarlton, Charles D. "'Azioni in modo l'una dall'altra: Action for Action's Sake in Machiavelli's *The Prince*." *History of European Ideas* 29, no. 2 (2003): 123–40.

– "*Fortuna* and the Landscape of Action in Machiavelli's *Prince*." *New Literary History* 30, no. 4 (1999): 737–55.

– "Machiavelli's Burden: *The Prince* as Literary Text." In *Seeking Real Truths: Multidisciplinary Perspectives on Machiavelli*, edited by Patricia Vilches and Gerald Seaman, 43–68. Leiden: Brill, 2007.

Terray, Emmanuel. "An Encounter: Althusser and Machiavelli." In *Postmodern Materialism and the Future of Marxist Theory: Essays in the Althusserian*

Tradition, edited and translated by Antonio Callari and David F. Ruccio, 257–77. Hanover: Wesleyan University Press, 1996.

Tinkler, John F. "Praise and Advice: Rhetorical Approaches in More's *Utopia* and Machiavelli's *The Prince*." *Sixteenth Century Journal* 19, no. 2 (1988): 187–207.

Torres, Sebastián. "Tempo e politica: una lettura materialista di Machiavelli." In *The Radical Machiavelli: Politics, Philosophy, and Language*, edited by Filippo Del Lucchese, Fabio Frosini, and Vittorio Morfino, 174–89. Leiden: Brill, 2015.

Turner, Brandon. "Private Vices, Public Benefits: *Mandragola* in Machiavelli's Political Theory." *Polity* 48, no. 1 (2016): 109–32.

Van Parijs, Philippe. *Just Democracy: The Rawls-Machiavelli Programme*. Colchester: ECPR Press, 2011.

Vatter, Miguel. *Between Form and Event: Machiavelli's Theory of Political Freedom*. Dordrecht: Kluwer Academic Publishers, 2000.

– *Machiavelli's The Prince*. London: Bloomsbury, 2013.

Viroli, Maurizio. *From Politics to Reasons of State: The Acquisition and Transformation of the Language of Politics, 1250–1600*. Cambridge: Cambridge University Press, 1992.

– *Machiavelli*. Oxford: Oxford University Press, 1998.

– "Machiavelli and the Republican Idea of Politics." In *Machiavelli and Republicanism*, edited by Gisela Bock, Quentin Skinner, and Maurizio Viroli, 143–71. Cambridge: Cambridge University Press, 1990.

– *Machiavelli's God*. Translated by Anthony Shugaar. Princeton: Princeton University Press, 2010.

– "Machiavelli's Realism." *Constellations* 14, no. 4 (2007): 466–82.

– *Niccolò's Smile: A Biography of Machiavelli*. Translated by Antony Shugaar. New York: Hill and Wang, 2000.

– *Redeeming The Prince: The Meaning of Machiavelli's Masterpiece*. Princeton: Princeton University Press, 2014.

Visentin, Stefano. "The Different Faces of the People: On Machiavelli's Political Topography." In *The Radical Machiavelli: Politics, Philosophy, and Language*, edited by Filippo Del Lucchese, Fabio Frosini, and Vittorio Morfino, 368–89. Leiden: Brill, 2015.

Von Vacano, Diego A. *The Art of Power: Machiavelli, Nietzsche, and the Making of Aesthetic Political Theory*. Lanham: Lexington, 2007.

Vujadinovic, Dragica. "Machiavelli's Republican Political Theory." *Philosophy and Social Criticism* 40, no. 1 (2014): 43–68.

Waley, Daniel. "The Primitivist Element in Machiavelli's Thought." *Journal of the History of Ideas* 31, no. 1 (1970): 91–8.

Walsh, Mary. "Historical Reception of Machiavelli." In *Seeking Real Truths: Multidisciplinary Perspectives on Machiavelli*, edited by Patricia Vilches and Gerald Seaman, 273–302. Leiden: Brill, 2007.

Walzer, Michael. *The Revolution of the Saints*. Cambridge: Harvard University Press, 1965.

Weil, Eric. "Machiavel aujourd'hui." In *Essais et conférences*, vol. 2: *Politique*, 189–217. Paris: Librairie Philosophique J. Vrin, 1991.

Weil, Simone. "A Proletarian Uprising in Florence." In *Selected Essays: 1934–43*, translated by Richard Rees, 55–72. Oxford: Oxford University Press, 1962.

Wenman, Mark. *Agonistic Democracy: Constituent Power in the Era of Globalisation*. Cambridge: Cambridge University Press, 2013.

Whitfield, J.H. "Machiavelli's Use of Livy." In *Livy*, edited by T.A. Dorey, 73–96. Toronto: University of Toronto Press, 1971.

– "On Machiavelli's Use of *Ordini*." *Italian Studies*, no. 10 (1955): 19–39.

Winter, Yves. "Necessity and Fortune: Machiavelli's Politics of Nature." In *Second Nature: Rethinking the Natural through Politics*, edited by Crina Archer, Laura Ephraim, and Lida Maxwell, 26–45. New York: Fordham University Press, 2013.

– "Plebeian Politics: Machiavelli and the Ciompi Uprising." *Political Theory* 40, no. 6 (2012): 736–66.

– "The Prince and His Art of War: Machiavelli's Military Populism." *Social Research* 81, no. 1 (2014): 165–91.

Wolin, Sheldon. *Politics and Vision: Continuity and Innovation in Western Political Thought*. Princeton: Princeton University Press, 2004.

Wood, Neal. "Machiavelli's Humanism of Action." In *The Political Calculus: Essays on Machiavelli's Political Philosophy*, edited by Anthony Parel, 33–58. Toronto: University of Toronto Press, 1972.

– "Some Common Aspects of the Thought of Seneca and Machiavelli." *Renaissance Quarterly* 21, no. 1 (1968): 11–23.

– "Some Reflections on Sorel and Machiavelli." *Political Science Quarterly* 83, no. 1 (1968): 76–91.

– "The Value of Asocial Sociability: Contributions of Machiavelli, Sidney, and Montesquieu." *Bucknell Review* 16, no. 3 (1966): 1–22.

Yoran, Hanan. "Machiavelli's Critique of Humanism and the Ambivalences of Modernity." *History of Political Thought* 31, no. 2 (2010): 247–82.

Zerba, Michelle. *Doubt and Skepticism in Antiquity and the Renaissance*. Cambridge: Cambridge University Press, 2012.

– "The Frauds of Humanism: Cicero, Machiavelli, and the Rhetoric of Imposture." *Rhetorica: A Journal of the History of Rhetoric* 22, no. 3 (2004): 215–40.

Zerilli, Linda. "Machiavelli's Sisters: Women and 'The Conversation' of Political Theory." *Political Theory* 19, no. 2 (1991): 252–76.

Zmora, Hillay. "Love of Country and Love of Party: Patriotism and Human Nature in Machiavelli." *History of Political Thought* 25, no. 3 (2004): 424–45.

Zuckert, Catherine. "Machiavelli and the End of Nobility in Politics." *Social Research* 81, no. 1 (2014): 85–106.

– *Machiavelli's Politics*. Chicago: University of Chicago Press, 2017.

– "The Life of Castruccio Castracani: Machiavelli as Literary Artist." *History of Political Thought* 31, no. 4 (2010): 577–603.

Index